Handbook of
Secondary
Dementias

Handbook of Secondary Dementias

edited by

Roger Kurlan
University of Rochester Medical Center
Rochester, New York, U.S.A.

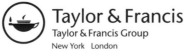

Taylor & Francis
Taylor & Francis Group
New York   London

Published in 2006 by
Taylor & Francis Group
270 Madison Avenue
New York, NY 10016

International Standard Book Number-10: 0-8247-5433-6 (Hardcover)
International Standard Book Number-13: 978-0-8247-5433-4 (Hardcover)
Library of Congress Card Number 2005056855

Library of Congress Cataloging-in-Publication Data

Handbook of secondary dementias / edited by Roger Kurlan.
      p. ; cm. -- (Neurological disease and therapy ; v. 82)
    Includes bibliographical references and index.
    ISBN-13: 978-0-8247-5433-4 (alk. paper)
    ISBN-10: 0-8247-5433-6 (alk. paper)
    1. Dementia--Handbooks, manuals, etc. 2. Neuropsychiatry--Handbooks, manuals, etc.
    I. Kurlan, Roger, 1952- II. Series.
    [DNLM: 1. Dementia--etiology. 2. Cognition Disorders--etiology. 3. Dementia--therapy. WM 220 H23696 2006]

    RC521.H3642 2006
    616.8'3--dc22   2005056855

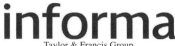

Preface

Those disorders in which dementia tends to be the presenting and predominant neurologic feature have been referred to as the "primary dementias." The primary dementias, such as Alzheimer's disease and frontotemporal dementia, have experienced an explosive rise in prevalence as the population ages. These are neurodegenerative diseases characterized by an inexorable loss of cerebral neurons and synapses, progressive cognitive decline, and behavioral disturbances despite available therapies. Although recent scientific findings such as those related to amyloid and tau protein metabolism have greatly advanced our understanding of mechanisms of neurodegeneration, the primary dementias remain incurable.

There is another group of disorders in which dementia occurs as part of a more diverse spectrum of clinical abnormalities and is viewed as being related to another neurologic or medical condition. These are the so-called "secondary dementias." While the primary dementias have been the subject of many books and monographs, the secondary dementias have received inadequate coverage. There are a number of reasons why the secondary dementias deserve the careful attention of clinicians. Most importantly, *secondary dementias are potentially reversible*; therefore, they should be the focus of any clinical evaluation for a patient presenting with memory loss or other cognitive impairment. One would not want to treat a patient for the symptoms of dementia with memory-enhancing cholinesterase inhibitors or antipsychotic agents while missing an opportunity to correct an underlying cause of the dementia. *Specific, effective therapies are sometimes available to treat dementia when secondary to other causes.* Just like the primary forms, the secondary dementias are increasing rapidly in frequency as the population ages and as therapeutic advances allow patients to live longer with their primary disorders.

Thus, *patients with a secondary dementia will commonly be encountered in clinical practice*.

This is a particularly opportune time to review the secondary dementias since there has been an explosion of new knowledge in this field with specialists who specifically focus on the cognitive and behavioral aspects of a variety of medical and neurological disorders.

I am very fortunate that many of the world's best experts have agreed to convey this new knowledge to you by serving as chapter authors and I greatly appreciate their superb contributions; I think you will as well.

Roger Kurlan

Contents

Contributors

Mindy Aisen   *Veteran's Health Administration, Rehabilitation Research and Development Service, Washington, D.C., U.S.A.*

Denise Burton   *Veteran's Health Administration, Rehabilitation Research and Development Service, Washington, D.C., U.S.A.*

Peter G. Como   *Department of Neurology, University of Rochester Medical Center, Rochester, New York, U.S.A.*

David J. Gill   *Department of Neurology, University of Rochester Medical Center, Rochester, New York, U.S.A.*

William D. Graf   *Section of Neurology, Children's Mercy Hospitals and Clinics, University of Missouri-Kansas City, Kansas City, Missouri and Department of Neurology, University of Kansas School of Medicine, Kansas City, Kansas, U.S.A.*

Simon Hawke   *Brain and Mind Research Institute, University of Sydney, Sydney, New South Wales, Australia*

Roger Kurlan   *Department of Neurology, University of Rochester Medical Center, Rochester, New York, U.S.A.*

Mark Mapstone   *Department of Neurology, University of Rochester Medical Center, Rochester, New York, U.S.A.*

Peter Mariuz   *Department of Infectious Diseases, University of Rochester Medical Center, Rochester, New York, U.S.A.*

Giovanni Meola   *University of Milan, San Donato Hospital, Milan, Italy*

Irene Hegeman Richard   *Department of Neurology, University of Rochester Medical Center, Rochester, New York, U.S.A.*

Gustavo C. Román *University of Texas Health Science Center at San Antonio and the Audie L. Murphy Memorial Veterans Hospital, Geriatric Research Education and Clinical Center, San Antonio, Texas, U.S.A.*

Valeria Sansone *University of Milan, San Donato Hospital, Milan, Italy*

Randolph B. Schiffer *Texas Tech University Health Sciences Center, Lubbock, Texas, U.S.A.*

Giovanni Schifitto *Department of Neurology, University of Rochester Medical Center, Rochester, New York, U.S.A.*

Larry E. Tune *Department of Psychiatry and Behavioral Sciences, Emory University School of Medicine, Atlanta, Georgia, U.S.A.*

1

Dementia in Cerebrovascular Disease (Vascular Dementia; VaD)

Gustavo C. Román

*University of Texas Health Science Center at San Antonio and the
Audie L. Murphy Memorial Veterans Hospital, Geriatric Research Education
and Clinical Center, San Antonio, Texas, U.S.A.*

INTRODUCTION

Vascular dementia (VaD) due to cerebrovascular disease (CVD) and ischemic brain injury from cardiovascular disease is the most common of the secondary dementias. Cognitive changes occurring after a stroke have been described since the seventeenth century (1).

In 1672, the English physician Thomas Willis (Fig. 1) provided the first accurate clinical observations of patients developing dementia post-apoplexy in his book *De Anima Brutorum*. The clinical picture of progressive cognitive decline ("dullness of mind and forgetfulness") accompanied by hemiparesis, sometimes with recovery or "partial resolution" of a motor deficit, most likely corresponds to instances of VaD.

The prevalence of CVD in the elderly is so prominent that for most of the last century it was widely held that "atherosclerotic dementia" was the etiology of senile dementia (1). It is currently accepted that a neurodegenerative condition—Alzheimer's disease (AD)—is the primary cause of dementia in the aged. Nevertheless, epidemiological and clinical evidence gathered during the last two decades have shown that CVD is an important contributor to the clinical expression of AD and other primary dementias (2,3).

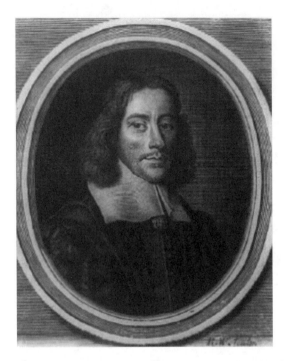

Figure 1   Thomas Willis (1621–1675) described in 1672 the first accurate clinical observations of patients with post-stroke VaD.

The considerable progress achieved in the understanding and treatment of stroke, in the prevention of recurrent stroke, and in the management of vascular risk factors, grants new hope for the prevention of VaD. In addition, encouraging results from controlled clinical trials for the pharmacologic treatment of VaD suggest that effective therapies are possible. This chapter provides an overview of the magnitude of the problem, pathogenesis, clinical manifestations, treatment, and prevention of VaD.

DEFINITIONS

VaD: This is a secondary dementia that includes several clinical and pathological forms of severe cognitive impairment resulting from ischemic or hemorrhagic stroke and CVD, or from ischemic-hypoperfusive brain lesions of cardiovascular origin (Table 1).

Post-stroke VaD: This term refers to acute-onset forms of VaD occurring after ischemic or hemorrhagic stroke (4). Dementia may result from a single stroke interrupting brain circuits important for memory and cognition (*strategic stroke VaD*) or from multiple strokes (*multi-infarct*

Table 1   Clinical and Pathological Forms of VaD

Large-Vessel Dementia (Mechanisms: Artery-to-artery embolism; thrombosis/ occlusion of extracranial or intracranial cerebral arteries; cardiogenic embolism)
- MID: Multiple large complete infarcts, cortico-subcortical in location, usually with perifocal incomplete infarction involving the white matter
- Strategic Infarct Dementia: Single brain infarct in functionally critical areas of the brain (angular gyrus, thalamus, basal forebrain, posterior cerebral artery, and anterior cerebral artery territories)

Small-Vessel Dementia
- SIVD: Binswanger's disease; CADASIL; lacunar dementia or lacunar state (état lacunaire); multiple lacunes with extensive perifocal incomplete infarction
- Cortical–Subcortical: Hypertensive and arteriolosclerotic angiopathy; CAA; other hereditary forms; collagen-vascular disease with dementia; moyamoya; cerebral sinus/venous thrombosis

Ischemic-Hypoperfusive Dementia
- Border-Zone Infarction: Restricted injury due to selective vulnerability; incomplete white matter infarction
- Hemorrhagic Dementia: Traumatic subdural hematoma; subarachnoid hemorrhage; cerebral hemorrhage; hematological factors

---

Abbreviations: CADASIL, cerebral autosomal dominant arteriopathy with subcortical infarcts and leukoencephalopathy; VaD, vascular dementia; MID, multi-infarct dementia; SIVD, subcortical ischemic vascular dementia; CAA, cerebral amyloid angiopathy.
Source: From Ref. 102.

dementia or MID). Post-stroke dementia is ascertained by performing neuropsychological tests after stroke (typically, at three months post-ictus).

Pre-stroke dementia: Not every patient with onset or worsening of dementia after stroke qualifies for a diagnosis of post-stroke VaD. Careful questioning of patients and relatives using tests, such as the Informant Questionnaire on Cognitive Decline in the Elderly (5) can separate patients with pre-existing memory loss and probable AD (pre-stroke dementia) from pure cases of post-stroke VaD. The prevalence of pre-stroke dementia in cases initially diagnosed as post-stroke dementia ranges from 9% in Taiwan (6) to 15–16% in Europe (7–9). Most cases of pre-stroke dementia have dual pathology, such as AD or dementia with Lewy bodies and CVD.

Subcortical ischemic VaD (SIVD): This is a form of VaD caused by small-vessel disease characterized by subacute onset and the presence of white matter ischemic lesions and lacunes (10). The term "subcortical" refers both to the location of the lesions and to the clinical features of the dementia with preponderant executive dysfunction.

Vascular cognitive impairment (VCI): By analogy with the concept of mild cognitive impairment (MCI)—currently considered the earliest clinical manifestation of AD—the term VCI refers to patients with classic vascular risk factors or CVD and some degree of cognitive loss short of dementia. This term was introduced to enhance recognition of the damaging cognitive effects of vascular burden on the brain preceding the development of VaD. Although appealing, this concept has been difficult to implement due to lack of a strict definition and diagnostic criteria. Furthermore, Ballard et al. (11) recently demonstrated that half of the stroke survivors older than 75 years of age improved in global cognitive tests 15 months after the stroke, in comparison with scores obtained three months post-ictus.

MAGNITUDE OF THE PROBLEM

Projected figures for stroke and CVD indicate a worldwide increase in their prevalence. Therefore, VaD may become the most common form of dementia in the elderly, both by itself and as an enhancing factor of primary degenerative dementias (12). Currently, about 20% of the 5.6 million cases of dementia in the United States or 1.1 million cases are vascular in origin. The situation in Europe is similar: about 800,000 people have a diagnosis of VaD out of 3,286,000 with clinical dementia (13). Considering that 26% of older stroke patients may develop severe cognitive impairment, an estimated 140,000 new cases of post-stroke VaD may occur in Europe out of 536,000 strokes per year (13). In the United States, with over 750,000 first-ever stroke cases, VaD cases may reach 200,000 per year.

Prevalence

Population-based epidemiological studies of VaD are difficult to implement due to lack of recognition of subcortical VaD using criteria based on the MID model, the need for expensive imaging studies in large populations, and shortage of bedside tests of executive dysfunction. The most recent population-based studies are those of the European collaboration in dementia (EURODEM) (14). Autopsy-confirmed cases from the Rochester (Minnesota) database (15) recently found the following etiologies: AD 51%, pure VaD 13%, and combined AD plus CVD 12%, resulting in an overall prevalence of VaD of 25%. In a few prevalence studies from South America (Uruguay, Argentina, Brazil, and Venezuela), VaD is the second most common form of dementia (16). VaD remains the first cause of dementia in Japan (17).

A meta-analysis of 47 international prevalence studies (18) found that VaD prevalence increases exponentially with age and is more prevalent than AD in subjects older than 85 years of age. Prevalence rates for VaD double every 5.3 years, compared with 4.5 years for Alzheimer's disease. Prevalence rates range from about $1.5/100$ at ages 70–75 years to $14–16/100$ at 80 years of age and above. VaD has a peculiar geographical (racial) variation, being more prevalent in Asian, Black, and mixed races than in Caucasian populations. This is probably due to the preponderance of small-vessel disease in these races. However, the prevalence of Alzheimer's disease versus VaD tends to increase among ethnic Japanese who migrated to Hawaii (19), indicating environmental interaction on genetic susceptibility.

Incidence

Incidence data for VaD from longitudinal cohort studies are rather limited. In a meta-analysis of 11 VaD studies, Jorm and Jolley (20) provide age-specific incidence data. Recent EURODEM incidence rates (21) range from 0.7 per 1000 person-years at ages 65–69 to 8.1 at age 90+. Table 2 summarizes incidence data for VaD in pooled population-based studies in Europe (21). Notice that in all age groups, VaD is more common in men, in contrast to AD that predominates in women. Dubois and Herbert (22) used age-standardized incidence ratios (SIR) to analyze data from 10 incidence studies in comparison with the Canadian Study of Health and Aging. SIRs ranged from 0.42 to 2.68, confirming a wide geographical variation. These variations may be due to genetic, environmental, or methodological differences between studies.

Risk Factors for VaD

As discussed in the following, anatomical location of the stroke is more relevant for a dementia outcome than the volume of the lesion (4). For this reason, infarctions in the territory of the anterior cerebral artery (ACA) and posterior cerebral artery (PCA), in the thalamus or the caudate nucleus result more often in VaD than lesions in other territories. These lesions disrupt the structures underlying memory and executive function. In addition, a number of factors, such as

Table 2 Incidence of VaD in Europe: Pooled Rates by Age Group and Sex Per 1000 Person-Years

Age group (yr)	Male, rate (95% CI)	Female, rate (95% CI)	Total, rate (95% CI)
65–69	1.2 (0.3–3.1)	0.3 (0.01–1.4)	0.7 (0.2–1.6)
70–74	1.6 (0.7–3.2)	0.8 (0.2–1.6)	1.2 (0.6–1.9)
75–79	3.9 (2.3–6.2)	3.2 (1.8–4.5)	3.5 (2.1–4.3)
80–84	8.3 (4.5–11.1)	4.5 (2.9–6.8)	5.9 (4.0–7.4)
85–89	6.2 (1.9–9.9)	6.1 (3.0–8.9)	6.1 (3.3–7.9)
90+	10.9 (2.0–18.6)	7.0 (2.0–10.0)	8.1 (2.8–9.9)

Abbreviation: VaD, vascular dementia; CI, confidence interval.
Source: From Ref. 21.

Table 3   Main Risk Factors Post-Stroke VaD

Age: Older age
Education: Lower educational level
Personal Factors: Lower income, current smokers
Genetic Factors: Family history of dementia
Stroke Type: Recurrent strokes
Stroke Location: Left-sided lesions, "strategic strokes" (i.e., posterior association areas,
    such as gyrus angularis; posterior cerebral artery territories including paramedian
    thalamic artery territory, inferomedial temporal lobes, and hippocampus; watershed or
    border-zone infarcts mainly involving superior frontal and parietal regions; bilateral
    anterior cerebral artery territories, anterior choroidal artery strokes, and basal forebrain
    lesions; and frontal white matter lesions). Inferior capsular genu stroke producing
    diaschisis of frontal lobes and cerebellum
Stroke Volume: Lesions larger than 50–100 mL of tissue destruction, large perilesional
    incomplete ischemic areas involving white matter, larger periventricular white matter
    ischemic lesions
Stroke Complications: Hypoxic and ischemic complications of acute stroke (i.e., seizures,
    cardiac arrhythmias, aspiration pneumonia, hypotension)
Stroke Manifestations: Dysphagia, gait limitations, urinary impairment

---

Abbreviation: VaD, Vascular dementia.
Source: From Ref. 4.

age, left hemisphere location, recurrent stroke, and degree of white matter ischemia also increase the likelihood of developing dementia after a stroke (Table 3).

Patients with large *lesions of the left (dominant) hemisphere* have almost a fivefold risk of developing post-stroke dementia, an effect not explained by aphasia (23). The left-sided predominance of lesions in demented patients with large-vessel stroke in the ACA and PCA territories has been repeatedly demonstrated (23–27). Recently, progressive decline in cognitive function was described in participants in the Cardiovascular Health Study who had stenosis of the left internal carotid artery (ICA), but not in those with stenosis of the right ICA, in the absence of stroke or CVD (28). Possible explanations include the fact that the left hemisphere has a larger cholinergic innervation than the right one and that tests such as the Mini Mental State Examination (MMSE) rely heavily on language functions.

Moroney et al. (29) found that hypoxic and ischemic complications of acute stroke (e.g., seizures, cardiac arrhythmias, aspiration pneumonia, etc.) are strong and independent risk factors for post-stroke dementia, increasing more than fourfold the risk of developing post-stroke dementia (OR 4.3, 95% CI 1.9–9.6, after adjustment for demographic factors, recurrent stroke, and baseline cognitive function). Hypoxic and ischemic complications of acute stroke may result in border-zone infarcts and may cause Binswanger-type ischemic periventricular white matter lesions. The latter occur with higher frequency in subjects with orthostatic hypotension (30).

Dementia is a predictor of poor outcome in patients with stroke (31–33). In Rochester (Minnesota), 10% of 482 incident cases of dementia had onset or worsening of the dementia within three months of a stroke (34). Overall, patients with VaD had worse mortality than matched subjects [relative risk (RR), 2.7], particularly among cases of post-stroke VaD (RR, 4.5).

PATHOPHYSIOLOGY

Volume loss was the first explanation proposed for the pathogenesis of VaD. In 1970, Tomlinson, Blessed, and Roth (35) demonstrated that the loss of more than 50–100 mL of brain tissue from large-vessel strokes resulted in dementia. Based on their findings, the term multi-infarct dementia (MID) was coined for this condition (36). However, careful neuropathological correlation studies pioneered by T. Del Ser et al. (37) demonstrated that dementia could occur with very small lesion volumes. Thereafter, stroke location became a priority factor in VaD. In 1988, Brun and Gustafson (38,39) coined the name "strategic infarcts" for these lesions. With the advent of new-generation computerized tomography (CT) and magnetic resonance imaging (MRI) of the brain, the important role of ischemic-hypoperfusive lesions of the periventricular white matter in the pathogenesis of VaD was recognized. Román (40) proposed the name *senile dementia of the Binswanger type* for cases of VaD with preponderant white-matter lesions. More recently, neuropathological studies have shown that cortical microinfarcts increase the risk of dementia significantly (41,42). Finally, the role of cholinergic denervation from ischemic brain lesions became relevant following positive trials of cholinergic medications in VaD. The main mechanisms involved in the pathogenesis of VaD are reviewed in the following paragraphs.

VaD from Large-Vessel Disease

In 1962, J. Delay and S. Brion (43) described three possible locations for strokes producing VaD: (i) A posterior form, with infarction in the territory of the PCA, involving the ventral-medial temporal lobe, occipital structures, and thalamus. (ii) An anterior form, with infarction in the ACA territory and medial frontal lobe lesions. (iii) A basal form, with bilateral involvement of the basal ganglia and thalamus. The common element of lesions in these regions is the involvement of the memory circuit. Amnesia results from interruption by ischemic injury of any portion of the circuit comprising the hippocampus, fornix, mamillary body, mammillo-thalamic tract, anterior thalamus, and cingulate cortex.

Memory impairment is a requirement for the diagnosis of dementia in all current definitions (which are based on the paradigm of AD), but amnesia may be also prominent in patients with VaD, as described next.

PCA Lesions

About 25% of patients with infarctions in the PCA territory present with amnesia (44) as a result of damage to the hippocampus, isthmus, entorhinal and perirhinal cortex, and parahippocampal gyrus (Fig. 2). Smaller lesions occur with strokes of the anterior or posterior choroidal arteries.

Unilateral lesions cause verbal amnesia with left-sided lesions; loss of visuospatial memory and memory for locations with lesions on the right side, and global amnesia with bilateral damage. These patients present episodic anterograde amnesia—similar to that of AD—and are unable to encode and consolidate new verbal material, facts, events, stories, names, or concepts, but working memory and procedural memory are intact (45) and confabulations are rare. More than 80% of the patients with PCA strokes have visual signs (44), including homonymous hemianopsia, color agnosia, and visual agnosia. Other findings may include transcortical sensory aphasia, pure alexia or alexia without agraphia with left-sided lesions, and spatial disorientation with right-sided ones. Bilateral occipital lesions cause Anton's syndrome (cortical blindness with anosognosia for blindness) or Balint's syndrome (simultagnosia, optic ataxia, and ocular apraxia) with bilateral parieto-occipital infarctions above the calcarine fissure. Prosopagnosia occurs with bilateral occipital ischemia below the calcarine fissure.

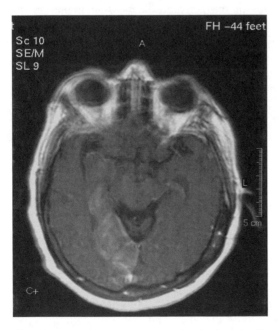

Figure 2 Infarction of the right PCA territory leading to amnesia as a result of damage to the hippocampus, isthmus, entorhinal and perirhinal cortex, and parahippocampal gyrus as shown in this diffusion-weighted brain MRI.

Basal Forebrain Infarction

Ischemic injury of the cholinergic nuclei in the basal forebrain may occur with subarachnoid hemorrhage from ruptured aneurysms of the anterior communicating artery (AComA), usually after surgical repair (46,47). Perforating branches of the AComA or of the proximal ACA may be damaged at the time of surgery. Phillips et al. (48) found severe anterograde amnesia for verbal and visuospatial material in a patient after surgical repair of an aneurysm of the AComA. The patient also had severe apathy, lack of initiative and spontaneity, and executive dysfunction. On post-mortem neuropathological examination it was found that the lesions had damaged midline basal areas, rostral to the anterior commisure and lamina terminalis, destroying the medial septal nuclei (Ch1), the vertical portion (Ch2) of the nucleus of the diagonal band of Broca (ndbB), the nucleus accumbens, and adjacent areas. Damage to the cholinergic neurons in the septal nucleus and ndbB appears to determine the persistence of the amnesia.

Thalamic VaD

In 1966, Castaigne et al. (49,50) first described a dramatic form of VaD occurring after paramedian thalamic ischemic strokes involving the anterior thalamus. The polar thalamic artery, a branch of the posterior communicating artery, irrigates these territories.

Symptoms also occur with lesions of the medial and central thalamus (Fig. 3) involving the dorsomedial nucleus (DMn) and the mamillothalamic

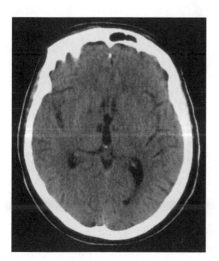

Figure 3 Lesions of the medial and central thalamus are shown, which caused thalamic VaD. Paramedian thalamic ischemic strokes involving the anterior thalamus, dorsomedial nuclei or the mamillothalamic tract also may cause thalamic VaD.

tract (51,52). The paramedian thalamic artery, a branch of the basilar communicating artery of Percheron (53), irrigates the latter two structures.

Damage to the mamillothalamic tract is the critical lesion in thalamic amnesia affecting episodic long-term memory, with relative sparing of short-term memory and intellectual capacities (51,54). The mamillothalamic tract projects into the anterior nuclei of the thalamus and then into the cingulate cortex. Using MRI, Van der Werf et al. (54) also demonstrated that lesions in the DMn midline nuclei and intralaminar nuclei are manifested by executive dysfunction with reduced processing speed. Severe attention deficits occur with lesion of the intralaminar nuclei.

Anterior thalamic stroke patients typically present with fluctuating hypersomnolence or a depressed level of consciousness that gradually improves over days to weeks to reveal impairments in attention, motivation, initiative, executive functions, memory, as well as dramatic verbal and motor slowness, apathy, and perseverative behavior (55).

Gaze abnormalities are common and include vertical gaze paresis, medial rectus paresis, and absent convergence. Dysarthria and mild hemiparesis may be present when the lesions extend to the subthalamic and midbrain tegmentum irrigated by the superior paramedian mesencephalic artery (53).

VaD from Small-Vessel Disease

A lacunar stroke may rarely produce dramatic changes in personality and cognition, often considered psychiatric in nature until brain imaging demonstrates the strategically located vascular lesion capable of producing this clinical picture. The acute, apoplectiform onset of the deficit reveals its vascular nature. Such highly symptomatic solitary lacunes have been localized in the dorsal intralaminar nuclei of the thalamus (56), or in the inferior genu of the internal capsule, as described later.

However, there is increased recognition of a form of VaD characterized by slow onset and gradual progression of cognitive decline. This form is called SIVD (10), because the lesions are subcortical in location and because the clinical deficits conform to the clinical picture of the subcortical dementias (in contrast with the cortical dementias exemplified by AD). The lesions of SIVD include *incomplete white matter ischemia*, *lacunar strokes*, and areas of *microinfarction*. Each one of these three elements is independently associated with increased risk of dementia (57–60).

Inferior Genu Lacunar Stroke

In 1992, Tatemichi et al. (61,62) described in patients with lacunar infarction involving the inferior genu of the internal capsule a typical lacunar syndrome manifested by sudden changes in cognitive function, fluctuating attention, confusion, abulia, striking psychomotor retardation, executive dysfunction, and other features of frontal lobe dysfunction but with mild focal findings such as hemiparesis or dysarthria. Memory loss was present in all cases but left-sided infarcts had severe verbal memory loss and right-sided ones had visuospatial memory loss (63,64).

This lacunar stroke of the inferior genu of the internal capsule, by a postulated mechanism of diaschisis, causes ipsilateral blood flow reduction to the inferior and medial frontal cortex and to the ipsilateral temporal lobe and contralateral cerebellar hemisphere (65). Inferior genu stroke is closely related to thalamic VaD because the lesion may sever corticothalamic and thalamocortical fibers in the thalamic peduncles.

Caudate Nucleus Stroke

Caudate strokes may also present with memory loss characterized by recall difficulties even with cues but with normal recognition (66). These features, along with the typical abulia (67,68), are probably due to interruption of frontal connections. There are important frontal lobe connections relevant to memory.

Subacute Ischemic VaD

In contrast with the acute onset of lacunar strokes, patients with SIVD present a subacute, slowly progressive course. Lesions result from non-occlusive small-vessel disease affecting periventricular white matter (Binswanger's disease); stepwise worsening may occur when small-vessel occlusion leads to recurrent lacunar strokes. This pattern is typical of CADASIL (cerebral autosomal dominant arteriopathy with subcortical infarcts and leukoencephalopathy), a genetic form of VaD (69,70). The main forms of SIVD are lacunar state (*état lacunaire*), Binswanger's disease, CADASIL, and some forms of cerebral amyloid angiopathy (CAA).

Lacunar state (*état lacunaire*):   In 1901, Pierre Marie (71) described this clinicopathological syndrome in the elderly, emphasizing the presence of multiple lacunes in basal ganglia, pons, and white matter. Numerous clinical lacunar syndromes occur; however, most lacunes are clinically silent. Traditionally considered benign lesions, lacunes actually have excess risk of death after five years, increased risk of recurrence, and high risk of cognitive impairment and dementia (72). Interruption of cortico-subcortical circuits critical for memory, cognition, and behavior may result in VaD. In the Nun Study (73) lacunes increased about 20 times the risk of clinical expression of dementia in subjects with AD lesions. In population-based studies, silent lacunes doubled the risk of dementia in the elderly (74). Lacunes are a reliable marker of small-vessel disease of the brain.

Senile dementia of the Binswanger type: In 1894, Binswanger (75) described as the hallmark of this condition the presence of an ischemic periventricular leukoencephalopathy that typically spares the arcuate subcortical U fibers. Binswanger's disease is often seen in patients with long-standing, poorly treated hypertension, or with other forms of small-vessel disease, such as diabetes. Therefore, multiple lacunes often coexist with white-matter lesions.

Patients with Binswanger's disease present a cognitive and motor syndrome with executive dysfunction, loss of verbal fluency, slowing of motor function with perseveration, impersistence, inattention, difficulties with set shifting, and abnormal Luria's kinetic melody tests (40). Memory difficulties consist of poor retrieval with intact recognition. Apathy, depression, and behavioral problems are common. Mild residual hemiparesis or other discrete focal findings are often found, as well as a peculiar short-stepped gait *(marche à petits pas)*, dysarthria, and pseudobulbar palsy. Extrapyramidal features, such as inexpressive facies, slowness of movement, axial rigidity, loss of postural reflexes, and frequent falls are common; there is also increased urinary frequency and nocturia.

CADASIL: A major advance in the field of VaD was the clinical and genetic description of CADASIL, an autosomal dominant disorder of cerebral small-vessels mapped to chromosome 19q12 (69). Clinical manifestations (70) include TIAs and strokes (80%), cognitive deficits leading to subcortical VaD (50%), migraine with focal deficits (40%), mood disorders (30%), and epilepsy (10%). Onset occurs in early adulthood (mean age: 46 years) with absence of risk factors. Usually, there is an absence of risk factors for vascular disease. Patients with CADASIL usually have a downhill clinical course that culminates in dementia and death some 20 years after the onset of symptoms.

Clinically, the dementia of CADASIL is identical to that of sporadic Binswanger's disease with slow onset, frontal subcortical features, prominent executive dysfunction, abnormal gait, urinary disturbances, and pseudobulbar palsy. MRI reveals a combination of small lacunar lesions and diffuse white-matter abnormalities; the latter are often present in asymptomatic relatives.

The vascular lesion in CADASIL is a unique non-amyloid non-atherosclerotic microangiopathy involving arterioles (100–400 μ in diameter) and capillaries, primarily in the brain but also in other organs (76). The vessels show typical deposits of eosinophilic, PAS-positive material in the arterial media. Under an electron microscope, these are granular osmiophilic deposits with accumulation of the ectodomain of the *Notch3* receptor in the basal lamina of degenerated smooth muscle cells. Genetic tests or a typical skin biopsy immunostained with a *Notch3* monoclonal antibody (77) confirms the diagnosis.

CAA: CAA is characterized by deposition of amyloid in the walls of leptomeningeal and cerebral cortical blood vessels, with recurrent, multiple lobar hemorrhages and cognitive deterioration leading to death or VaD. MRI displays diffuse white-matter abnormalities along with ischemic or hemorrhagic focal brain lesions. There are sporadic and autosomal dominant forms of CAA. A-β, the major amyloid component of AD, also occurs in sporadic CAA and in familial forms of the Dutch-, Flemish-, and Iowa-type. Familial British dementia (FBD) is an autosomal dominant CAA due to a point mutation in the BRI gene, characterized by progressive spastic paraparesis and cerebellar ataxia with onset in the sixth decade (78). Brain MRI shows Binswanger-type deep white-matter hyper-intensities and lacunar infarcts without intracerebral hemorrhages; the corpus callosum is involved and atrophic (78). Plaques and tangles are present in the brain but the amyloid subunit (ABri) is different and unrelated to other amyloid proteins. FBD combines neurodegeneration and dementia with systemic amyloid deposition (79).

Hypoperfusion

The elderly are particularly prone to hypoperfusive brain lesions due to two main reasons: (i) Normal aging affects the autonomic control of cardiovascular function resulting in *decreased vagal control* of cardiac frequency, favoring the development of cardiac arrhythmias, and in *sympathetic system alterations* of resistance and capacitance vessels predisposing the elderly to orthostatic hypotension. Furthermore, congestive heart failure (CHF) and cardiac disease are common among them. (ii) The anatomical and physiological changes of cerebral vasculature occurring with aging increase the susceptibility of certain brain regions to hypoperfusion (80).

A review of the mechanisms and pathology of central autonomic cardiovascular control is beyond the limits of this chapter but excellent reviews are available (81,82). The name "neurocardiovascular instability" (NCVI) is used for neurally mediated forms of hypotension with or without bradycardia, manifested as dizziness, syncope, or falls (83,84). According to Kenny (83), NCVI includes carotid sinus syndrome, orthostatic hypotension, and vasovagal syndrome. Kenny, Kalaria and Ballard (85) found a prevalence of NCVI of about 70% among patients presenting with frequent falls, with cognitive impairment or dementia. Multifactorial interventions, including treatment of NCVI, significantly reduced falls and syncope. Cardio-inhibitory carotid sinus hypersensitivity, bradycardia, and hypotension were particularly high in Lewy body dementia. Deep white-matter hyperintensities on MRI correlated with systolic fall during carotid sinus stimulation ($R = 0.58$; $p < 0.005$), suggesting a possible causal association between hypotension induced by bradyarrhythmias. NCVI is a reversible cause of falls and syncope, and repeated hypotensive episodes may exaggerate cognitive decline in these patients. Treatment with L-DOPS, a norepinephrine precursor, appears promising in some patients with neurogenic orthostatic hypotension (86). The changes in brain vessels with aging, and the main lesions associated with hypoperfusion, are described in the following sections.

Hypoperfusive Brain Lesions

The main hypoperfusive brain lesions are border zone strokes, incomplete white-matter infarction, and hippocampal sclerosis.

Watershed or boundary zone infarcts: These lesions occur in relentless and prolonged hypotension or in patients with impaired collateral circulation due to severe, extensive, or multiple atheromatous stenoses of the cerebral arteries.

Lesions typically affect areas at the junction of large-vessel arterial territories. For instance, in the cortex posterior to the interparietal sulcus at the boundaries between the ACA and middle cerebral artery in cases of extracranial internal carotid artery occlusion; or in the center of the white matter, between the deep territories of the ACA and middle cerebral artery; as well as in the periventricular white matter fed by long-penetrating end-arterioles.

Incomplete white matter infarction: This is a frequent hypoperfusive brain lesion often resulting from cardiac failure or hypotension in the elderly. Lesions are identical to those of Binswanger's disease and similar to that observed at the penumbra of large infarcts (87). Moody et al. (88) performed a careful study of the anatomical patterns of microcirculation that explains the susceptibility of certain cerebral areas to hypoperfusion. According to these authors, brain areas irrigated by short penetrating arteries can tolerate better hypotension and hypoperfusion (88). These resistant areas include cerebral cortex, the subcortical arcuate fibers, and the corpus callosum. In addition, the claustrum, the external and extreme capsules, receive dual circulation and are resistant to hypotensive and hypoperfusive injuries (88). In contrast, the white matter in the centrum semiovale, as well as the periventricular white matter, are distal watershed territories irrigated by long, penetrating medullary arteries; these are highly sensitive to hypoperfusion (88), particularly in the elderly. Likewise, the distal territories of the lenticulostriate arteries in the basal ganglia are affected selectively by lacunar strokes.

Hippocampal sclerosis: This is a localized form of ischemia and atrophy observed in very old demented subjects (89–92), particularly in those with cardiac disease (90). The particular vascular supply of the hippocampus (93) probably explains the development of this lesion. The hippocampal arteries arise mainly from the PCA and anterior choroidal artery, a branch of the internal carotid artery. Straight arteries from the hippocampal arteries enter Ammon's horn through the dentate gyrus and then branch out at right angles in a rake-like pattern. As a result, the CA1 sector is poorly vascularized (93). Hippocampal sclerosis was originally described in patients with epilepsy and with perinatal injury. Hippocampal sclerosis in the elderly may be caused by systemic hypoperfusion or from ischemia due to intrinsic CVD (89,91,94).

Aging Vascular Changes: *État Criblé* and Arteriolosclerosis

The most important vascular changes with age are lengthening and tortuosity of the medullary and cortical arterioles. This process leads to dilatation of the perivascular spaces of Virchow-Robin (95) causing *état criblé* (cribriform or sieve-like state), which interferes with metabolic exchanges between blood and neural tissue. These vessels undergo progressive thickening of the vessel walls with reduction of the lumen due to arteriolosclerosis (96), a concentric deposition of lamellar collagen fibers, and accumulation of a fibrohyaline substance in the subadventitia, with minimal changes in median and intima. Arteriolosclerosis is a common change in the elderly beginning late in the fourth decade, increasing in severity after age 65. It is more prominent in the frontal lobes, followed by the parietal, occipital, and temporal lobes. The cause is unknown but endothelial reaction to shear, stretch stress, and oxidation are some possible causes. Vessels become elongated, tortuous, narrow, often calcified, and unreactive to vasodilatation.

According to Poiseuille's law, a major decrease in flow occurs in small vessels with decrease in caliber (radius) and with increase in vessel length. Thus, flow in distal white-matter territories depends almost exclusively on perfusion pressure and blood viscosity. Therefore, arteriolosclerosis of the medullary vessels and elongation increase the risk of hypoperfusion and ischemia in the distal white-matter territories irrigated by these arteries. This explains the presence of ischemic periventricular white-matter lesions in elderly subjects with CHF, cardiac arrhythmias, or orthostatic hypotension. Furthermore, increasing degrees of arteriolosclerosis in the elderly correlate with greater severity of lesions of Binswanger-type periventricular incomplete ischemia (96).

In addition, the deleterious effects of hypertension, diabetes, smoking, and other risk factors that cause endothelial damage increase the morphological damage of the cerebral microcirculation.

Vascular Effects of Cholinergic Denervation

In the experimental animal, stimulation of the cholinergic nucleus basalis of Meynert produces extensive cortical vasodilatation (97). In the human, cholinergic deficits are well documented in patients with VaD, independently of any concomitant AD pathology (98). Cholinergic structures in the basal forebrain and their projections in the deep white matter and the periventricular regions are highly vulnerable to ischemic damage (99,100). Mesulan et al. (101) demonstrated cholinergic denervation from ischemic lesions in a young patient with CADASIL. Decreased cholinergic innervation and decreased vasodilatation probably enhance the risk of hypotensive and hypoperfusive brain injuries.

CLINICAL FORMS OF VaD

From the clinical viewpoint, Román (102) divides the clinical syndromes of VaD into two main groups, *acute* and *subacute* (Table 4), according to the temporal profile of clinical presentation.

Acute Onset VaD

This group includes patients with new-onset dementia after a clinically eloquent acute ischemic event, either from a single strategic stroke resulting from occlusion (or rupture) of a large-size vessel, from recurrent strokes (MID), or after a symptomatic lacunar stroke caused by small-vessel disease.

Table 4   Clinical Forms of VaD

Location	Vascular lesion	Clinical manifestations
Acute-onset VaD		
PCA territory	Ventral-medial temporal lobe, hippocampus, occipital lobe, thalamus	Anterograde amnesia, aphasia, visuospatial difficulties, constructional apraxia
ACA territory (AcoA aneurysm)	Medial frontal lobe lesions, basal nucleus of Meynert	Amnesia, abulia, inattention, executive dysfunction
Angular gyrus	Left *angular gyrus*	Right–left disorientation, finger agnosia, acalculia, dysgraphia aphasia and constructional difficulties
	Right *angular gyrus*	Hemispatial neglect, visuospatial or visuo-constructive disturbances
Thalamus	Anterior (polar), medial, and central thalamus involving DMn and mamillothalamic tract	Initial unconsciousness, then inattention, amotivation, loss of initiative, executive dysfunctions, memory loss, verbal and motor slowness and apathy, gaze problems
Inferior genu internal capsule	Lacunar stroke in territory of anterior perforators arising from ICA or ACA	Confusion, abulia, striking psychomotor retardation, inattention, executive dysfunction
Caudate nucleus	Ischemic stroke or hemorrhage in head of the caudate	Abulia, recall problems, frontal signs
Subacute-onset VaD		
Lacunar state (état lacunaire)	Lacunes in putamen, globus pallidus, thalamus, frontal white matter, pons	Subcortical dementia: slow mentation, gait problems, incontinence
Binswanger's disease	Periventricular white matter ischemia sparing arcuate fibers plus lacunes	Subcortical dementia
CADASIL	Leukoencephalopathy, lacunes, typical small-artery lesions, *Notch 3* gene	Depression, migraines, subcortical dementia

Abbreviations: VaD, vascular dementia; PCA, posterior cerebral artery; ACA, anterior cerebral artery; AcoA, anterior communicating artery; DMn, dorsomedial nucleus; ICA, internal carotid artery; CADASIL, cerebral autosomal dominant arteriopathy with subcortical infarcts and leukoencephalopathy.
Source: From Ref. 102.

Table 5 provides a summary of ischemic cortical strokes with behavioral and cognitive manifestations. As described earlier, single large-vessel stroke in one of the following locations may produce VaD:

1. PCA territory involving ventral-medial temporal lobe, hippocampus, occipital structures, and thalamus; patients present with anterograde amnesia, aphasia, visuospatial difficulties, or constructional apraxia.
2. ACA territory and medial-frontal lobe lesions, often from an ACA aneurysm rupture, causing ischemia of the basal nucleus of Meynert resulting in cholinergic deficit.
3. Infarction of the left *angular gyrus* presenting with right–left disorientation, finger agnosia, acalculia, dysgraphia, aphasia, and constructional difficulties; on the right side hemispatial neglect, visuo-spatial, or visuo-constructive disturbances may occur.

The most frequent location of lacunar strokes resulting in dementia include:

1. *Thalamus*: Thalamic VaD is caused by butterfly-shaped bilateral paramedian polar thalamic artery infarcts.
2. Some cases of *caudate* stroke.
3. *Capsular genu infarction*: A characteristic syndrome manifested by sudden change in cognitive function, with fluctuating attention, memory loss, confusion, abulia, striking psychomotor retardation, inattention, and other features of frontal lobe dysfunction but with mild focal findings, such as hemiparesis or dysarthria. The usual cause is a lacune involving the inferior genu of the internal capsule, causing ipsilateral blood flow reduction to the inferomedial frontal cortex by a mechanism of diaschisis. This is a thalamo-cortical disconnection syndrome.

Subacute-Onset (Subcortical) VaD

The temporal profile of presentation of these forms of VaD is typically subacute, with a chronic course marked by fluctuations and progressive worsening that is usually inconsistent with an acute stroke. This group is characterized clinically by a subcortical dementia with frontal lobe deficits, executive dysfunction, slow information processing, impaired memory, inattention, depressive mood changes, motor involvement, parkinsonian features, urinary disturbances, and pseudobulbar palsy. Subcortical VaD is common and results from small-vessel disease with lacunes and white-matter lesions that damage structures of the prefrontal–subcortical circuits (caudate nucleus, globus pallidus, thalamus, and connecting fibers). The frontal cortical–subcortical circuits underlie executive functions, as well as motivation and social behaviors. These are parallel anatomic circuits linking regions of the frontal cortex (dorsolateral prefrontal region, lateral orbitofrontal area, and anterior cingulate cortex) to the striatum

Table 5 Cortical Strokes with Behavioral and Cognitive Manifestations

Stroke location	Executive dysfunction	Delirium	Aphasia	Abulia	Agnosia	Neglect	Amnesia
ACA[a]	+	+	+L	+		+	
AChA[b]					+	+	
MCA[c]			+L(Br)		+	+	
Orbitofrontal[d]	+		+L	+			
Precentral[e]	+						
Central sulcus[f]			+L				
Anterior parietal[g]		+	+L			+R	
Posterior parietal[h]		+	+L(W)		+	+R	
Angular[i]		+	+L(W)		+	+R	
Temporal[j]		+R	+L(W)		+	+R	
Caudate[k]	+	+		+		+R	+
PCA[l]		+	+L		+		+

[a]Lower limb paresis, sensory loss, grasp, transcortical aphasia (L), mutism, neglect (R, L, B), callosal disconnection syndrome (L), confusion, euphoria, disinhibition, laughing (Witzelsucht), abulia (R, L), akinetic mutism (B). Similar syndromes with head of the caudate stroke; [b]Hemiplegia, hemianesthesia, hemianopsia or superior quadrantanopsia, visual neglect, anosognosia, apraxia, gaze preference; [c]Massive hemiplegia, hemianesthesia, hemianopsia, gaze deviation, aphasia (L), dressing and constructional apraxia, neglect, anosognosia, prosopagnosia, stupor, coma; [d]Luria's prefrontal syndrome: dysexecutive, loss of programming abilities, imitation behavior, perseveration, grasp, apathy, abulia; [e]Proximal brachial paresis, Luria's dysexecutive premotor syndrome, loss of kinetic melody, motor impersistence. Transcortical motor aphasia (L); [f]Faciobrachial sensorimotor deficit, rare cheiro-oral sensory loss (posterior operculum syndrome), Broca's aphasia (L), pseudobulbar palsy (B); [g]Pseudothalamic sensory loss (faciobrachiocrural), hemisensory and spatial neglect (R), conduction aphasia (L), ideomotor apraxia (L); [h]Supramarginal gyrus: Cortical sensory loss (astereognosia, agraphestesia, propioceptive loss). Wernicke's aphasia (L), Gerstmann's syndrome (L): right–left disorientation, finger agnosia, acalculia, agraphia. Spatial neglect, extinction (R); [i]Supramarginal and gyrus angularis: Hemianopsia or inferior quadrantanopsia, mild hemiparesis. L-lesions: Gerstmann's ± Wernicke's; transcortical sensory/anomic aphasia. R-lesions: Extinction, spatial neglect, asomatognosia, constructional apraxia. Bilateral lesions: Balint's syndrome (psychic gaze paralysis, optic ataxia, visual inattention); [j]Contralateral hemianopsia, superior quadrantanopsia, transient hemi-sensorimotor deficit. L-lesion: Wernicke's aphasia. R-lesion: Extinction, spatial neglect, constructional apraxia, agitated delirium. Bilateral lesions: Pure word deafness, cortical deafness; [k]Dysexecutive syndrome (impaired planning and sequencing), inattention, decreased recall episodic/verbal memory; abulia, lack of drive and motivation. L-lesions: nonfluent/transcortical aphasia; R-lesions: neglect; [l]Headache, homonymous hemianopsia, superior quadrantanopsia, visual hallucination in hemianopic field, hemichromatopsia, palinopsia, arm-face sensory loss, mild hemiparesis. L-lesions: alexia without agraphia; transcortical aphasia (fluent, jargon, paraphasias, impaired comprehension, preserved repetition); anomia, color anomia, visual agnosia; verbal memory learning impairment; delirium. R-lesions: visual neglect, visual amnesia, spatial disorientation, delirium, confusion. Bilateral lesions: Anton's syndrome (cortical blindness with anosognosia (denial of the blindness); agitated delirium, severe amnesia, Balint's syndrome (simultagnosia, optic ataxia, ocular apraxia), prosopagnosia.
Abbreviations: ACA, anterior cerebral artery; AChA, anterior choroidal artery; MCA, middle cerebral artery; PCA, posterior cerebral artery; W, Wernicke's aphasia; Br, Broca's aphasia; B, bilateral lesions; L, left-side lesion; R, right-side lesion.
Source: From Ref. 102.

(caudate/putamen), globus pallidus/substantia nigra, and thalamus, with thalamo-cortical connections closing the loop. Interruption at any portion of the loop of the dorsolateral prefrontal circuit results in executive dysfunction, orbitofrontal circuit lesions are manifested by uninhibited behaviors, and anterior cingulate circuit lesions result in apathy. Not surprisingly, executive dysfunction, apathy, mood changes, and uninhibited behaviors are frequently observed in patients with VaD.

Cardiogenic Dementia

The term cardiogenic dementia (103) may be used for cases of subcortical VaD in elderly patients with CHF and hypotension; the cognitive decline usually remains undiagnosed in these patients. Cognitive deterioration may occur also following recurrent episodes of cardiac arrhythmias or heart disease (103). In a recent Italian study, Zuccalà et al. (104) demonstrated cognitive impairment in 26% of patients discharged from hospitals after treatment for CHF. Worse cognitive function correlates with lower degrees of left ventricular dysfunction and with systolic blood pressure levels below 130 mm Hg (105–108). Hypoperfusion from left ventricular failure appears to be the most significant risk factor for cognitive decline in these elderly subjects (108).

Atrial fibrillation is a well recognized and important cause of recurrent embolic stroke, leading sometimes to MID. Patients with atrial fibrillation also have increased severity of ischemic periventricular white-matter lesions (109) and decreased cognitive performance (110). Brain hypoperfusion from pump failure has been invoked as an explanation for these findings.

Hypotension and Dementia

Population-based epidemiological studies in many parts of the world have long recognized an increase risk of dementia in hypertensive subjects (111–113). More recent evidence, however, indicates that hypotension also carries an increase (about 1.5 times) in risk of dementia (114–117). Qiu et al. (118) have shown that poor cerebral perfusion is related to decreased pulse pressure. Recently, Duschek et al. (119) found reduced cognitive performance and prolonged reaction time in nondemented subjects with moderate hypotension.

Coronary Artery Bypass Graft

Patients with post-coronary artery bypass graft (CABG) present transient cognitive decline in over 60% of the cases (120). Permanent deficits leading to VaD may also occur. Other neurological complications include delirium and stroke (121–123). A meta-analysis (124) of 176 studies involving 205,717 post-CABG patients showed the following average in-hospital incidence of major adverse effects: death (1.7%), non-fatal myocardial infarction (2.4%), and non-fatal stroke (1.3%). Risk factors were age more than 70 years, female sex, low ejection fraction, history of stroke, myocardial infarction, or heart surgery, and presence of diabetes or hypertension (124).

Cognitive deficits probably result from hypoperfusion and cerebral microemboli (120,125). Postmortem studies show ischemic neuronal damage and neuronal loss in the cerebral and cerebellar cortex, and basal ganglia, along with watershed infarctions. These lesions may result from the postulated loss of cerebral autoregulation in the elderly, worsened by the use of the cardiopulmonary bypass circuit.

In addition to cerebral hypoperfusion, embolism is an important factor. Restrepo et al. (126), using diffusion-weighted MRI, showed that a significant number of patients suffer silent embolic strokes in the post-operative period, increasing thereby the risk of VaD. Myriads of microemboli in small brain capillaries and arterioles have been demonstrated in patients who undergo autopsy after long CABG surgery performed under extra-corporeal circulation (127,128). Aortic cannulation in preparation for cardiopulmonary bypass is the moment of surgery with highest risk of embolism (128). CABG surgeries performed without the pump (Off-pump CABG or OPCABG) (129,130) has lower rates of embolism and less cognitive decline. Newman et al. (131) studied the long-term (5-year) incidence of cognitive effects of CABG surgery and found that close to half of the patients (42%) had significant long-term cognitive dysfunction, compared with 53% at hospital discharge. Significantly better results, however, are obtained with coronary stent placement (132).

Cognitive Decline After Major Surgery in the Elderly

In addition to post-CABG subjects, patients with subcortical VaD may be found in rehabilitation services among patients recovering from stroke, or undergoing cardiac rehabilitation post-myocardial infarction (133), or in convalescence units after major surgery, in particular post-coronary CABG and after hip fracture repair. The International Study of Postoperative Cognitive Dysfunction (134,135) found that 26% of patients aged 60 years and older undergoing major abdominal or orthopedic surgery had short-term cognitive dysfunction. A common risk factor for post-operative cognitive decline in the elderly is cerebral hypoperfusion.

In summary, a number of cardiovascular conditions in the elderly are associated with cerebral hypoperfusion, development of vascular cognitive impairment, and VaD. The most important cardiogenic sources are CHF, cardiac arrhythmias, orthostatic hypotension, CABG, and other major surgeries in the elderly.

In addition to the morphological factors resulting from aging, damage from recurrent or prolonged hypoperfusion depends on differences in oxygen and glucose requirements of individual brain cells and duration of hypoperfusion. Compensatory autoregulatory changes intervene when cerebral perfusion pressure falls (136–138). Initially, blood vessels dilate to increase blood volume and to maintain blood flow. The effects of aging, as described previously, limit these protective responses. With blood flow decline, oxygen extraction fraction increases to maintain cerebral oxygen metabolism. If decline in perfusion pressure exceeds compensatory mechanisms, oxygen metabolism is compromised, leading to oxidative stress. Neuronal–glial interaction is lost, there is uncoupling of metabolism, and altered DNA and protein synthesis occur.

Regardless of the cellular mechanisms, these cardiac and circulatory conditions result in localized brain injury affecting the periventricular white matter, basal ganglia, and the hippocampus, leading to frequent and under diagnosed forms of cognitive decline in the elderly.

DIAGNOSTIC CRITERIA FOR VaD

The NINDS–AIREN criteria (Table 6) proposed by Román et al. (139) have the highest specificity of all available criteria and offer an operative approach to the basic elements needed for a diagnosis of VaD: (i) *cognitive loss*—often a subcortical form of dementia; (ii) *cerebrovascular lesions* demonstrated by brain imaging (CT, MRI); (iii) *exclusion of other causes of dementia*, such as AD; and (iv) a *logical link* between the vascular lesions and the dementia. A temporal relationship, that is, development of dementia within three months after a stroke, has proven to be more difficult to fulfill, particularly in patients with silent strokes or subcortical VaD.

Separating AD from VaD may be a frequent problem in patients with pre-existing and progressive memory loss worsened by an acute vascular episode. This combination is called AD + CVD (or "mixed" dementia). Careful interview of relatives and caregivers allows a successful diagnosis of pre-stroke dementia when the family confirms that the patient had worsening memory deficit prior to the stroke. Despite a number of similarities with AD, patients with VaD have relatively superior function in verbal long-term memory and more impairment of frontal executive function (140,141). Therefore, these patients require the use of tests for sub-cortical dysfunction, such as the drawing of a clock on command (142), and other executive function tests (141).

PREVENTION

Major advances have been made in the prevention of stroke. Although age, gender, ethnicity, and genetic factors are non-modifiable stroke risk factors, there is clear Class I evidence for primary and secondary prevention of stroke and VaD. The term "secondary prevention" indicates the need to prevent further ischemic episodes after the occurrence of first stroke or myocardial infarction in order to halt the development of VaD. Primary prevention is directed to the control of vascular risk factors in an effort to prevent stroke and ischemic heart disease.

Table 6 NINDS–AIREN Diagnostic Criteria for Vascular Dementia

I. The criteria for the diagnosis of *probable* VaD include *all* of the following:
  1. Dementia: Impairment of memory and two or more cognitive domains (including executive function), interfering with ADLs and not due to physical effects of stroke alone. Exclusion criteria: Alterations of consciousness, delirium, psychoses, severe aphasia or deficits precluding testing, systemic disorders, AD, or other forms of dementia.
  2. Cerebrovascular disease: Focal signs on neurological examination (hemiparesis, lower facial weakness, Babinski sign, sensory deficit, hemianopia, dysarthria) consistent with stroke (with or without history of stroke, and evidence of relevant CVD by brain CT or MRI including *multiple large-vessel infarcts* or a *single strategically placed infarct* (angular gyrus, thalamus, basal forebrain, or PCA or ACA territories), as well as *multiple basal ganglia* and *white matter lacunes* or *extensive periventricular white matter lesions*, or combinations thereof. Exclusion criteria: Absence of cerebrovascular lesions on CT or MRI.
  3. A relationship between the above two disorders: Manifested or inferred by the presence of one or more of the following:
     (a) Onset of dementia within three months following a recognized stroke.
     (b) Abrupt deterioration in cognitive functions; or fluctuating, stepwise progression of cognitive deficits.
II. Clinical features *consistent* with the diagnosis of *probable* VaD include the following:
  1. Early presence of gait disturbances (small step gait or marche à petits pas, or magnetic, apraxic-ataxic or parkinsonian gait).
  2. History of unsteadiness and frequent, unprovoked falls.
  3. Early urinary frequency, urgency, and other urinary symptoms not explained by urologic disease.
  4. Pseudobulbar palsy.
  5. Personality and mood changes, abulia, depression, emotional incontinence, or other deficits including psychomotor retardation and abnormal executive function.
III. Features that make the diagnosis of VaD uncertain or unlikely include:
  1. Early onset of memory deficit and progressive worsening of memory and other cognitive functions, such as language (transcortical sensory aphasia), motor skills (apraxia), and perception (agnosia), in the absence of corresponding focal lesions on brain imaging.
  2. Absence of focal neurological signs, other than cognitive disturbances.
  3. Absence of CVD on CT or MRI.

Abbreviations: ACA, anterior cerebral artery; ADLs, activities of daily living; CT, computerized tomography; CVD, cerebrovascular disease; MRI, magnetic resonance imaging; PCA, posterior cerebral artery; VaD, vascular dementia; AD, Alzheimer's disease.
Source: From Ref. 139.

Secondary Prevention

Optimal management of acute stroke and implementation of secondary prevention is mandatory in patients with stroke to prevent VaD (143–147). The treatment of *hypertension* reduces the risk of recurrent stroke by 28%. Likewise, using statins to decrease by 25% *low-density lipoprotein (LDL) cholesterol* reduces stroke risk up to 30%. *Antiplatelet medications* reduce the risk of recurrent stroke by 17% with aspirin and 25% with ticlopidine; clopidogrel is a safe and effective alternative to ticlopidine but is not superior to aspirin; dipyridamole in combination with aspirin appears to be superior to aspirin alone. *Anticoagulation* with warfarin (INR = 2–3) in patients with atrial fibrillation is highly efficacious in preventing recurrent stroke (about 70% risk reduction). For patients with more than 75% *carotid artery stenosis*, surgery reduces recurrent stroke by 51%.

In the PROGRESS study (148), lowering blood pressure in patients with previous stroke or TIA reduced the incidence of secondary stroke by 28%, of major vascular events by 26% and of major coronary events by 26%. These reductions were all magnified by approximately 50% in a subgroup of patients in whom the angiotensin-converting enzyme (ACE)-inhibitor perindopril was routinely combined with the diuretic indapamide (148). This condition alone could reduce the burden of stroke and could avert between 0.5 and one million strokes each year, worldwide.

Primary Prevention

It is clear that control of a number of traditional and newer risk factors, such as inflammation and endothelial injury, effectively prevents stroke and heart disease (149–153). Of significant public health interest are the observations that in the elderly the treatment of hypertension and the use of statins have been associated with decreased incidence of dementia. For instance, Murray et al. (154) found that antihypertensive treatment reduced the odds of incident cognitive impairment by 38% in a cohort of elderly African-Americans. Antihypertensive therapy was associated with a 28% reduction in the risk of recurrent stroke and a 38–55% reduction in the risk of dementia.

Preventive measures to decrease the vascular burden on the brain must be implemented (155), including control of hypertension and cardiac disease, lowering lipids with the use of statins, decreasing homocysteine with oral folate and parenteral B_{12} supplementation, with smoking cessation and a Mediterranean diet rich in fruits and antioxidants, among other factors.

In subcortical VaD, control of hemorheological factors that increase blood viscosity becomes important in subjects with small-vessel disease and disturbances of the microcirculation. Control of diabetes, hyperlipidemia, polycytemia, hyperfibrinogenemia, and hyperviscosity are required. Orthostatic hypotension, cardiac arrhythmias, CHF, and obstructive sleep apnea must be identified and treated appropriately.

DRUG TREATMENTS FOR VaD

Currently there are no officially approved treatments for VaD. However, the following agents have demonstrated efficacy in randomized controlled clinical trials of VaD (Class I evidence) (156–160):

Calcium Channel Blockers

Nimodipine and nicardipine have shown moderate efficacy in tests of attention and psychomotor performance in the subcortical (small-vessel) form of VaD (161,162). These agents have effects on autoregulation of cerebral blood flow, and block L-type calcium receptors providing some degree of neuroprotection.

Neuroprotective (Nootropic) Agents

Piracetam, oxiracetam,and nicergoline appear to be safe and modestly effective in MID. Citicoline (CDP-choline) has positive short-term effects on memory and behavior (163). Citicoline activates the biosynthesis of structural phospholipids in the neuronal membranes, increases cerebral metabolism, and increases noradrenaline and dopamine levels in the CNS.

Pentoxifylline

This is a xanthine derivative with hemorheological and immunomodulatory properties that shows significant cognitive improvement in MID. Pentoxifylline treatment lowers fibrinogen and TNF-α levels in patients with VaD.

Antiplatelet Agents

Aspirin, triflusal (165), and *Ginkgo biloba* (166) showed very modest results, using the MMSE as the primary endpoint for cognitive evaluation.

Memantine

This agent is a non-competitive antagonist of the *N*-methyl-D-aspartate (NMDA) receptor with nootropic properties. Memantine is well tolerated and useful in severe dementia. Two randomized, placebo-controlled 6-month trials (167,168) studied memantine (20 mg per day) in patients with mild to moderate probable VaD according to NINDS–AIREN criteria. After 28 weeks, there was cognitive improvement relative to placebo. Other behavioral scales showed no significant difference between the two groups. Memantine was well tolerated in the two studies.

Cholinesterase Inhibitors (AChEI)

Encouraging results have been obtained with the use of AChEIs in VaD. All the available cholinergic agents approved for the treatment of AD: donepezil hydrochloride (Aricept®), rivastigmine tartrate (Exelon®), and galantamine hydrobromide (Reminyl®, Razadyne®) have been used in patients with VaD.

Donepezil

Two large, 24-week, multicenter, randomized, placebo-controlled international trials of donepezil in VaD (169,170) randomized 1219 subjects with mild to moderate VaD, selected according to the NINDS-AIREN criteria. Compared with placebo, significant cognitive improvement was noted, with beneficial effects on activities of daily living and global scores. Patients on the 5-mg dose tolerated the drug better than those on the high dose of 10 mg/day. Donepezil-treated patients remained above baseline in the instrumental activities of daily living, suggesting that the beneficial effect of donepezil may be related to improvement or stabilization of executive function (171). Donepezil was well tolerated, even in patients on multiple cardiovascular medications and anticoagulation.

Galantamine

This modulates central nicotinic receptors to increase cholinergic neurotransmission. In a 6-month, multicenter, randomized, controlled clinical trial (172), patients diagnosed with probable VaD, or with AD combined with CVD, received galantamine 24 mg/day or placebo. Primary endpoints were cognition and global function. Secondary endpoints included assessments of activities of daily living and behavioral symptoms. In analyses of both groups as a whole, galantamine demonstrated efficacy on all outcome measures. Galantamine was well tolerated. In an open-label extension (173), the original galantamine group of patients with probable VaD or AD + CVD showed similar sustained benefits in terms of maintenance of or improvement in cognition, functional ability, and behavior after 12 months, although the study was not designed to detect differences between subgroups.

Rivastigmine

This is an AChEI and butirylcholinesterase inhibitor; its effects on VaD remain to be established (174). In a small open-label study of patients with subcortical VaD (175), rivastigmine improved cognition, decreased caregiver stress, and improved behavior.

Other Agents

Atypical antipsychotic drugs, such as risperidone and olanzapine, have been useful in the treatment of agitation and disruptive behaviors. Often, the use of cholinergic medications controls these problems.

For some patients with depression and anxiety, the use of antidepressants, such as the SSRIs citalopram or sertraline, may be required. The use of tricyclic antidepressants in elderly patients with VaD is discouraged, because of anticholinergic effects and orthostatic hypotension.

SUMMARY

VaD is the most common secondary dementia and the second most common cause of dementia in the elderly after AD. VaD is defined as the severe loss of cognitive function resulting from ischemic, ischemic-hypoxic, or hemorrhagic brain lesions due to CVD and cardiovascular pathology. Diagnosis requires: (i) cognitive loss—often predominantly subcortical, (ii) vascular brain lesions demonstrated by imaging, and (iii) exclusion of other causes of dementia, such as AD. VaD may be caused by multiple strokes (MID or post-stroke dementia), but also by single-strategic strokes, multiple lacunes, and hypoperfusive lesions, such as border-zone infarcts and ischemic periventricular leukoencephalopathy (Binswanger's disease). Primary and secondary prevention of stroke and cardiovascular disease decrease the burden of VaD. Genetic advice is needed in patients with familial forms, such as CADASIL and familial amyloid angiopathies. Cholinergic medications used for AD are also useful in VaD, and atypical antipsychotic agents and antidepressants (SSRIs) may be required in some patients. Prevention of VaD requires control of risk factors.

REFERENCES

1. Román GC. A historical review of the concept of vascular dementia: lessons from the past for the future. Alzheimer Dis Assoc Disord 1999; 13(suppl 3):S4–S8.
2. Skoog I, Gustafson D. Hypertension and related factors in the etiology of Alzheimer's disease. Ann NY Acad Sci 2002; 977:29–36.
3. Jellinger KA. Alzheimer disease and cerebrovascular pathology: an update. J Neural Transm 2002; 109:813–836.
4. Román GC. Vascular dementia revisited: diagnosis, pathogenesis, treatment, and prevention. Med Clin N Am 2002; 86:477–499.
5. Jorm AF. A short form of the Informant Questionnaire on Cognitive Decline in the Elderly (IQCODE): development and cross-validation. Psychol Med 1994; 24:145–153.
6. Lin JH, Lin RT, Tai CT, Hsieh CL, Hsiao SF, Liu CK. Prediction of poststroke dementia. Neurology 2003; 61:343–348.
7. Hénon H, Pasquier F, Durieu I, et al. Pre-existing dementia in stroke patients: baseline frequency, associated factors and outcome. Stroke 1997; 28:2429–2436.
8. Hénon H, Durieu I, Guerouaou D, et al. Post-stroke dementia: incidence and relationship to pre-stroke cognitive decline. Neurology 2001; 57:1216–1222.
9. Barba R, Castro MD, del Mar Morin M, Rodriguez-Romero R, Rodriguez-Garcia E, Canton R, Del Ser T. Prestroke dementia. Cerebrovasc Dis 2001; 11:216–224.
10. Román GC, Erkinjuntti T, Wallin A, Pantoni L, Chui HC. Subcortical ischaemic vascular dementia. Lancet Neurol 2002; 1:426–436.
11. Ballard C, Rowan E, Stephens S, Kalaria R, Kenny RA. Prospective follow-up study between 3 and 15 months after stroke: improvements and decline in cognitive function among dementia-free stroke survivors >75 years of age. Stroke 2003; 34:2440–2444.

12. Román GC. Vascular dementia may be the most common form of dementia in the elderly. J Neurol Sci 2002; 203–204:7–10.
13. Launer LJ, Hofman A. Frequency and impact of neurologic diseases in the elderly of Europe: a collaborative study of population-based cohorts. Neurology 2000; 54 (suppl 5):S1–S3.
14. Lobo A, Launer LJ, Fratiglioni L, et al. Prevalence of dementia and major subtypes in Europe: a collaborative study of population-based cohorts. Neurology 2000; 54(suppl 5):S4–S9.
15. Knopman DS, Parisi JE, Boeve BF, Cha RH, Apaydin H, Salviati A, Edland SD, Rocca WA. Vascular dementia in a population-based autopsy study. Arch Neurol 2003; 60:569–575.
16. Arizaga RL, Mangone CA, Allegri RF, Ollari JA. Vascular dementia: The Latin American perspective. Alzheimer Dis Assoc Disord 1999; 13(suppl 3):S201–S215.
17. Fujishima M, Kiyohara Y. Incidence and risk factors of dementia in a defined elderly Japanese population: the Hisayama study. Ann NY Acad Sci 2002; 977:1–8.
18. Jorm AF, Korten AE, Henderson AS. The prevalence of dementia: a quantitative integration of the literature. Acta Psychiatr Scand 1987; 76:465–479.
19. Petrovitch H, White LR, Ross GW, et al. Accuracy of clinical criteria for AD in the Honolulu-Asia Aging Study, a population-based study. Neurology 2001; 57:226–234.
20. Jorm AF, Jolley D. The incidence of dementia: a meta-analysis. Neurology 1998; 51:728–733.
21. Fratiglioni L, Launer LJ, Andersen K, Breteler MMB, Copeland JRM, Dartigues J-F, Lobo A, Martinez-Lage J, Soininen H, Hofman A, for the Neurologic Diseases in the Elderly Research Group. Incidence of dementia and major subtypes in Europe: A collaborative study of population-based cohorts. Neurology 2000; 54(suppl 5):S10–S15.
22. Dubois MF, Hebert R. The incidence of vascular dementia in Canada: a comparison with Europe and East Asia. Neuroepidemiology 2001; 20:179–187.
23. Tatemichi TK, Desmont DW, Paik M, et al. Clinical determinants of dementia related to stroke. Ann Neurol 1993; 33:568–575.
24. Leys D, Pasquier F: How can cerebral infarcts and hemorrhages lead to dementia? J Neural Transm 2000; 59(suppl):31–36.
25. Liu CK, Miller BL, Cummings JL, et al. A quantitative MRI study of vascular dementia. Neurology 1991; 42:138–143.
26. Gorelick PB, Chatterjee A, Patel D, et al. Cranial computed tomographic observations in multi-infarct dementia: a controlled study. Stroke 1992; 23:804–811.
27. Engstad T, Almkvist O, Viitanen M, Arnesen E. Impaired motor speed, visuospatial episodic memory and verbal fluency characterize cognition in long-term stroke survivors: The Tromso Study. Neuroepidemiology 2003; 22:326–331.
28. Johnston SC, O'Meara ES, Manolio TA, Lefkowitz D, O'Leary DH, Goldstein S, Carlson MC, Fried LP, Longstreth WT. Cognitive impairment and decline are associated with carotid artery disease in patients without clinically evident cerebrovascular disease. Ann Intern Med 2004; 140:237–247.
29. Moroney JT, Bagiella E, Desmond DW, et al. Risk factors for incident dementia after stroke. Role of hypoxic ischemic disorders. Stroke 1996; 27:1283–1289.
30. Longstreth WT Jr, Manolio TA, Arnold A, et al. Clinical correlates of white matter findings on cranial magnetic resonance imaging of 3301 elderly people. The Cardiovascular Health Study. Stroke 1996; 27:1274–1282.

31. Desmond DW, Moroney JT, Bagiella E, et al. Dementia as a predictor of adverse outcomes following stroke. An evaluation of diagnostic methods. Stroke 1998; 29:69–74.
32. Barba R, Martinez-Espinosa S, Rodriguez-Garcia E, et al. Post-stroke dementia. Clinical features and risk factors. Stroke 2000; 31:1494–1501.
33. Linden T, Skoog I, Fagerberg B, Steen B, Blomstrand C. Cognitive impairment and dementia 20 months after stroke. Neuroepidemiology 2004; 23:45–52.
34. Knopman DS, Rocca WA, Cha RH, Edland SD, Kokmen E. Survival study of vascular dementia in Rochester, Minnesota. Arch Neurol 2003; 60:85–90.
35. Tomlinson BE, Blessed G, Roth M: Observations on the brains of demented old people. J Neurol Sci 1970; 11:205–242.
36. Hachinski V, Lassen N, Marshall J. Multi-infarct dementia: a cause of mental deterioration in the elderly. Lancet 1974; 14:207–210.
37. del Ser T, Bermejo F, Portera A, Arredondo JM, Bouras C, Constantinidis J. Vascular dementia. A clinicopathological study. J Neurol Sci 1990; 96:1–17.
38. Brun A, Gustafson L. Zerebrovaskuläre Erkrankungen. In: Kisker KP, Lauter A, Meyer J-E, Müller E, Strömgren E, eds. Psychatrie der Gegenwart. Vol. 6, Organische Psychosen. Berlin-Heidelberg: Springer-Verlag, 1988:253–297.
39. Brun A: Pathology and pathophysiology of cerebrovascular dementia: pure subgroups of obstructive and hypoperfusive etiology. Dementia 1994; 5:145–147.
40. Román GC: Senile dementia of the Binswanger type: a vascular form of dementia in the elderly. JAMA 1987; 258:1782–1788.
41. Kovari E, Gold G, Herrmann FR, Canuto A, Hof PR, Michel JP, Bouras C, Giannakopoulos P. Cortical microinfarcts and demyelination significantly affect cognition in brain aging. Stroke 2004; 35:410–414.
42. White L, Petrovitch H, Hardman J, Nelson J, Davis DG, Ross GW, Masaki K, Launer L, Markesbery WR. Cerebrovascular pathology and dementia in autopsied Honolulu-Asia Aging Study participants. Ann NY Acad Sci 2002; 977:9–23.
43. Delay J, Brion S. Les Démences Tardives. Paris: Masson et Cie, 1962.
44. Brandt T, Steinke W, Thie A, Pessin MS. Posterior cerebral artery territory infarcts: clinical features, infarct topography, causes and outcome. Multicenter results and a review of the literature. Cerebrovasc Dis 2000; 10:170–182.
45. von Cramon DY, Hebel N, Schuri U. Verbal memory and learning in unilateral posterior cerebral infarction. A report of 30 cases. Brain 1988; 111:1061–1077.
46. Richardson JT. Cognitive performance following rupture and repair of intracranial aneurysms. Acta Neurol Scand 1991; 83:110–122.
47. von Cramon DY, Markowitsch HJ. Human memory dysfunctions due to septal lesions. In: Numan R, ed. The Behavioral Neuroscience of the Septal Region. New York: Springer, 2000:380–413.
48. Phillips S, Sangalang V, Sterns G. Basal forebrain infarction. A clinicopathologic correlation. Arch Neurol 1987; 44:1134–1138.
49. Castaigne P, Buge A, Cambier J, Escourolle R, Brunet P, Degos JD. Démence thalamique d'origine vasculaire par ramollissement bilatéral, limité au territoire du péduncule retromamillaire. A propos de deux observations anatomo-cliniques. Rev Neurol (Paris) 1966; 114:89–107.
50. Castaigne P, Lhermitte F, Buge A, et al. Paramedian thalamic and midbrain infarcts: clinical and neuropathological study. Ann Neurol 1981; 10:127–148.

51. von Cramon DY, Hebel N, Schuri U. A contribution to the anatomical basis of thalamic amnesia. Brain 1985; 108:993–1008.
52. Van der Werf Y, Witter MP, Uylings HB, Jolles J. Neuropsychology of infarctions in the thalamus: a review. Neuropsychologia 2000; 38:613–627.
53. Percheron G. Les artères du thalamus humain: II. Artères et territoires thalamiques paramedians de l'artère basilaire communicante. Rev Neurol (Paris) 1976; 132:309–324.
54. Van der Werf YD, Scheltens P, Lindeboom J, Witter MP, Uylings HB, Jolles J. Deficits of memory, executive functioning and attention following infarction in the thalamus: A study of 22 cases with localized lesions. Neuropsychology 2003; 41:1330–1344.
55. Ghika-Schimid F, Bogousslavsky J. The acute behavioral syndrome of anterior thalamic infarction: a prospective study of 12 cases. Ann Neurol 2000; 48:220–227.
56. Van den Werf YD, Weerts JG, Jolles J, Witter MO, Lindneboom J, Scheltens P. Neuropsychological correlates of a right unilateral lacunar thalamic infarction. J Neurol Neurosurg Psych 1999; 66:36–42.
57. Kovari E, Gold G, Herrmann FR, Canuto A, Hof PR, Michel JP, Bouras C, Giannakopoulos P. Cortical microinfarcts and demyelination significantly affect cognition in brain aging. Stroke 2004; 35:410–414.
58. White L, Petrovitch H, Hardman J, Nelson J, Davis DG, Ross GW, Masaki K, Launer L, Markesbery WR. Cerebrovascular pathology and dementia in autopsied Honolulu-Asia Aging Study participants. Ann NY Acad Sci 2002; 977:9–23.
59. De Groot JC, De Leeuw FE, Oudkerk M, Van Gijn J, Hofman A, Jolles J, Breteler MM. Periventricular cerebral white matter lesions predict rate of cognitive decline. Ann Neurol 2002; 52:335–341.
60. Pasquier F, Henon H, Leys D. Relevance of white matter changes to pre- and poststroke dementia. Ann NY Acad Sci 2000; 903:466–469.
61. Tatemichi TK, Desmont DW, Prohovnik I, et al. Confusion and memory loss from capsular genu infarction: a thalamocortical disconnection syndrome? Neurology 1992; 42:1966–1979.
62. Tatemichi TK, Desmont DW, Prohovnik I, et al. Strategic infarcts in vascular dementia. A clinical and imaging experience. Arzneimittel-Forschung/Drug Research 1995; 45:371–385.
63. Madureira S, Guerreiro M, Ferro JM. A follow-up study of cognitive impairment due to inferior capsular genu infarction. J Neurol 1999; 246:764–769.
64. Pantoni L, Basile AM, Romanelli M, et al. Abulia and cognitive impairment in two patients with capsular genu infarct. Acta Neurol Scand 2001; 104:185–190.
65. Chukwudelunzu FE, Meschia JF, Graff-Radford NR, Lucas JA. Extensive metabolic and neuropsychological abnormalities associated with discrete infarction of the genu of the internal capsule. J Neurol Neurosurg Psych 2001; 71:658–662.
66. Ferro JM. Hyperacute cognitive stroke syndromes. J Neurol 2001; 248:841–849.
67. Caplan LR, Schmahmann JD, Kase CS, et al. Caudate infarcts. Arch Neurol 1990; 47:133–143.
68. Kumral E, Evyapan D, Balkir K. Acute caudate vascular lesions. Stroke 1999; 30:100–108.
69. Tournier-Lasserve E, Iba-Zizen MT, Romero N, Bousser M-G: Autosomal dominant syndrome with stroke-like episodes and leukoencephalopathy. Stroke 1991; 22:1297–1302.

70. Dichgans M, Mayer M, Uttner I, et al. The phenotypic spectrum of CADASIL: clinical findings in 102 cases. Ann Neurol 1998; 44:731–739.

71. Marie P. Des foyers lacunaires de désintégration et de différents autres états cavitaires du cerveau. Revue de Médecine (Paris) 1901; 21:281–298.

72. Norrving B. Long-term prognosis after lacunar infarction. Lancet Neurol 2003; 2:238–245.

73. Snowdon DA, Kemper SJ, Mortimer JA, Greiner LH, Wekstein DR, Markesbery WR. Brain infarction and the clinical expression of Alzheimer's disease. JAMA 1996; 275:528–532.

74. Vermeer SE, Prins ND, den Heijer T, et al. Silent brain infarcts and the risk of dementia and cognitive decline. N Engl J Med 2003; 348:1215–1222.

75. Binswanger O. Die Abgrenzung der allgemeinen progressiven Paralyse (Referat, erstattet auf der Jahres versammlung des Vereins Deutscher Irrenärtzte zu Dresden am 20 Sept. 1894). Berl Klin Wochenschr 1894; 31:1103–1105, 1137–1139, 1180–1186.

76. Ruchoux MM, Guerouaou D, Vandenhaute B, et al. Systemic vascular smooth muscle impairment in cerebral autosomal dominant arteriopathy with subcortical infarcts and leukoencephalopathy. Acta Neuropathol (Berl) 1995; 89:500–512.

77. Joutel A, Favrole P, Labauge P, et al. Skin biopsy immunostaining with a Notch3 monoclonal antibody for CADASIL diagnosis. Lancet 2001; 358:2049–2051.

78. Mead S, James-Galton M, Revesz T, et al. Familial British dementia with amyloid angiopathy: early clinical, neuropsychological and imaging findings. Brain 2000; 123:975–991.

79. Ghiso JA, Holton J, Miravalle L, et al. Systemic amyloid deposits in familial British dementia. J Biol Chem 2001; 276:43909–43914.

80. Roman GC. Brain hypoperfusion: A critical factor in vascular dementia. Neurological Research 2004; 26:454–458.

81. Loewy AD, Spyer KM, eds. Central Regulation of Autonomic Functions. Oxford: Oxford University Press, 1990.

82. Benarroch EE. The central autonomic network: Functional organization, dysfunction, and perspective. Mayo Clin Proc 1993; 68:988–1001.

83. Kenny RA. Syncope in the elderly: diagnosis, evaluation, and treatment. J Cardiovasc Electrophysiol 2003; 14(suppl):S74–S77.

84. Kaufmann H, Bhattacharya K. Diagnosis and treatment of neurally mediated syncope. Neurologist 2002; 8:175–185.

85. Kenny RA, Kalaria R, Ballard C. Neurocardiovascular instability in cognitive impairment and dementia. Ann NY Acad Sci 2002; 977:183–195.

86. Kaufmann H, Saadia D, Voustianiouk A, Goldstein DS, Holmes C, Yahr MD, Nardin R, Freeman R. Norepinephrine precursor therapy in neurogenic hypotension. Circulation 2003; 108:724–728.

87. Pantoni L, Garcia JH, Gutierrez JA. Cerebral white matter is highly vulnerable to ischemia. Stroke 1996; 27:1641–1647.

88. Moody DM, Bell MA, Challa VR. Features of cerebral vascular pattern that predict vulnerability to perfusion or oxygenation deficiency: an anatomical study. Am J Neuroradiol 1990; 11:431–439.

89. Dickson DW, Davies P, Bevona C, Van Hoeven KH, Factor SM, Grober E, Aronson MK, Crystal HA. Hippocampal sclerosis: a common pathological feature

of dementia in very old (greater than 80 years of age) humans. Acta Neuropathol 1994; 88:212–221.

90. Corey-Bloom J, Sabbagh MN, Bondi MW, Hansen L, Alford MF, Masliah E, Thal LJ. Hippocampal sclerosis contributes to dementia in the elderly. Neurology 1997; 48:154–160.

91. Crystal HA, Dickson DW, Sliwinski MJ, Lipton RB, Grober F, Marks-Nelson H, Antis P. Pathological markers associated with normal aging and dementia in the elderly. Ann Neurol 1993; 34:566–573.

92. Leverenz JB, Agustin CM, Tsuang D, Peskind ER, Edland SD, Nochlin D, DiGiacomo L, Bowen JD, McCormick WC, Teri L, Raskind MA, Kukull WA, Larson EB. Clinical and neuropathological characteristics of hippocampal sclerosis. Arch Neurol 2002; 59:1099–1106.

93. Duvernoy HM. The Human Hippocampus: Functional Anatomy, Vascularization and Serial Sections with MRI. Second edition. Berlin: Springer-Verlag, 1998.

94. Vinters HV, Ellis WG, Zarow C, Zaias BW, Jagust WJ, Mack WJ, Chui HC. Neuropathologic substrates of ischemic vascular dementia. J Neuropathol Exp Neurol 2000; 59:931–945.

95. Awad IA, Johnson PC, Spetzler RF, Modak JA. Incidental subcortical lesions identified on magnetic resonance imaging in the elderly: II. Postmortem pathological correlation. Stroke 1986; 17:1090–1092.

96. van Swieten JC, van den Hout JH, van Ketel BA, Hijdra A, Wokke JH, van Gijn J. Periventricular lesions in the white matter on magnetic resonance imaging in the elderly. A morphometric correlation with arteriolosclerosis and dilated periventricular spaces. Brain 1991; 114:761–774.

97. Sato A, Sato Y, Uchida S. Regulation of regional cerebral blood flow by cholinergic fibers originating in the basal forebrain. Int J Dev Neurosci 2001; 19:327–337.

98. Court JA, Perry EK, Kalaria RN. Neurotransmitter control of the cerebral vasculature and abnormalities in vascular dementia. In: Erkinjuntti T, Gauthier S, eds. Vascular Cognitive Impairment. London: Martin Duniz Ltd., 2002:167–185.

99. Selden NR, Gitelman DR, Salamon-Murayama N, Parrish TB, Mesulam MM. Trajectories of cholinergic pathways within the cerebral hemispheres of the human brain. Brain 1998; 121:2249–2257.

100. Bocti C, Swartz RH, Gao FQ, Sahlas DJ, Behl P, Black SE. A new visual rating scale to assess strategic white matter hyperintensities within cholinergic pathways in dementia. Stroke 2005; 36:2126–2131. Epub 2005 Sep 22.

101. Mesulam M, Siddique T, Cohen B. Cholinergic denervation in a pure multi-infarct state. Observations on CADASIL. Neurology 2003; 60:1183–1185.

102. Román GC. Managing Vascular Dementia: Concepts, Issues, and Management London: Science Press, 2003.

103. Editorial. Cardiogenic dementia. Lancet 1981; 2:1171.

104. Zuccalà G, Onder G, Pedone C, et al. for the GIFA-ONLUS Study Group [Grupo Italiano di Farmacoepidemiologia nell'Anzanio].: Hypotension and cognitive impairment: Selective association in patients with heart failure. Neurology 2001; 57:1986–1992.

105. Zuccalà G, Cattel, Manes-Gravina E, Di Niro MG, Cocchi A, Bernabei R. Left ventricular dysfunction: a clue to cognitive impairment in older patients with heart failure. J Neurol Neurosurg Psych 1997; 63:509–512.

106. Cacciatore F, Abete P, Ferrara N, et al. Congestive heart failure and cognitive impairment in an older population. J Am Geriatr Soc 1998; 46:1343–1348.
107. Pullicino P, Mifsud V, Wong E, Graham S, Ali I, Smajlovic D. Hypoperfusion-related cerebral ischemia and cardiac left ventricular systolic dysfunction. J Stroke Cerebrovasc Dis 2001; 10:178–182.
108. Pullicino PM, Hart J: Cognitive impairment in congestive heart failure? Embolism vs. hypoperfusion. Neurology 2001; 57:1945–1946.
109. de Leeuw FE, de Groot JC, Ouderk M, et al. Atrial fibrillation and the risk of cerebral white matter lesions. Neurology 2000; 54:1795–1801.
110. O'Connell JE, Gray CS, French JM, Robertson IH. Atrial fibrillation and cognitive function: case-control study. J Neurol Neurosurg Psych 1998; 65:386–389.
111. Piguet O, Grayson DA, Creasey H, Bennett HP, Brooks WS, Waite LM, Broe GA. Vascular risk factors, cognition and dementia incidence over 6 years in the Sydney Older Persons Study. Neuroepidemiology 2003; 22:165–171.
112. Manolio TA, Olson J, Longstreth WT. Hypertension and cognitive function: pathophysiologic effects of hypertension on the brain. Curr Hypertens Rep 2003; 5:255–261.
113. Hanon O, Seux ML, Lenoir H, Rigaud AS, Forette F. Hypertension and dementia. Curr Cardiol Rep 2003; 5:435–440.
114. Verghese J, Lipton RB, Hall CB, Kuslansky G, Katz MJ. Low blood pressure and the risk of dementia in very old individuals. Neurology 2003; 61:1667–1672.
115. Pandav R, Dodge HH, DeKosky ST, Ganguli M. Blood pressure and cognitive impairment in India and the United States: a cross-national epidemiological study. Arch Neurol 2003; 60:1123–1128.
116. Guo Z, Viitanen M, Fratiglioni L, Winblad B: Low blood pressure and dementia in elderly people: The Kungsholmen project. Br Med J 1996; 312:805–808.
117. Qiu C, von Strauss E, Fastbom J, Winblad B, Fratiglioni L. Low blood pressure and risk of dementia in the Kungsholmen project: a 6-year follow-up study. Arch Neurol 2003; 60:223–228.
118. Qiu C, Winblad B, Viitanen M, Fratiglioni L. Pulse pressure and risk of Alzheimer disease in persons aged 75 years and older: a community-based, longitudinal study. Stroke 2003; 34:594–599.
119. Duschek S, Weisz N, Schandry R. Reduced cognitive performance and prolonged reaction time accompany moderate hypotension. Clin Auton Res 2003; 13:427–432.
120. Mark DB, Newman MF. Protecting the brain in coronary artery bypass graft surgery. JAMA 2002; 287:1448–1450.
121. Roach GW, Kanchuger M, Mangano CM, et al. Adverse cerebral outcomes after coronary bypass surgery. N Eng J Med 1996; 335:1857–1853.
122. McKhann GM, Grega MA, Borowicz LM Jr, Bechamps M, Selnes OA, Baumgartner WA, Royall RM. Encephalopathy and stroke after coronary artery bypass grafting: incidence, consequences, and prediction. Arch Neurol 2002; 59:1422–1428.
123. Scarborough JE, White W, Derilus FE, Mathew JP, Newman MF, Landolfo KP. Neurologic outcomes after coronary artery bypass grafting with and without cardiopulmonary bypass. Semin Thorac Cardiovasc Surg 2003; 15:52–62.
124. Nalysnyk L, Fahrbach K, Reynolds MW, Zhao SZ, Ross S. Adverse events in coronary artery bypass graft (CABG) trials: a systematic review and analysis. Heart 2003; 89:767–772.

125. Scarborough JE, White W, Derilus FE, Mathew JP, Newman MF, Landolfo KP. Neurologic outcomes after coronary artery bypass grafting with and without cardiopulmonary bypass. Semin Thorac Cardiovasc Surg 2003; 15:52–62.
126. Restrepo L, Wityk RJ, Grega MA, Borowicz L Jr, Barker PB, Jacobs MA, Beauchamp NJ, Hillis AE, McKhann GM. Diffusion- and perfusion-weighted magnetic resonance imaging of the brain before and after coronary artery bypass grafting surgery. Stroke 2002; 33:2909–2915.
127. Brown WR, Moody DM, Challa VR, et al. Longer duration of cardiopulmonary bypass is associated with greater numbers of cerebral microemboli. Stroke 2000; 31:707–713.
128. Sylivris S, Levi C, Matalanis G, et al. Pattern and significance of cerebral microemboli during coronary artery bypass grafting. Ann Thorac Surg 1998; 66:1674–1678.
129. Sharony R, Bizekis CS, Kanchuger M, Galloway AC, Saunders PC, Applebaum R, Schwartz CF, Ribakove GH, Culliford AT, Baumann FG, Kronzon I, Colvin SB, Grossi EA. Off-pump coronary artery bypass grafting reduces mortality and stroke in patients with atheromatous aortas: a case control study. Circulation 2003; 108 (suppl 1):II15–II20.
130. Schmitz C, Weinreich S, Schneider R, Schneider D, Speth I, Schulze-Rauschenbach C, Pohl C, Welz A. Off-Pump versus on-pump coronary artery bypass: can OPCAB reduce neurologic injury? Heart Surg Forum 2003; 6:127–130.
131. Newman MF, Kirchner JL, Phillips-Bute B, et al. Longitudinal assessment of neurocognitive function after coronary artery bypass surgery. N Eng J Med 2001; 344:395–402.
132. Jaroszewski DE, Restrepo L. Cognitive dysfunction after coronary artery bypass graft surgery. Seminars in Cerebrovascular Diseases and Stroke 2004; 4:109–116.
133. Barclay LL, Weiss EM, Mattis S, Bond O, Blass JP. Unrecognized cognitive impairment in cardiac rehabilitation patients. J Am Geriatr Soc 1988; 36:22–28.
134. Moller JT, Cluitmans P, Rasmussen LS, et al. Long-term postoperative cognitive dysfunction in the elderly ISPOCD1 study: International study of postoperative cognitive dysfunction. Lancet 1998; 351:857–861.
135. Abildstrom H, Rasmussen LS, Rentowl P, et al. Cognitive dysfunction 1–2 years after non-cardiac surgery in the elderly: International study of post-operative cognitive dysfunction. Acta Anaesthesiol Scand 2000; 44:1246–1251.
136. Baron JC. Perfusion thresholds in human cerebral ischemia: historical perspective and therapeutic implications. Cerebrovasc Dis 2001; 11(suppl 1):2–8.
137. Strandgaard S, Paulson OB. Regulation of cerebral blood flow in health and disease. J Cardiovasc Pharmacol 1992; 19(suppl):S89–S93.
138. Powers WJ. Hemodynamics and metabolism in ischemic cerebrovascular disease. Neurologic Clinics 1992; 10:31–48.
139. Román GC, Tatemichi TK, Erkinjuntti T, et al. Vascular dementia: diagnostic criteria for research studies. Report of the NINDS-AIREN International Workshop. Neurology 1993; 43:250–260.
140. Royall DR. Executive cognitive impairment: a novel perspective in dementia. Neuroepidemiology 2000; 19:293–299.
141. Royall DR, Lauterbach EC, Cummings JL, Reeve A, Rummans TA, Kaufer D, La France, WC Jr., Coffey E. Executive control function: a review of its promise

and challenges for clinical research. A report from the committee on research of the American Neuropsychiatric Association. J Neuropsychiatry Clin Neurosci 2002; 14: 377–405.

142. Royall DR, Cordes JA, Polk M. CLOX: an executive clock drawing task. J Neurol Neurosurg Psychiatry 1998; 64:588–594.

143. Gueyffier F, Boissel J-P, Boutitie F, et al. Effect of antihypertensive treatment in patients having already suffered from stroke: Gathering the evidence. The INDANA (INdividual Data ANalysis of Antihypertensive intervention trials) Project Collaborators. Stroke 1997; 28:2557–2562.

144. Blauw GJ, Lagaay AM, Smelt AHM, et al. Stroke, statins and cholesterol: a meta-analysis of randomized, placebo-controlled, double-blind trials with HMG-CoA reductase inhibitors. Stroke 1997; 28:946–950.

145. Majid A, Delanty N, Kantor J. Antiplatelet agents for secondary prevention of ischemic stroke. Ann Pharmacother 2001; 35:1241–1247.

146. Hart RG, Sherman DG, Easton D, Cairns JA. Prevention of stroke in patients with nonvalvular atrial fibrillation. Neurology 1998; 51:674–681.

147. Barnett HJM, Taylor DW, Eliasziw M, et al. Benefit of carotid endarterectomy in patients with symptomatic moderate or severe stenosis. N Eng J Med 1998; 339:1415–1425.

148. PROGRESS Collaborative Group. Randomized trial of perindopril-based blood pressure lowering regimen among 6105 individuals with prior stroke or transient ischemic attack. Lancet 2001; 358:1033–1041.

149. Gorelick PB. Can we save the brain from the ravages of midlife cardiovascular risk factors? Neurology 1999; 52:1114–1115.

150. Gorelick PB, Sacco RL, Smith DB, et al. Prevention of a first stroke. A review of guidelines and a multidisciplinary consensus statement from the National Stroke Association. JAMA 1999; 281:1112–1120.

151. Pearson TA, Blair SN, Daniels SR, et al. AHA guidelines for primary prevention of cardiovascular disease and stroke: 2002 update. Consensus panel guide to comprehensive risk reduction for adult patients without coronary or other atherosclerotic vascular disease. Circulation 2002; 106:388–391.

152. Sacco RL. Newer risk factors for stroke. Neurology 2001; 57(suppl 2):S31–S34.

153. Gorelick PB. Stroke prevention therapy beyond antithrombotics: Unifying mechanisms in ischemic stroke pathogenesis and implications for therapy. Stroke 2002; 33:862–875.

154. Murray MD, Lane KA, Gao S, Evans RM, et al. Preservation of cognitive function with antihypertensive medications: a longitudinal analysis of a community-based sample of African Americans. Arch Intern Med 2002; 162:2046–2052.

155. O'Brien JT, Erkinjuntti T, Reisberg B, Román G, Sawada T, Pantoni L, et al. Vascular cognitive impairment. Lancet Neurol 2003; 2:89–98.

156. Román GC: Perspectives in the treatment of vascular dementia. Drugs Today 2000; 36:641–653.

157. Román GC: Therapeutic strategies for vascular dementia. In: O'Brien J, Ames D, Burns A, eds. Dementia, 2nd ed. New York: Arnold, London/Oxford University Press: 2000:667–681.

158. Erkinjuntti T, Román GC, Gauthier S, Feldman H, Rockwood K. Emerging therapies for vascular dementia and vascular cognitive impairment. Stroke 2004; 35:1010–1017 (epub Mar 4).

159. Román GC, Rogers SJ. Donepezil: A clinical review of current and emerging indications. Exper Opin Pharmacother 2004; 5:161–180.
160. Román GC. Vascular dementia: Changing the paradigm. Curr Opin Psych 2003; 16:635–641.
161. Pantoni L, Rossi R, Inzitari D, et al. Efficacy and safety of nimodipine in subcortical vascular dementia: a subgroup analysis of the Scandinavian Multi-Infarct Dementia Trial. Journal of the Neurological Sciences 2000;175;124–134.
162. Pantoni L, Del Ser T, Soglina AG, et al. Efficacy and safety of nimodipine in subcortical vascular dementia: a randomized placebo-controlled trial. Stroke 2005; 36:619–624.
163. Fioravanti M, Yanagi M. Cytidinediphosphocholine (CDP-choline) for cognitive and behavioural disturbances associated with chronic cerebral disorders in the elderly. Cochrane Database of Systematic Reviews 2005 Apr 18;(2):CD000269.
164. European Pentoxifylline Multi-Infarct Dementia Study: The European pentoxifylline multi-infarct dementia study. European Neurology 1996; 36:315–321.
165. López-Pousa S, Mercadal-Dalmau J, Marti-Cuadros AM, et al. Triflusal in the prevention of vascular dementia. Revista de Neurologia 1997; 25:1525–1528.
166. Evans JG, Grimley EV, Van Dongen M. *Ginkgo biloba* for cognitive impairment and dementia. Cochrane Database of Systematic Reviews 2002; (4):CD003120.
167. Orgogozo J-M, Rigaud AS, Stoffler A, et al. Efficacy and safety of memantine in patients with mild to moderate vascular dementia: a randomized, placebo-controlled trial (MMM 300). Stroke 2002; 33:1834–1839.
168. Wilcock G, Möbius HJ, Stoffler A, and the MMM 500 group. A double-blind, placebo-controlled multicentre study of memantine in mild to moderate vascular dementia (MMM 500). International Clinical Psychopharmacology 2002; 17:297–305.
169. Black S, Román GC, Geldmacher DS, et al. for the Donepezil 307 Vascular Dementia Study Group. Efficacy and tolerability of donepezil in vascular dementia: positive results of a 24-week, multicenter, international, randomized, placebo-controlled clinical trial. Stroke 2003; 34:2323–2330. Epub 2003 Sep 11.
170. Wilkinson D, Doody R, Helme R, et al. for the Donepezil 308 Vascular Dementia Study Group. Donepezil in vascular dementia: a randomized, placebo-controlled study. Neurology 2003; 61:479–486.
171. Román GC, Wilkinson D, Doody R, Salloway SP, Schindler RJ. Donepezil in vascular dementia: combined analysis of two large-scale clinical trials. Dementia and Geriatric Cognitive Disorders 2005, 20:338–44. Epub 2005 Sep 23.
172. Erkinjuntti T, Kurz A, Gauthier S, et al. Efficacy of galantamine in probable vascular dementia and Alzheimer's disease combined with cerebrovascular disease: a randomised trial. Lancet 2002; 359:1283–1290.
173. Kurz A, Erkinjuntti T, Small GW, Lilienfeld S, Damaraju CR. Long-term safety and cognitive effects of galantamine in the treatment of probable vascular dementia or Alzheimer's disease with cerebrovascular disease. European Journal of Neurology 2003; 10:633–640.
174. Román GC. Rivastigmine for subcortical vascular dementia. Expert Review in Neurotherapeutics 2005; 5:309–313.
175. Moretti R, Torre P, Antonello RM, Cazzato G, Bava A. Rivastigmine in vascular dementia. Expert Opinion in Pharmacotherapy 2004; 5:1399–1410.

2

HIV-1-Associated Dementia (HAD)

Giovanni Schifitto

*Department of Neurology, University of Rochester Medical Center,
Rochester, New York, U.S.A.*

Peter Mariuz

*Department of Infectious Diseases, University of Rochester Medical Center,
Rochester, New York, U.S.A.*

INTRODUCTION

Infection with the human immunodeficiency virus type 1 (HIV-1) is frequently associated with neurological complications involving both the central and peripheral nervous system. Among these, HIV-1-associated dementia (HAD) is the most common sequela affecting the central nervous system (CNS). Before focusing on HAD, we will briefly review HIV infection epidemiology, viral cycle, and treatment.

As of December 31, 2001 the cumulative total of AIDS cases reported to the Centers for Disease Control (CDC) was 816,149. Total deaths of persons reported with AIDS were 467,910 (1). Worldwide, since the onset of the HIV/ adult immune deficiency syndrome (AIDS) epidemic, more than 47 million people have been infected and there were 3.1 million deaths in 2000.

AIDS-related mortality and morbidity from opportunistic infections and Kaposi's sarcoma have decreased dramatically since the introduction of highly active antiretroviral therapy (HAART) in 1996. AIDS is the end-stage disease of HIV-1 infection and is defined as the development of specific opportunistic infections, tumors, dementia, or CD4 white blood cell count below 200 cells/mm^3 or CD4 percentage less than 14% (2). Without specific therapy, once AIDS has developed, the disease progresses rapidly and patients die on average in approximately 2–3 years (3).

Most HIV-infected individuals develop AIDS within a median time of 7–10 years after the initial infection (typical progressors). Approximately 5–10% of the individuals, however, will develop AIDS within 2–3 years (rapid progressors). In contrast, less than 5% of the individuals will be AIDS-free 20 years after primary infection (nonprogressors).

HIV-1 enters the CNS soon after primary infection, likely by the ingress of infected macrophages into the CNS (4,5). Macrophages and microglia are the reservoir of HIV infection within the nervous system as neurons are not infected.

HIV LIFE CYCLE AND ANTIRETROVIRAL THERAPY

HIV is an enveloped RNA virus belonging to the lentivirus genus of retroviruses. The genome contains three primary genes: *gag, pol, env*, which encode for the major structural proteins (gag), enzymatic proteins (pol), and envelope (env). Other genes (*tat, nef, rev, vpu, vif*) regulate expression of proteins, viral assembly and release from infected cells. HIV binds to the CD4 molecule present on cells of the monocyte/macrophage lineage and CD4 T-lymphocytes (T-helper cells) via surface glycoprotein 120 (gp120) (Fig. 1). Fusion of the viral envelope with the cell membrane occurs by the interaction of HIV fusion protein (gp41) and a coreceptor on the host cell membrane. The viral genome (two single strands of RNA) is released into the cytoplasm. After entry, the viral genome is uncoated and undergoes reverse transcription (catalyzed by HIV reverse transcriptase) to double stranded DNA. Viral DNA is integrated into the host genome to form a provirus. After appropriate host cell stimulation, transcription of proviral DNA

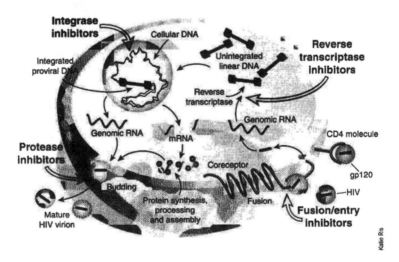

Figure 1   The replication cycle of HIV and targets for antiretroviral therapy. *Source:* From Ref. 86.

takes place resulting in the formation of new virions. These are assembled in the cytoplasm and mature only after budding through the cell membrane. HIV protease mediates final viral maturation by cleaving first itself and then the other viral proteins from a precursor polyprotein.

Remarkable advances have been made in the last 20 years in the treatment of HIV infection. Currently, five classes of drugs are available, acting against three different steps of viral entry and replication (Fig. 1). These include nucleoside reverse transcriptase inhibitors (NRTIs), nucleotide reverse transcriptase inhibitors (NtRTI), non-nucleoside reverse transcriptase inhibitors (NNRTIs), protease inhibitors (PIs), and fusion inhibitors (FI) (Table 1).

Quantitative HIV-RNA PCR are used to determine both the concentration of plasma viremia (viral load or burden) and CD4 lymphocyte counts to initiate therapy and to monitor the efficacy of therapy. Viral load is the best surrogate marker of disease progression. The CD4 lymphocyte counts remain the gold standard test to determine the risk of specific opportunistic infections (OIs) and some malignancies and therefore to initiate prophylaxis against various OIs. The goal

Table 1 Currently Approved Antiretroviral Therapy

Nucleoside reverse transcriptase inhibitors (NRTIs)
Zidovudine (AZT, Retrovir)
Didanosine (ddI, Videx)
Stavudine (d4T, Zerit)
Lamivudine (3TC, Epivir)
Emtricitabine (Emtriva, ETC)
Zalcitabine (ddC, Hivid)
Abacavir (Ziagem)
Combivir (AZT + 3TC)
Trizivir (AZT + 3TC + Abacavir)
Non-nucleoside reverse transcriptase inhibitors (NNRTIs)
Efavirenz (Sustiva, EFV)
Nevirapine (Viramune, NVP)
Delavirdine (Rescriptor, DLV)
Protease inhibitors (PIs)
Saquinavir (Fortovase, Sqv)
Ritonavir (Norvir, RTV)
Indinavir (Crixivan, IND)
Nelfinavir (Viracept, NLV)
Amprenavir (Agenerase, APV)
Atazanavir (Rayataz, ATV)
Fosamprenavir (Lexiva)
Lopinavir/Ritonavir (Kaletra, LPV/RTV)
NtRTI
Tenofovir (Viread, TDF)
Fusion inhibitors (FI)
Enfuvirtide (Fuzeon, T-20)

of antiretroviral therapy is to achieve sustained maximal suppression of viral replication (defined as an undetectable viral load, using an assay with a threshold of 50 genome copies/mL). For most patients, sustained viral suppression has been associated with partial immune reconstitution or inhibition of further immunosuppression (reflected by increased or stable CD4 T-lymphocyte counts). The effectiveness of HAART in this regard has resulted in the marked decline in HIV/AIDS-associated mortality, morbidity, incidence of opportunistic infections and some malignancies, hospitalization rates, hospice use, skilled nursing, and home care needs (6,7). Recommended regimens for initial therapy include combinations of two NRTIs and a PI or two NRTIs and an NNRTI (8).

The ability of drugs to cross the blood–brain barrier is of particular importance in treating CNS infections. Significant factors include the plasma concentration of free unbound drug and the degree of lipid solubility (9). With antivirals, however, of much greater importance may be the cerebrospinal fluid (CSF) concentration, which a drug achieves relative to its IC50 (9). For example, the NNRTI efavirenz is highly protein bound (>95%) and its CSF-plasma concentration is low. However, in one study the mean CSF concentration was above the IC95 for HIV (10). On the other hand, it is not known how well CSF drug levels correlate with the levels achieved in CSF macrophages and other target cells. Among the NRTIs, AZT and d4T have the best CNS penetration. Among NNRTIs, Nevirapine has high CSF-Plasma ratio and CSF concentrations above the IC50 of HIV. The (PIs) as a group are highly protein bound in plasma and except for Indinavir have poor CNS penetration. Despite this, when PIs other than Indinavir have been given in combination with NRTIs, CSF HIV RNA levels can become undetectable (11,12). Until controlled prospective data is available upon which to base the selection of one drug regimen over another for the treatment of HIV-associated cognitive impairment, it would seem appropriate to use drugs with good CNS penetration whenever possible.

HAD NOMENCLATURE AND STAGING

In 1991 the American Academy of Neurology AIDS Task Force (13) developed a consensus nomenclature and case definition for HAD complex (Table 2); however, several terms are still used interchangeably, including AIDS dementia complex, HIV encephalopathy, HIV subacute encephalitis, and HAD. The severity of dementia in the consensus nomenclature (mild, moderate, and severe) reflects functional deficits that affect the activities of daily living.

A milder form of cognitive impairment, HIV-1-associated minor cognitive/motor disorder (MCMD), was also introduced (Table 3); however, it was not determined whether this represented an intermediate step in the progression to dementia. Subsequent research has shown that MCMD is a risk factor for HAD (14).

AIDS dementia complex (ADC), a definition and staging of dementia primarily based on functional disability, was proposed by Price and Brew (15) and is

Table 2 HIV-1-Associated Dementia Complex

Probable (must have each of the following):
1. a. Acquired abnormality in at least two of the following cognitive abilities (present for at least one month): Attention/concentration, speed of processing of information, abstraction/reasoning, visuospatial skills, memory/learning, and speech/language. The decline should be verified by reliable history and mental status examination. In all cases, when possible, history should be obtained from an informant, and examination should be supplemented by neuropsychological testing.
   b. Cognitive dysfunction causing impairment of work or activities of daily living (objectively verifiable or by report of a key informant). This impairment should not be attributable solely to severe systemic illness.
2. At least one of the following:
   a. Acquired abnormality in motor function or performance verified by clinical examination (e.g., slowed rapid movements, abnormal gait, limb incoordination, hyperreflexia, hypertonia, or weakness), neuropsychological tests (e.g., fine motor speed, manual dexterity, perceptual motor skills), or both.
   b. Decline in motivation or emotional control or change in social behavior. This may be characterized by any of the following: change in personality with apathy, inertia, irritability, emotional lability, or new onset of impaired judgment characterized by social inappropriate behavior or disinhibition.
3. Absence of clouding of consciousness during a period long enough to establish the presence of #1.
4. No evidence of another etiology, including active CNS opportunistic infection or malignancy, psychiatric disorders (e.g., depressive disorder), active alcohol or substance use, or acute or chronic substance withdrawal, must be sought from history, physical and psychiatric examination, and appropriate laboratory and radiologic investigation (e.g., lumbar puncture, neuroimaging). If another potential etiology (e.g., major depression) is present, it is not the cause of the above cognitive, motor, or behavioral symptoms and signs.

Possible (must have one of the following):
1. Other potential etiology present (must have each of the following):
   a. As above (see Probable) #1, 2, and 3.
   b. Other potential etiology is present but the cause of #1 above is uncertain.
2. Incomplete clinical evaluation (must have each of the following):
   a. As above (see Probable) #1, 2, and 3.
   b. Etiology cannot be determined (appropriate laboratory or radiologic investigations not performed).

The level of impairment due to cognitive dysfunction should be assessed as follows:
Mild: Decline in performance at work, including work in the home, that is conspicuous to others. Unable to work at usual job, although may be able to work at a much less demanding job. Activities of daily living or social activities are impaired but not to a degree making the person completely dependent on others. More complicated daily tasks or recreational activities cannot be undertaken. Capable of basic self-care,

(Continued)

Table 2 HIV-1-Associated Dementia Complex (*Continued*)

such as feeding, dressing, and maintaining personal hygiene, but activities such as
   handling money, shopping, using public transportation, driving a car, or keeping track of
   appointments or medications are impaired.
Moderate: Unable to work, including work in the home. Unable to function without some
   assistance of another in daily living, including dressing, maintaining personal hygiene,
   eating, shopping, handling money, and walking, but able to communicate basic needs.
Severe: Unable to perform any activities of daily living without assistance. Requires
   continual supervision. Unable to maintain personal hygiene, nearly or absolutely mute.

---

still frequently used. However, subjects with mild dementia are difficult to stage with the ADC scale. Recently, the ADC staging has been revisited by Marder et al. (16); in particular, functional deficits have been complemented with more specific cognitive deficits (Table 4). Similarly to the AAN classification for HAD and minor cognitive/motor disorders (14), Marder et al. have been able to generate a computerized algorithm for the ADC staging that would be particulary suitable for multicenter studies (16).

The neuropsychological test battery to assess HIV-associated cognitive impairment should include tests of attention, memory, psychomotor speed, and executive function. NIMH had originally recommended a long neuro-psychological battery that we find impractical for either clinical or research purposes (18). We routinely use the Rey auditory verbal learning test (attention and memory), Rey complex figure (visual memory, visuoconstruction function), grooved pegboard and symbol digit (psychomotor speed), CalCAP reaction time (speed of information processing), and verbal fluency (19) (executive function).

Epidemiology

HAD affects patients with moderate to severe immunosuppression. In the era before the introduction of HAART, HAD was reported in 7% of patients with AIDS (20) and up to 25% in longitudinal cohorts, such as the Multicenter AIDS Cohort Study (MACS) (21). Although the incidence of HAD has decreased significantly with the use of HAART (22) (Fig. 2), the prevalence of HAD may have actually increased, given the increased survival of HIV-infected individuals (23). In pre-HAART studies, in addition to low CD4 cell count, several other risk factors have been associated with the development of HAD, including lower hemoglobin, lower body mass index, older age, more systemic symptoms before the development of AIDS and HIV viral load (21,24–26). Since HAART has changed the natural history of HIV infection and related complications, it is not surprising that recent studies have shown a lack of association between baseline immunological and virological markers and HAD (27).

Table 3 HIV-1-Associated Minor Cognitive/Motor Disorder

Probable (must have each of the following):
1. Cognitive/motor/behavioral abnormalities (must have each of the following):
   a. At least two of the following acquired cognitive, motor, or behavioral symptoms (present for at least one month) verified by reliable history (when possible, from an informant):
      1) Impaired attention or concentration
      2) Mental slowing
      3) Impaired memory
      4) Slowed movements
      5) Incoordination
      6) Personality change, or irritability or emotional lability
   b. Acquired cognitive/motor abnormality verified by clinical neurologic examination or neuropsychological testing (e.g., fine motor speed, manual dexterity, perceptual motor skills, attention/concentration, speed of processing of information, abstraction/reasoning, visuospatial skills, memory/learning, or speech/language).
2. Disturbance from cognitive/motor/behavioral abnormalities (see #1) causes mild impairment of work or activities of daily living[a] (objectively verifiable or by report of a key informant).
3. Does not meet criteria for HAD complex or HIV-1-associated myelopathy.
4. No evidence of another etiology, including active CNS opportunistic infection or malignancy, or sever systemic illness determined by appropriate history, physical examination, and laboratory and radiologic investigation (e.g., lumbar puncture, neuroimaging). The above features should not be attributable solely to the effects of active alcohol or substance use, acute or chronic substance withdrawal, adjustment disorder, or other psychiatric disorders.

Possible (must have one of the following):
1. Other potential etiology present (must have each of the following):
   a. As above (see Probable) #1, 2, and 3.
   b. Other potential etiology is present and the cause of the cognitive/motor/behavioral abnormalities is uncertain.
2. Incomplete clinical evaluation (must have each of the following):
   a. As above (see Probable) #1, 2, and 3.
   b. Etiology cannot be determined (appropriate laboratory or radiologic investigations not performed).

---

[a]Able to perform all but the most demanding aspects of work or activities of daily living. Performance at work is mildly impaired but able to maintain usual job; social activities may be mildly impaired, but person is not dependent on others. Can feed self, dress, and maintain personal hygiene, handle money, shop, use public transportation, or drive a car, but complex daily tasks such as keeping track of appointments or medications may be occasionally impaired.
Abbreviation: HAD, HIV-1-associated dementia.

Table 4   Clinical Staging of HAD: NEAD Classification

ADC Stage[a]	New criteria: NEAD Modification	Characteristics
Stage 0 (normal)	NP impression = 0 EVEN IF cognitive complaints are present	Normal mental and motor function. No IADL functional impairments.
Stage 0.5 (subclinical or equivocal)	(1) NP impression = 0 AND any CNS neuro findings OR any IADL functional impairment (2) NP impression = 1 AND no IADL functional impairment	Either minimal/equivocal symptoms or motor dysfunction characteristic of HIV-D, or mild neurological signs (e.g., sout, slowed extremity movements), but without impairment of work or capacity of perform ADL.
Stage 1 (mild HIV-D)	(1) NP impression is 1 AND abnormalities in both CNS neurological exam AND IADL function (2) NP impression is 2 BUT no abnormalities in EITHER CNS neuro exam OR IADL function	Able to perform all but the more demanding aspects of work or ADL but with unequivocal evidence (has to include abnormal NP performance) of functional, intellectual or motor impairment. AND Can walk without assistance.
Stage 2 (moderate HIV-D)	(1) NP impression is 2 AND abnormalities in EITHER CNS neuro exam OR IADL function (2) NP impression is 2 AND mild to moderate abnormalities in BOTH CNS neuro exam AND IADL function, however neither severe	Able to perform basic activities of self-care but cannot work or maintain the more demanding aspects of daily life. AND Ambulatory, but may require a single prop or cane.
Stage 3 (severe HIV-D)	(1) NP impression is 2 AND severe abnormalities in BOTH CNS neuro exam AND IADL function	Major intellectual incapacity (cannot follow news or personal events, cannot sustain complex conversation, considerable slowing of all outputs). OR

(Continued)

Table 4   Clinical Staging of HAD: NEAD Classification (*Continued*)

	(2) NP impression is 2 AND mild to moderate abnormalities in CNS neuro exam AND severe IADL functional impairment AND severe gait impairment (3) NP impression is 3 AND gait is mild to moderately impaired	Motor disability (cannot walk unassisted, requiring walker or personal support, usually with slowing and clumsiness of arms as well).
Stage 4 (very severe/end stage HIV-D)	(1) Unable to perform NP testing because of cognitive-motor impairments (2) Unable to walk on CNS basis	Nearly vegetative. Intellectual and social comprehension and output are at a rudimentary level. Nearly or absolutely mute. Paraparetic or paraplegic with urinary and fecal incontinence.

[a]Developed at Memorial Sloan Kettering Center (17).
Abbreviations: NP, impression may be the neuropsychologist's global cognitive impression or the quantitative global neuropsychological impression (16); ADL, activities of daily living; IADL, instrumental activities of daily living.

Pathology

Macroscopically, the brain of patients with HAD appears atrophic (28). Although all areas of the brain can be affected, histological abnormalities are primarily seen

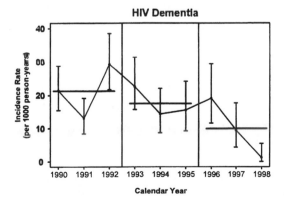

Figure 2   Incidence rate of HIV dementia per 1000 person years in the period 1990–1998. Note the decline in incidence of dementia with the introduction of HAART in 1996. *Source*: From Ref. 22.

in the white and subcortical gray matter (28,29). The histological hallmark of HAD is the presence of multinucleated giant cells (MNGCs), the syncytia of fused infected macrophages (30–32). MNGCs are found preferentially in pericapillary and perivenular areas of the centrum semiovale, basal ganglia, and pons. However, in clinical–pathological correlation studies, MNGCs were found in less than 40% of HAD patients (28,33). Less specific findings include perivascular lymphocytic and macrophagic infiltrate of the leptomeninges and brain parenchyma and microglia nodules (microglia cells and astrocytes) in cerebral cortex and basal ganglia.

The white matter appears pale, which is thought to be primarily the result of altered blood–brain barrier (34). Focal areas of vacuolation can be found in the centrum semiovale; infrequently these areas may become confluent. Additional vacuolation can be seen along the white matter tracts, the basal ganglia, the brain stem, and the cerebellum. The cerebral cortex is relatively spared compared to the basal ganglia and white matter; however, dendritic simplification and neuronal loss are often found (35–38).

PATHOGENESIS

The mechanisms of neuronal injury responsible for HAD are still unknown. HIV does not infect neurons. However, viral proteins, such as gp120 and tat, have been shown to be neurotoxic, both by directly altering the function of glia and neurons (39,40) and indirectly by stimulating the secretion of inflammatory products by macrophages (41,42).

Microglia and macrophages are particularly important not only because they are productively infected, representing the CNS viral reservoir (30,43) [astrocytes are not productively infected (44,45)], but also because they release numerous immune mediators when either infected or activated. In this regard, several products of immune activation, such as beta-2 microglobulin, neopterin, prostaglandins, and metalloproteinases (MMP), have been associated with HAD (46–50). Some products of immune activation, including quinolinic acid, platelet-activating factor (PAF), and tumor necrosis factor-alpha are by themselves potentially neurotoxic, in part via NMDA receptors stimulation (42,51–54). In addition, the state of immune activation triggered by HIV infection is associated with increased systemic and CNS oxidative stress (55,56). Oxidative stress and activation of N-methyl-D-ospontate (NMDA) receptors have been suggested to be an important intermediate step in the pathogenesis of neuronal dysfunction and death occurring in HAD (57).

CLINICAL PRESENTATION

The onset of HAD is usually subacute, developing over months. Forgetfulness and decreased attention and concentration are the most frequent early symptoms of HAD (58,59). As the ability to attend multiple tasks decreases, there is a concomitant decreased efficiency in performing the most demanding aspects of daily life.

Behavioral changes include irritability, apathy, reduced social contact, decreased libido, and altered sleeping patterns. Mild to moderate depressive symptoms may precede the onset of HAD (60); however, significant depression may confound the diagnosis of HAD and needs to be considered along with HAD since depressive symptoms can be ameliorated with both pharmacological and nonpharmacological intervention.

Patients with mild to moderate cognitive impairment often have a normal neurological exam. Early neurological findings include abnormal pursuit and saccadic eye movements and reduced rapid alternating and sequential hand movements. Later, patients develop hyperreflexia (ankle reflexes may be normal or reduced if HIV-associated neuropathy coexists) and postural instability. As HAD progresses, ataxia, tremor, hypertonia, and frontal release signs appear.

Atypical presentations of HAD have been described, presenting in the context of a manic episode (61), with a remitting and relapsing course (62), or rapid progression associated with focal neurological deficits (63). However, suspicion of other etiologies should be considered in such cases.

OPPORTUNISTIC CONDITIONS IN HAD: DIFFERENTIAL DIAGNOSIS

Several CNS infections and primary CNS lymphoma can have a subacute course, mimicking in part the clinical manifestaion of HAD. However, neuroimaging will usually help distinguish HAD from mass occupying lesions such as occur with *Toxoplasma gondii* infection and primary CNS lymphoma. The following are CNS infections that are not readily distinguishable from HAD by neuroimaging.

CMV encephalitis (CMVE) is often a subacute illness that can present with confusion, forgetfulness, and apathy (64,65). Focal neurological findings, including cranial neuropathies and gaze-evoked nystagmus, may be found in about 50% of the patients with CMVE (65). CMVE virtually always occurs in patients with severe immunosuppression (CD4 counts $<50/mm^3$) and is often associated with other organ involvement, for example, chorioretinitis.

Periventricular white matter abnormalities, often enhancing with contrast, are seen on brain MRI. Other areas that can be affected include the cerebellum and brain stem. CSF analysis is not diagnostic, but a negative CMV PCR is very helpful in excluding CMVE (66).

Papovavirus (JC virus) infection can result in progressive multifocal leukoencephalopathy (PML) (67,68). PML represents the reactivation of a latent infection (about 75% of the adult population have evidence of past infection with JC virus). JC virus infects both oligodendrocytes and astrocytes, but productive viral infection occurs only in oligodendrocytes.

Patients with PML can present with a variety of neurological symptoms from focal weakness to cognitive dysfunction. Brain MRI reveals asymmetric homogenous white matter lesions that have low signal, non-enhancing on T1-weighted images and without mass effect. Multiple areas may be involved including the cerebellum and brainstem. When lesions are confluent and involve the centrum semiovale, differentiation from white matter abnormalities seen in HAD may be difficult. However, T1 low-density signal is usually seen only in PML. Rarely, the MRI lesions may enhance or they may be confined to the posterior fossa (69). The cerebral cortex and deep nuclear structures may also be affected.

The diagnosis of PML is highly suggested by a focal neurological presentation and typical neuroimaging findings. The diagnosis is confirmed if CSF PCR for JC virus is also positive (70). If the PCR testing of CSF is negative a definitive diagnosis rests on brain biopsy.

Cryptococcal meningitis is caused by *Cryptococcus neoformans*, an encapsulated ubiquitous budding yeast. The clinical presentation of cryptococcal meningitis shows extreme variation ranging from complaints of a subtle headache to obtundation and death. Brain MRI may show punctate hyperintensities with or without contrast enhancement that correspond pathologically to dilated perivascular spaces and cryptococcomas (71). Rarely, cryptococcomas may present as larger intraparenchymal mass lesions. The gold standard diagnostic test for cryptococcal meningitis is culturing the organism from the CSF; however, assessing CSF cryptococcal antigen is a rapid and extremely reliable diagnostic test with a sensitivity of 93–99% (72,73).

Two additional CNS infections to consider are *Mycobacterium tuberculosis* meningitis and neurosyphillis. Although the clinical presentations of these infections do not differ between HIV-infected and HIV non-infected individuals, co-infection with HIV is not unusual in particular settings, and so these two conditions should be included in the differentiation of HAD.

DIAGNOSTIC EVALUATION

Patients with predominantly memory and concentration complaints are usually referred for neurological consultation to assess cognitive function. However, in our experience, those with more apathy and depressive symptoms are likely to be referred to a psychiatrist first and further work-up for a possible associated cognitive impairment may be delayed. Although patients with significant depression usually do respond to typical antidepressants (and should be treated appropriately), the co-existence of cognitive impairment should be suspected and a comprehensive neurological evaluation should be obtained.

Given that the neurological findings may be subtle early in the course of dementia, we routinely perform neuropsychological tests to assess cognitive performance, particularly if current CD4 cell count is <200 mm^3. This baseline assessment is useful to monitor progression and response to therapeutic intervention.

HAD is a diagnosis of exclusion. Therefore, opportunistic CNS infections and primary CNS lymphoma must first be excluded. Magnetic resonance imaging (MRI) is the neuroimaging study of choice in this regard. A brain MRI of a patient with HAD will typically show generalized atrophy and periventricular white matter changes (Fig. 3). Contrast enhancement is seen only in the rare instance when there are areas of necrosis at the white–gray matter junction. In this situation, other opportunistic conditions must be ruled out. Magnetic

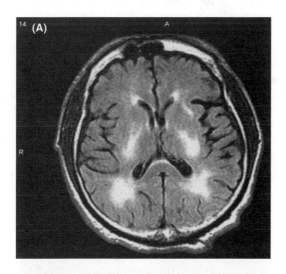

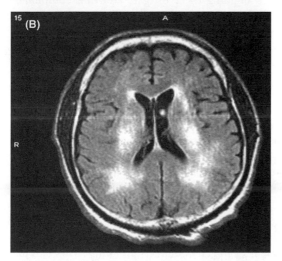

Figure 3 MRI scan (axial flair) of a patient presenting with dementia as the first sign of HIV infection. Note the diffuse, largely symmetric, periventricular white matter changes.

resonance spectroscopy (MRS) is primarily a research tool, but appears to be a promising technique to assess CNS injury. Concentrations of *N*-acetyl aspartate (NAA), a neuronal marker, are reduced in the basal ganglia and the concentrations of myoinositol (glia marker) are incresead in the centrum semiovale of patients with HAD (74,75). Furthermore, treatment with HAART tends to normalize the concentration of these metabolites (17).

Lumbar puncture is performed to exclude other etiologies. The CSF profile of patients with HAD is often indistinguishable from HIV-infected individuals without cognitive impairment. The nonspecific abnormalities may include mild elevated total protein and mild mononuclear pleocytosis.

Other laboratory testing should include: electrolytes, vitamin B12 levels, thyroid and liver function tests, a serological test for syphilis, cryptococcus serum antigen, and serum toxoplasma antibody titers. CSF analysis is particularly useful to evaluate CMVE and PML (by PCR) and chronic infections, such as cryptococcus meningitis, tuberculosis meningitis, and neurosyphilis.

TREATMENT

Thus far, the complex pathogenesis of HAD has prevented the development of effective treatment. There is evidence that antriretrovirals can improve cognitive deficits (76,77) and HAART has significantly decreased the incidence of HAD (22). Therefore, we maximize the use of potent antiretroviral therapy in patients with HAD with the objective of obtaining an undetectable plasma viral load. Although antiretrovirals differ in their ability to cross the blood–brain barrier, there is no strong evidence that one regimen is better than another (78). Efforts have been made (79–85) and are ongoing to investigate adjuvant compounds based on putative mechanisms that suggest NMDA receptors, oxidative stress, and cytokines are involved in neuronal injury.

REFERENCES

1. CDC. HIV/AIDS Surveillance Report, 2001. US Department of Health and Human Services C, editor 2001; 13(2): Atlanta, Georgia.
2. 1993 revised classification system for HIV infection and expanded surveillance case definition for AIDS among adolescents and adults. MMWR Morb Mortal Wkly Rep 1996; 41-RR-17.
3. Weiss RA. How does HIV cause AIDS. Science 1993; 260:1273–1279.
4. Chiodi F, Asjo B, Fanyo EM, Norkrans G, Hagberg L, Albert J. Isolation of HIV from cerebrospinal fluid of antibody-postive virus carrier without neurological symptoms. Lancet 1986; II:1276–1277.
5. Ho DD, Rota TR, Schooley RT. Isolation of HTLV-III from cerebrospinal fluid and neural tissues of patients with neurological syndromes related to the Acquired Immunodeficiency Syndrome. N Engl J Med 1985; 313:1493–1497.
6. World Health Organization. Report on the global HIV/AIDS epidemic, 2000; 1–115.

7. Palella FJ, Delaney KM, Moorman AC, Loveless MO, Fuhrer J, Satten GA, et al. Declining morbidity and mortality among patients with advance Human Immunodeficiency Virus infection. N Engl J Med 1998; 338(13):853–860.
8. Guidelines for the use of antiretroviral agents in HIV-1-infected adults and adolescents. DHHS, editor. 11-10-2003.
9. Enting RH, Hoetelmans RM, Lange JM, Burger DM, Beijnen JH, Portegies P. Antiretroviral drugs and the central nervous system. AIDS 1998; 12:1941–1955.
10. Tashima KT, Caliendo AM, Ahmad M, Gormley JM, Fiske WD, Brennan JM, et al. Cerebrospinal fluid Human Immunodeficiency Virus type 1 (HIV-1) suppression and Efavirenz drug concentrations in HIV-1-infected patients receiving combination therapy. J Infect Dis 1999; 180:862–864.
11. Gisolf E, Jurrians S, van der Ende M, Portegies P, Hoetelmans R, Danner S. The Prometheus Study: double protease inhibitor (PI) treatment only is unable to suppress detectable viral load in the CSF. 6th Conference on Retroviruses and Opportunistic Infections 1999; 1 (Abstract).
12. Aweeka F, Jayewardene A, Staprans S, Bellibas SE, Kearney B, Lizak P, et al. Failure to detect Nelfinavir in the cerebrospinal fluid of HIV-1-infected patients with and without AIDS dementia complex. JAIDS 1999; 20:39–43.
13. American Academy of Neurology AIDS Task Force. Nomenclature and research case definitions for neurologic manifestations of Human Immunodeficiency Virus-type 1 (HIV-1) infection. Neurology 1991; 41:778–785.
14. Marder K, Albert S, Dooneief G, Stern Y, Ramachandran G, Todak G, et al. Clinical confirmation of the American Academy of Neurology algorithm for IIIV-1 associated cognitive/motor disorder. Neurology 1996; 47:1247–1253.
15. Price RW, Brew BJ. The AIDS dementia complex. J Infect Dis 1988; 158:1079–1083.
16. Marder K, Albert SM, McDermott MP, McArthur JC, Schifitto G, Selnes OA, et al. Inter-rater reliability of a clinical staging of HIV-associated cognitive impairment. Neurology 2003; 60:1467–1473.
17. Chang L, Ernst T, Leonido-Yee M, Witt M, Speck O, Walot I, et al. Highly active antiretroviral therapy reverses brain metabolite abnormalities in mild HIV dementia. Neurology 1999; 53:782–789.
18. Butters N, Grant I, Haxby J, Judd LL, Martin A, McClelland J, et al. Assessment of AIDS-related cognitive changes: Recommendations of the NIMH workshop on neuropsychological assessment approaches. J Clin Exp Neuropsychol 1990; 12: 963–978.
19. Schifitto G, Kieburtz K, McDermott MP, McArthur J, Marder K, Sacktor N, et al. Clinical trials in HIV-associated cognitive impairment: Cognitive and functional outcomes. Neurology 2001; 56:415–418.
20. Janssen RS, Nwanyanwu OC, Selik RM, Stehr-Green JK. Epidemiology of Human Immunodeficiency Virus encephalopathy in the United States. Neurology 1992; 42:1472–1476.
21. McArthur JC, Hoover DR, Bacellar H, Miller EN, Cohen BA, Becker JT, et al. Dementia in AIDS patients: Incidence and risk factors. Neurology 1993; 43:2245–2252.
22. Sacktor N, Lyles RH, Skolasky R, Kleeberger C, Selnes OA, Miller EN, et al. HIV-associated neurologic disease incidence changes: Multicenter AIDS Cohort Study, 1990–1998. Neurology 2001; 56:257–260.

23. Dore GJ, Correll PK, Li Y, Kaldor JM, Cooper DA, Brew BJ. Changes to AIDS dementia complex in the era of highly active antiretroviral therapy. AIDS 1999; 13:1249–1253.

24. Childs EA, Lyles RH, Selnes OA, Chen B, Miller EN, Cohen BA, et al. Plasma viral load and CD4 lymphocytes predict HIV-associated dementia and sensory neuropathy. Neurology 1999; 52:607–613.

25. Ellis RJ, Hsia K, Spector SA, Nelson JA, Heaton RK, Wallace MR, et al. Cerebrospinal fluid Human Immunodeficiency Virus type 1 RNA levels are elevated in neurocognitively impaired individuals with Acquired Immunodeficiency Syndrome. Ann Neurol 1997; 42(5):679–688.

26. McArthur JC, McClernon DR, Cronin MF, Nance-Sproson TE, Saah AJ, St. Clair M, et al. Relationship between Human Immunodeficiency Virus-associated dementia and viral load in cerebrospinal fluid and brain. Ann Neurol 1997; 42(5):689–698.

27. McArthur J, McClernon D, McDermott M, Conant K, Kieburtz K, Marder K, et al. Viral load markers and neurological status: a report from the North-East Dementia Cohort. J NeuroVirol 2002; 8(suppl 1):10.

28. Navia BA, Cho E-S, Petito CK, Price RW. The AIDS dementia complex: II. Neuropathology. Ann Neurol 1986; 19:525–535.

29. Snider WD, Simpson DM, Nielsen S, Gold JWM, Metroka CE, Posner JB. Neurological complications of Acquired Immune Deficiency Syndrome: Analysis of 50 patients. Ann Neurol 1983; 14:403–418.

30. Budka H. Multinucleated giant cells in brain: A hallmark of the Acquired Immune Deficiency Syndrome (AIDS). Acta Neuropathol 1986; 69:253–258.

31. Koenig S, Gendelman HE, Orenstein JM, Dal Canto MC, Pezeshkpour GH, Yungbluth M, et al. Detection of AIDS virus in macrophages in brain tissue from AIDS patients with encephalopathy. Science 1986; 233:1089–1093.

32. Budka H, Wiley CA, Kleihues P, Artigas J, Asbury AK, Cho E-S, et al. HIV-associated disease of the nervous system: Review of nomenclature and proposal for neuropathology-based terminology. Brain Pathol 1991; 1:143–152.

33. Glass JD, Wesselingh SL, Selnes OA, McArthur JC. Clinical-neuropathologic correlation in HIV-associated dementia. Neurology 1993; 43:2230–2237.

34. Power C, Kong P-A, Crawford TO, Wesselingh SL, Glass JD, McArthur JC, et al. Cerebral white matter changes in Acquired Immunodeficiency Syndrome dementia: Alterations of the blood–brain barrier. Ann Neurol 1993; 34:339–350.

35. Gray F, Haug H, Chimelli L, Geny C, Gaston A, Scaravilli F, et al. Prominent cortical atrophy with neuronal loss as correlate of Human Immunodeficiency Virus encephalopathy. Acta Neuropathol 1991; 82(3):229–233.

36. Wiley CA, Masliah E, Morey M, Lemere C, DeTeresa R, Grafe M, et al. Neocortical damage during HIV infection. Ann Neurol 1991; 29(6):651–657.

37. Ketzler S, Weis S, Haug H, Budka H. Loss of neurons in the frontal cortex in AIDS brains. Acta Neuropathol 1990; 80:92–94.

38. Everall IP, Luthert PJ, Lantos PL. Neuronal loss in the frontal cortex in HIV infection. Lancet 1991; 3357:1119–1121.

39. Benos DJ, Hahn BH, Ghosh SK, Mashburn NA, Chaikin MA, Shaw GM, et al. Envelope glycoprotein gp120 of Human Immunodeficiency Virus type 1 alters ion transport in astrocytes: Implications for AIDS dementia complex. Proc Natl Acad Sci USA 1994; 91:494–498.

40. Magnuson DSK, Knudson BE, Geiger JD, Brownstone RM, Nath A. Human Immunodeficiency Virus Type 1 tat activates non-*N*-methyl-d-aspartate excitatory amino acid receptors and causes neurotoxicity. Ann Neurol 1995; 37:373–380.

41. Epstein LG, Gendelman HE. Human Immunodeficiency Virus Type 1 infection of the nervous system: Pathogenetic mechanisms. Ann Neurol 1993; 33:429–436.

42. Lipton SA, Gendelman HE. Dementia associated with the Acquired Immunodeficiency Syndrome. N Engl J Med 1995; 332:934–940.

43. Brinkman R, Schwinn A, Narayan O, Zink C, Kreth HW, Roggendorf W, et al. Human Immunodeficiency Virus infection in microglia: Correlation between cells infected in the brain and cells cultured from infectious brain tissue. Ann Neurol 1992; 31:361–365.

44. Tornatore C, Chandra R, Berger JR, Major EO. HIV-1 infection of subcortical astrocytes in the pediatric nervous system. Neurology 1994; 44:481–487.

45. Saito Y, Sharer LR, Epstein LG, Michaels J, Mintz M, Louder M, et al. Overexpression of nef as a mark for restricted HIV-1 infection of astrocytes in postmortem pediatric central nervous tissues. Neurology 1994; 44:474–481.

46. McArthur JC, Nance-Sproson TE, Griffin DE, Hoover D, Selnes OA, Miller EN, et al. The diagnostic utility of elevation in cerebrospinal fluid β_2-microglobulin in HIV-1 dementia. Neurology 1992; 42:1707–1712.

47. Heyes MP, Brew BJ, Martin A, Price RW, Salazar AM, Sidtis JJ, et al. Quinolinic acid in cerebrospinal fluid and serum in HIV-1 infection: Relationship to clinical and neurological status. Ann Neurol 1991; 29:202–209.

48. Brew BJ, Bhalla RB, Paul M, Gallardo H, McArthur JC, Schwartz MK, et al. Cerebrospinal fluid neopterin in Human Immunodeficiency Virus Type 1 infection. Ann Neurol 1990; 28:556–560.

49. Griffin DE, Wesselingh SL, McArthur JC. Elevated central nervous system prostaglandins in Human Immunodeficiency Virus-associated dementia. Ann Neurol 1994; 35(5):592–597.

50. Conant K, McArthur JC, Griffin DE, Sjulson L, Wahl LM, Irani DN. Cerebrospinal fluid levels of MMP-2, 7, and 9 are elevated in association with Human Immunodeficiency Virus dementia. Ann Neurol 1999; 46:391–398.

51. Wilt SG, Milward E, Zhou JM, Nagasato K, Patton H, Rusten R, et al. In vitro evidence for a dual role of tumor necrosis factor-a in Human Immunodeficiency Virus Type 1 encephalopathy. Ann Neurol 1995; 37:381–394.

52. Talley AK, Dewhurst S, Perry SW, Dollard SC, Gummuluru S, Fine SM, et al. Tumor necrosis factor alpha-induced apoptosis in human neuronal cells: protection by the antioxidant *N*-acetylcysteine and the genes bcl-2 and crmA. Mol Cell Biol 1995; 15:2359–2366.

53. Gelbard HA, Dzenko KA, DiLoreto D, del Cerro M, Epstein LG. Neurotoxic effects of tumor necrosis factor alpha in primary human neuronal cultures are mediated by activation of the glutamate AMPA receptor subtype: Implications for AIDS neuropathogenesis. Dev Neurosci 1993; 15:417–422.

54. Gelbard HA, Nottet HS, Swindells S, Jett M, Dzenko KA, Genis P, et al. Plateletactivity factor: a candidate Human Immunodeficiency Virus type 1-induced neurotoxin. J Virol 1994; 68:4628–4635.

55. Herzenberger LA, deRosa SC, Dubs JG, Roederer M, Anderson MT, Ela SW, et al. Glutathione deficiency is associated with impaired survival in HIV disease. Proc Natl Acad Sci USA 1997; 94:1967–1972.

56. Turchan J, Pocernich CB, Gairola C, Chauhan A, Schifitto G, Butterfield DA, et al. Oxidative stress in HIV demented patients and protection ex vivo with novel anti-oxidants. Neurology 2003; 60:307–314.

57. Rausch DM, Davis MR. HIV in the CNS: Pathogenic relationships to systemic HIV disease and other CNS diseases. J NeuroVirol 2001; 7:85–96.

58. Navia BA, Jordan BD, Price RW. The AIDS Dementia Complex: I. Clinical Features. Ann Neurol 1986; 19:517–524.

59. McArthur JC. Neurologic manifestations of AIDS. Medicine 1987; 66:407–437.

60. Stern Y, McDermott MP, Albert S, Palumbo D, Selnes OA, McArthur J, et al. Factors associated with incident Human Immunodeficiency Virus-dementia. Arch Neurol 2001; 58:473–479.

61. Lyketsos CG, Hanson AL, Fishman M, Rosenblatt A, McHugh PR, Treisman GJ. Manic syndrome early and late in the course of HIV. Am J Psych 1993; 150:326–327.

62. Berger JR, Tornatore C, Major EO, Bruce J, Shapshak P, Yoshioka M, et al. Relapsing and remitting Human Immunodeficiency Virus-associated leukoencephalomyelopathy. Ann Neurol 1992; 31:34–38.

63. von Giesen H-J, Arendt G, Neuen-Jacob E, Prestien K, Jablonowski H, Freund HJ. A pathologically distinct new form of HIV associated encephalopathy. J Neurol Sci 1994; 121:215–221.

64. Fiala M, Singer EJ, Graves MC, Tourtellotte WW, Stewart JA, Schable CA, et al. AIDS dementia complex complicated by cytomegalovirus encphalopathy. J Neurol 1993; 240:223–231.

65. Kalayjian RC, Cohen ML, Bonomo RA, Flanigan TP. Cytomegalovirus ventriculo-encephalitis in AIDS, a syndrome with distinct clinical and pathologic features. Medicine 1993; 72:67–77.

66. Sindic CJM, Van Antwerpen MP, Goffette S. Clinical relevance of polymerase chain reaction (PCR) assays and antigen-driven immunoblots for the diagnosis of neurological infectious diseases. Brain Res Bull 2003; 61(3):299–308.

67. Hall CD, Dafni U, Simpson D, Clifford D, Wetherill PE, Cohen B, et al. Failure of cytarabine in progressive multifocal leukonencephalopathy associated with Human Immunodeficiency Virus infection. N Engl J Med 1998; 338:1345–1351.

68. Clifford DB, Yiannoutsos C, Glicksman M, Simpson DM, Singer EJ, Piliero PJ, et al. HAART improves prognosis in HIV-associated progressive multifocal leukoencephalopathy. Neurology 1999; 52:623–625.

69. Whiteman ML, Post MJ, Berger JR, Tate LG, Bell MD, Limonte LP. Progressive multifocal leukoencephalopathy in 47 HIV-seropositive patients: neuroimaging with clinical and pathologic correlation. Radiology 1993; 187(1):233–240.

70. Antinori A, Ammassari A, De Luca A, Cingolani A, Murri R, Scoppettuolo G, et al. Diagnosis of AIDS-related focal brain lesion: A decision-making analysis based on clinical and neuroradiologic characteristics combined with polymerase chain reaction assays in CSF. Am Acad Neurol 1997; 48:687–694.

71. Mathews VP, Alo PL, Glass JD, Kumar AJ, McArthur JC. AIDS-related CNS crypto-coccosis: radiologic-pathologic correlation. Ajnr: American Journal of Neuroradiology 1992; 13(5):1477–1486.

72. Gade W, Hinnefeld SW, Babcock LS, Gilligan P, Kelly W, Wait K, et al. Comparison of the PREMIER cryptococcal antigen enzyme immunoassay and the latex agglutination assay for detection of cryptococcal antigens. [comment]. J Clin Microbiol 1991; 29(8):1616–1619.

73. Saag MS, Powderly WG, Cloud GA, Robinson P, Grieco MH, Sharkey PK, et al. Comparison of amphotericin B with fluconazole in the treatment of acute AIDS-associated cryptococcal meningitis. The NIAID Mycoses Study Group and the AIDS Clinical Trials Group. [comment]. N Eng J Med 1992; 326(2):83–89.

74. Tracey I, Carr CA, Guimaraes AR, Worth JL, Navia BA, Gonzalez RG. Brain choline-containing compounds are elevated in HIV-positive patients before the onset of AIDS dementia complex: A proton magnetic resonance spectroscopic study. Neurology 1996; 46:783–788.

75. Chang L, Ernst T, Leonido-Yee M, Walot I, Singer E. Cerebral metabolite abnormalities correlate with clinical severity of HIV-1 cognitive motor complex. Neurology 1999; 52:100–108.

76. Sidtis JJ, Gatsonis C, Price RW, Singer EJ, Collier AC, Richman DD, et al. Zidovudine treatment of the AIDS dementia complex: results of a placebo-controlled trial. Ann Neurol 1993; 33:343–349.

77. Sacktor NC, Lyles RH, Skolasky RL, Anderson DE, McArthur JC, McFarlane G, et al. Combination antiretroviral therapy improves psychomotor speed performance in HIV-Seropositive homosexual men. Neurology 1999; 52:1640–1647.

78. Sacktor N, Tarwater PM, Skolasky RL, McArthur JC, Selnes OA, Becker J, et al. CSF antiretroviral drug penetrance and the treatment of HIV-associated psychomotor slowing. Neurology 2001; 57:542–544.

79. Navia BA, Dafni U, Simpson D, Tucker T, Singer E, McArthur JC, et al. A phase I/II Trial of Nimodipine for the treatment of neurological manifestations associated with HIV infection, including AIDS dementia complex and peripheral neuropathy. Neurology 1998; 51:221–228.

80. Sacktor N, Schifitto G, McDermott MP, Marder K, McArthur JC, Kieburtz K. Transdermal selegiline in HIV-associated cognitive impairment: pilot placebo-controlled study. Neurology 2000; 54:233–235.

81. Schifitto G, Sacktor N, Marder K, McDermott MP, McArthur JC, Kieburtz K, et al. Randomized trial of the platelet-activating factor antagonist lexipafant in HIV-associated cognitive impairment. Neurology 1999; 53:391–396.

82. The Dana Consortium. Safety and tolerability of the antioxidant OPC-14117 in HIV-associated cognitive impairment. Neurology 1997; 49:142–146.

83. The Dana Consortium on the Therapy of HIV Dementia and Related Cognitive Disorders. Safety and tolerability of thioctic acid and deprenyl in HIV dementia. Neurology 1998; 50:645–651.

84. Heseltine PNR, Goodkin K, Atkinson JH, Vitiello B, Rochon J, Heaton RK, et al. Randomized double-blind placebo-controlled trial of peptide T for HIV-associated cognitive impairment. Arch Neurol 1998; 55:41–51.

85. Navia BA, Yiannoutsos CT, Change L, Marra CM, Miller E, Nath A, et al. ACTG 301: A phase II randomized, double-blind, placebo-controlled trial of memantine for AIDS dementia complex. Neurology 2001; 56(suppl 3):A474–A475.

86. Fauci A. Nature Medicine 200; 9:839–843.

3

Dementia in Prion Disorders

Simon Hawke

*Brain and Mind Research Institute, University of Sydney,
Sydney, New South Wales, Australia*

INTRODUCTION

Prion diseases or transmissible spongiform encephalopathies are the most feared and fulminant of the dementias. Often rapidly fatal and without effective therapy, the disorders are also transmissible by exposure to infectious tissues or body fluids, raising major public health concerns. The prion diseases comprise sporadic, inherited, and iatrogenic subtypes (for reviews see Refs. 1–4) and include Creutzfeldt-Jakob disease (CJD), the most common of the human prion diseases, and animal diseases, such as scrapie of sheep and goats, and bovine spongiform encephalopathy (BSE or mad cow disease) (reviewed in 5). Scrapie is endemic in many countries and has been recognized for over 200 years (reviewed in 6). Other prion disorders, such as BSE, variant CJD, and the so-called exotic ungulate encephalopathies have only recently emerged as disease entities. Other rarer human prion diseases include Kuru, which is confined to the Fore tribe in the highlands of New Guinea, Gerstmann-Straussler-Scheinker (GSS) disease, and fatal familial (FFI) and sporadic fatal insomnia (FI) (Table 1).

Prion diseases have characteristic neuropathology, with spongiform degeneration of neurones and a marked astrocytic reaction in the brains of affected humans and animals, the extent of which varies between the disease subtypes. A hallmark of prion diseases is the deposition of an abnormally folded isoform (designated PrP^{Sc} or PrP^{res}) of a cell-surface sialoglycoprotein, cellular prion protein or PrP^C. PrP^C is expressed to high levels in neurones and glia and also outside the central nervous system (CNS) on diverse cell types. It is

Table 1 Transmissible Spongiform Encephalopathies or Prion Diseases

	Disease	Mechanism of disease
Human	Kuru	Ritualistic cannibalism
	Iatrogenic CJD	Dura mater grafts, contaminated hGH, other
	vCJD	Infection from BSE prions
	Familial CJD, GSS, FFI	Germline mutations in *PRNP*
	Sporadic CJD, FI	Infection, somatic mutation or spontaneous conversion of PrP^C into PrP^{Sc}
Animal	Scrapie in sheep and goat	Sporadic/spontaneous infection in genetically susceptible animals
	BSE	Infection with contaminated feed—cause of epidemic
	Transmissible mink encephalopathy	Infection from BSE prions
	Feline spongiform encephalopathy	Infection from BSE prions
	Exotic ungulate encephalopathy (including kudu, nyala, oryx)	Infection from BSE prions
	Chronic wasting disease (mule, deer, elk)	Unknown

Abbreviations: CJD, Creutzfeldt-Jakob disease; vCJD, variant CJD; BSE, bovine spongiform encephalopathy; hGH, human growth hormone; GSS, Gerstmann-Sträussler-Scheinker disease; FFI, fatal familial insomnia; FI, sporadic fatal insomnia.
Source: From Ref. 1.

largely alpha helical and detergent soluble without a well characterized function, and refolds without post-translational modification into the pathogenic isoform, PrP^{Sc}. PrP^{Sc} is the biochemical signature of protein misfolding and segregates strongly with disease. It is detectable as a disease marker in tissue homogenates and sections, because of its detergent insolubility and resistance to degradation by proteases and physical denaturation.

Unlike other disorders of protein misfolding, such as Alzheimer-type dementia and the various tauopathies, prion diseases are unique in that tissues and body fluids derived from affected animals or humans are infectious, particularly those derived from the CNS. Initially the resistance of the infectious agent to irradiation (7) led Griffith (8) to propose that it was a protein. Prusiner and colleagues then found that PrP^{Sc} and infectivity co-purified (9) and the "prion hypothesis" was proposed arguing that the transmissible agent is wholly composed of an infectious protein (a protein-only infectious agent or prion), devoid of nucleic acid (10). Although PrP^{Sc} is a marker of disease, it is also a marker of infectivity. In fact given that PrP^{Sc} has not been identified in any other context, its detection must be taken as indicative of infectivity similar to the polymerase chain reaction (PCR), virus cultures or EM studies used to determine the presence of virus infection. In some prion disorders, for example, variant CJD (vCJD) and scrapie in sheep, PrP^{Sc} also replicates outside the CNS where it may be detectable allowing antemortem diagnosis (reviewed in 2). Otherwise definitive diagnosis requires biopsy of brain tissue or must await post-mortem confirmation. PrP^{C} expression is necessary for prion replication (11) and stabilizing PrP^{C} using antibodies inhibits prion replication both in vitro (12–14) and in vivo (15).

For bacterial or virus infection, phenotypic variability is encoded by nucleic acid sequence mutations and with prion infection, variability is thought to be enciphered within the structure of prion protein itself. Structural or conformational dissimilarities between prions must therefore produce the observable variation in clinical phenotype, incubation period, biochemical and neuropathological characteristics that define a stable prion "strain." Although recent data by Soto and colleagues go some way to establishing proof of the prion hypothesis (16), to date it has not been possible to show beyond doubt that chemically synthesized prions cause prion disease.

DISEASE MECHANISMS

Normal cellular prion protein is encoded by a single copy gene *PRNP*, which in humans is located on chromosome 20. Human PrP is 253 amino acids in length prior to cleavage of a 22 amino acid signal peptide. There is a repeating octapeptide sequence within residues 51–91, and following translation, the protein is modified by N-linked glycosylation at residues 181 and 197. The glycans attached at these sites can be occupied or not and hence three major PrP^{C} glycoform bands are revealed in western blots with anti-PrP antibodies. On cells as diverse as lymphocytes and neurons, PrP^{C} is attached to the cell membrane via a GPI linkage that unusually is sialyated. The protein is expressed widely throughout the nervous system with the highest expression on neurones. There is considerable heterogeneity in the expression of PrP^{C} fragments and glycoforms in different brain regions (17). In the periphery many different cell types express PrP^{C}, particularly in the lymphoreticular system and on virtually every circulating cell in the blood (our unpublished observations). The function of PrP^{C} is unknown, but it is likely to be involved in signaling particularly through associated kinases (18).

Analyses of PrP^{C} and PrP^{Sc} fail to find any consistent differences in terms of primary amino acid structure, reflecting transformation occurring after post-translational modification. There are two main theories of prion propagation: The first called "template-directed refolding," postulates that a thermodynamically unfavorable barrier prevents the direct conversion of PrP^{C} into PrP^{Sc}, PrP^{C} transformation occurring via an intermediate isoform, PrP* with or without the association of another factor or protein called protein X, catalyzing the formation of a homodimer of PrP^{Sc} that joins an ordered aggregate. The second, called the "seeding" model, states that PrP^C and PrP^{Sc} are in reversible thermodynamic equilibrium that favors the PrP^C state. Thus small amounts of PrP^{Sc} are slowly produced under normal circumstances and are metabolized, and that other unknown factors, most probably interaction with other prions, allow the seed to rapidly induce aggregate formation (reviewed in 19). It has been postulated that mono or oligomeric folding intermediates exist, for example, PrP^* or beta PrP, that then aggregate to form conglomerates of poly-meric protein, some with characteristics of amyloid. PrP^C is necessary for prion propagation and mice that have been engineered not to express the PrP^C, are resistant to disease (11). Furthermore, very recent work indicates that disease, but not infectivity or PrP^{Sc} accumulation is dependent on PrP^C being anchored to the cell surface via its GPI linkage (20). The exact disease-associated isoform, which is infectious remains to be determined. An earlier work indicated that one infectious unit was comprised of 10^5 PrP molecules (21). Recently it has been shown however, that 17–27 nm (300–600 kDa; equivalent to 14–28 PrP molecules) particles are the most infectious and not PrP^{Sc} oligomers (<5 nm) or fibrillar aggregates (22). Oligomers of course may be the more neurotoxic. Clearly the disease can transmit in the absence of the detectable PrP^{Sc} (23), and it has been shown that PrP^{Sc} deposition and even neuronal degeneration can occur in the absence of the disease (24). Asymptomatic life-long carriers of disease are therefore likely to exist. Proof that protein alone is sufficient for infec-tivity requires that artificially produced protein can be shown to be infectious. Yet it is still impossible to refold denatured prions and restore their infectivity.

A recent report indicates that truncated mouse recombinant prion protein folded into an aggregated state can transmit infectivity to transgenic mice expres-sing a truncated and mutated form of prion protein (25). Furthermore, Soto et al., using a method of in vitro amplication of the disease associated PrP^{Sc} isoforms, have proved that under laboratory conditions infectious prions can apparently be synthesized (16). These two studies provide further support for the prion replication hypothesis (for review see Ref. 26).

After exposure to infectious material, there is usually a long asymptomatic incubation period, which for humans can be measured in years. Experimentally after intracerebral inoculation, rodents remain without signs for months and then come down with disease with remarkably similar incubation periods, after which the animals rapidly succumb to disease. Factors influencing the incubation period include the strain type, the host genotype, the route of infection, associated illness, and the infectious dose. Sequential pathological studies in rodents after peripheral inoculation show that prion infection spreads slowly from the periph-ery and then into the thoraco-lumbar spinal cord and then into the brain, most likely via autonomic afferent nerves. Direct hematogenous spread has been pos-tulated, and small amounts of infectivity are measurable in the blood (reviewed in 27). Although prions are able to accumulate for years prior to the onset of clinical symptoms, data from cell lines that are permissive for prion replication suggest that the cellular machinery for metabolizing disease-associated prion protein exists and when measured, the half-life of PrP^{Sc} is only 3–5-fold longer than that of normal cellular prion protein (28). What causes clinical disease remains to be determined. The scant evidence that is available indicates that it is not due to the accumulation of PrP^{Sc}, or even infectivity (29).

During the 1980s and early 1990s it is estimated that over one million BSE-infected cattle entered the human food chain in northern Europe, largely in the United Kingdom. As these BSE prions have jumped across species to produce vCJD in humans (30) and also feline spongiform encephalopathy and the so-called exotic ungulate encephalopathies in animals that were unwittingly fed BSE prion-contaminated food, our concept of species barrier has been refined. We now recognize the term strain barrier (reviewed in 2), where one strain can passage with differing efficiency into the same or alternate species depending on host-prion protein genotype and other factors. From these and other studies, we also recognize that the transmission of prions within and/or across species can induce sub-clinical infection (24), posing further difficult questions for public health.

The efficiency of transmission between or across species can be quantitated in laboratory mice by assessing clinical, neuropathological, and biochemical characteristics emerging after primary and secondary passage. When fixed, these characteristics define a given prion strain. There is a great deal of variation between species with regard to how permissive each is for prion replication, and some species are resistant. Humans clearly permit the replication of several prion strains, in sheep many different strains can be identified, and in cattle only a single strain, the BSE agent has been identified. BSE prions appear to be particularly promiscuous, numerous species being susceptible to them. The prion hypothesis contends that strain characteristics are solely encoded by the protein itself. Biochemically, different prion strains show well-defined differences in fragment length, and glycosylation status on western blotting (called molecular strain typing), presumably largely indicative of the strain's particular folding characteristics or conformation. These conformational changes also presumably direct the strain's predominant sites of replication leading to anatomical variation where the major pathological changes occur.

HUMAN SPONGIFORM ENCEPHALOPATHIES

Creutzfeldt-Jakob disease, the most common human prion disease has sporadic, inherited, and iatrogenic forms. Sporadic CJD (sCJD) is by far the most common with a world-wide prevalence of 1–2 per million individuals distributed evenly across geographical and racial groups. About 10% of cases are associated with mutations in the coding region of the *PRNP* gene. A small proportion of CJD cases (<5%) result from an individual's exposure to infectious prions. These include the oral ingestion of BSE prions, thought to be the cause of variant CJD (30,31), exposure to CJD prion–contaminated human pituitary extracts or human gonadotrophin, exposure to CJD prion–contaminated dura mater used in neurosurgery, and a few cases caused by exposure to CJD prions contaminating corneal grafts and EEG depth electrodes used in mapping epileptogenic foci (32). Where it can be reliably determined, the clinical onset of disease may occur long after exposure to the infectious agent. For iatrogenic CJD resulting from treatment with pituitary derived hormones the incubation periods can be as long as 20 years.

The cause of sporadic CJD is unknown. Some epidemiological studies implicate exposure to environmental agents; there is an increased prevalence among farm workers and individuals that have had multiple surgical procedures, but the increased risk is small (33). Of particular importance is the lack of association between the prevalence of scrapie in sheep and goats and sCJD; countries such as Australia and New Zealand that are free of scrapie have similar rates of sCJD to other countries where scrapie is endemic. A major influence on disease susceptibility is polymorphism of *PRNP*, the prion protein gene, where at codon 129, the population is homozygous or heterozygous for methionine (M) or valine (V) (see Table 2 for allele frequencies). MM homozygotes are significantly overrepresented in the sCJD group, and MV heterozygosity appears to be protective. This effect is greatest in the vCJD population where almost all patients have the MM genotype (reviewed in 3). It is likely that genes at other loci also influence disease susceptibility (34).

Spontaneous disease resulting from rare stochastic events seems the most plausible explanation for disease occurrence, perhaps paralleling the rare cases of BSE in animals without known exposure to BSE prions. From the biochemical point of view, in spontaneous and inheritable prion disease, PrP^C may continually interconvert into more protease-resistant conformations, though unfavorable thermodynamics are likely to make these rare events. Certainly refolding of recombinant proteins with PrP^C-like qualities into so-called beta PrP isoforms was relatively straightforward in vitro (35).

Clinical Features

Human spongiform encephalopathies are characterized clinically by progressive cognitive decline associated with pyramidal, extrapyramidal, and cerebellar dysfunction of varying degrees, and movement disorder. The onset of symptoms to death, usually by secondary infection when subjects have become akinetic and mute can be very rapid indeed in sCJD, and in some patients, the clinical course is measurable in weeks. Considerable variation in the clinical features between different human prion strains occurs. GSS is usually a slowly progressive ataxia with cognitive decline occurring late. Similarly in Kuru, where ataxia predominates and cognition may be less affected. Variant CJD affects younger individuals and has a less rapid clinical course than patients with sCJD. Neuropsychiatric symptoms commonly occur early in vCJD. Nevertheless, in individual patients diagnostic confusion can occur. Perhaps some of the clinical differences between vCJD and sCJD may be related to prion disease occurring in the younger

Table 2 Disease Characteristics of Variant CJD and Sporadic CJD in Young Adults

	Variant CJD[a]	Sporadic CJD	
Mean age at onset (range) M:F	26 (12–74) years	≤50 years[b]	>50 years
Median duration of illness (range)	13 (6–39) months	16 (2–76) months	6 (1–39) months
Common clinical features at onset	Purely psychiatric symptoms at onset in 63% BUT neurological symptom presentation in 15%; combined psychiatric/ neurological in 22%	Dementia at onset (56%); visual disorders (29%); affective disorder at onset (35%) Cerebellar features and myoclonus less common	Rapidly progressive dementia with myoclonus Variants presenting with cerebellar syndrome (10%) or isolated visual disturbance (Heidenhain's variant)
Clinical course	If psychiatric presentation, slow progression to signs of neurological dysfunction	If psychiatric presentation, rapid progression to signs of neurological dysfunction	Rapid progression to akinetic mutism and death, often in 2–3 months
PrP codon 129 genotype[c]	MM 100%	MM 52% MV 15% VV 33%	MM 68% MV 16% VV 16%
EEG (% with PSWCs)	0	24	66
14-3-3	50	92	94
MRI	70 (pulvinar sign)	40 (basal ganglia hyperintensition)	63 (basal ganglia hyperintensities)

[a]Based on the analysis of the first 100 patients with vCJD (55).
[b]Based on the analysis of 52 young onset sCJD patients (36).
[c]Allele frequency in the normal (UK) population for comparison: MM: 37%; VV: 12%; MV: 51% (56).

as opposed to the aged brain (36). Table 2 highlights clinical similarities and differences between vCJD and sCJD occurring in younger patients. In addition to a more prolonged clinical course, younger sCJD patients have a greater prevalence of psychiatric symptoms than older patients with sCJD, although in comparison to vCJD, a progressive neurological syndrome rapidly ensues. In recent years subtypes of CJD have been identified representing infection by alternative prion strains and definable by their biochemical signature. Molecular strain typing reveals the existence of five CJD PrP^{Sc} types (37). Type I pattern PrP^{Sc} on western blotting tends to be associated with more rapidly progressive CJD. The type 4 pattern, is seen exclusively in variant CJD and also interestingly in BSE and other of the so-called exotic ungulate encephalopathies that all arose (or for BSE the numbers were amplified) by the same mechanism, namely, by the ingestion of BSE prions (reviewed in 2). Critics of this adherence to the biochemical characteristics of PrP^{Sc} point out that more than one biochemical pattern can be observed in the same brain, though interestingly, this has not been observed for the BSE prion–induced diseases.

Diagnosis

Sporadic Creutzfeldt-Jakob disease is usually considered in the clinical setting of a rapidly progressive dementia in late middle age and is often associated with ataxia and myoclonus. Occasionally the onset can be abrupt and stroke-like, though a relentlessly progressive course will ensue. Some patients present with a progressive cerebellar syndrome, or progressive visual failure due to cortical blindness (Heidenhain variant) (38). Other focal neurological features can be seen in the early stages. However, in sCJD it will not be long before other worrying neurological symptoms and signs supervene. In most cases a firm diagnosis can be made on clinical grounds given a compatible course, EEG abnormalities, and an elevated CSF 14-3-3 protein. MRI is particularly useful, not only to exclude structural disease, for example, tumors or strokes, but recently abnormalities have been observed in both sporadic and vCJD on standard MRI sequences. In sCJD, high signal in the head of caudate nucleus was initially observed with T2 weighted images, now more apparent with FLAIR and DWI (39,40). In vCJD some patients have increased signal in the pulvinar nuclei of the thalamus, the so-called pulvinar sign (41) and this has now been incorporated into diagnostic clinical criteria for vCJD (http://www.cjd.ed.ac.uk/criteria.htm). There are only a few reports of the use of other diagnostic imaging modalities. Imaging of cerebral glucose metabolism using 18F FDG positron emission tomography not unexpectedly shows perfusion abnormalities (42).

Abnormal EEG and CSF 14-3-3 protein seem to correlate with a rapid clinical course. The classical EEG abnormality in sCJD, periodic sharp-wave complexes (PSWC) (Fig. 1), is present during the course of the disease in 64% of patients (giving a sensitivity and specificity of 64% and 94%, respectively) (43). PSWC are not seen in the more indolent vCJD and are observed at lower frequencies in younger sCJD patients at least early in the clinical course (36). PSWC are occasionally seen in other types of dementia, for example, Alzheimer-type and multi-infarct dementia as well (43).

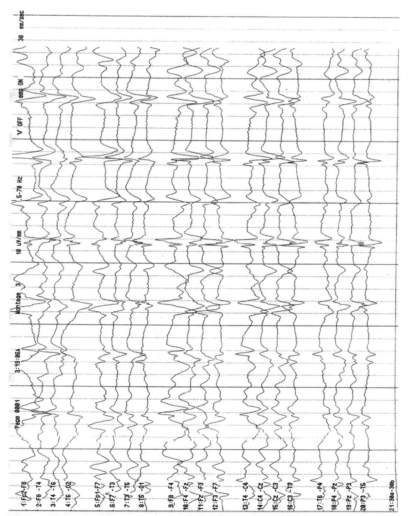

Figure 1 EEG from a patient with sporadic CJD showing periodic complexes. *Source:* Courtesy of Dr. S. Hammond and Justin Stent.

The 14-3-3 protein is a normal neuronal protein with no part in prion pathogenesis, which is released by dying neurones. Not specific to CJD, it is positive in any condition in which there is rapid neuronal degeneration or injury [e.g., meningitis (44)]. In patients in whom experienced clinicians have a high index of suspicion for CJD, 14-3-3 testing has a high sensitivity and specificity (>90%) (45). Of course patients with other neurological conditions such as meningitis or rapidly progressive Alzheimer-type dementia may have a positive CSF 14-3-3, raising unfounded suspicion of CJD. Nevertheless, 14-3-3 has been included in CJD diagnostic criteria (http://www.cjd.ed.ac.uk/criteria.htm). Most experts advocate sequencing the prion (*PRNP*) gene to exclude familial CJD and, as is common with other genetic neurological diseases, the clinical spectrum of the disorders associated with mutations of the prion gene is wide (reviewed in 46). No specific diagnostic tests for CJD have been developed that are applicable to tissues outside the CNS or prior to death. The one exception to this is in the setting of vCJD where prion replication occurs outside the CNS, particularly in lymphoreticular tissue. In fact vCJD prion accumulation has now been documented in a diverse range of organs (47) and tonsilar biopsy is now routinely performed where the index of suspicion for vCJD is high. The abnormal PrP^{Sc} can be visualized by both sensitive western blotting techniques and by standard immunohistochemistry (48). Tonsilar biopsy has no place in the antemortem diagnosis of other CJD subtypes.

Is it likely that a blood-based diagnostic test for CJD will become available? Most infections are diagnosed by detecting an immune response to the invading pathogen. For prion diseases, the widespread expression of PrP^C in the lymphoreticular system and in the bone marrow causes profound T cell tolerance to both normal and disease-associated PrP and no antibody response is measurable at any stage of the disease. Detection of PrP^{Sc} first requires the complete digestion of PrP^C followed by antibody detection of residual PrP after a denaturation step. The challenge for PrP^{Sc} detection in blood is depleting the proportionally huge excess of PrP^C present. It is also worth remembering that there is only a 300-fold differential sensitivity to proteinase K between PrP^C and PrP^{Sc}. Low femtomolar PrP^{Sc} concentrations are now detectable in blood in some experimental systems. However, technology will need to reach atomolar sensitivity to achieve reliable detection and even then such methods are not likely to be applicable to sCJD as prion replication seems to occur largely in the CNS. Nevertheless, many workers still believe detection of disease-associated isoforms will be possible if reagents can be developed that bind specifically to PrP^{Sc} with high affinity. Of course, detecting viruses or bacteria now often depends on nucleic acid amplification using PCR and recently methods of amplifying tiny quantities of PrP^{Sc} in a test tube have become available. In so-called PMCA (protein misfolding cyclic amplification), PrP^C is transformed into PrP^{Sc} in vitro using PrP^{Sc} present in the starting sample as template (16). Very encouragingly, Soto and colleagues have detected PrP^{Sc} in blood (49) using this method. It remains to be determined, if it can be used for amplifying the disease-associated PrP undoubtedly present in the blood of vCJD patients (50).

Other approaches to diagnostics include identifying surrogate markers of disease in blood. However, despite a lot of effort nothing has emerged that is diagnostically useful.

TREATMENT OF PRION DISEASES

Many different classes of drugs have been assessed for their effects on prion replication in various systems (reviewed in 51). Generally, it is easier to show suppressive effects in cell culture models. However, translating these results to the in vivo situation has been far more challenging and generally disappointing. Perhaps the most promising results came from the work in a murine model of scrapie (16). In these experiments, monoclonal antibodies raised against recombinant human PrP were passively transferred into mice challenged with RML prions. Even though treatment was delayed until significant prion replication had occurred in the periphery, satisfactory disease suppression was achieved, and, in fact, the onset of disease was indefinitely delayed in one group. It is important to point out, however, that monoclonal antibody therapy had no effect once clinical signs of scrapie had developed in the mice. Huge doses of highly purified monoclonal antibodies were also used to achieve the results. It remains to be shown if by bypassing the blood–brain barrier, which of course excluded most of the inhibiting antibodies, an effect on CNS disease can be achieved. Prion replication in terminally differentiated neurones and glia may not be amenable to inhibition by large molecules such as antibodies.

The enthusiasm for this therapeutic approach was soon dampened by Solforosi et al. (52) who, in elegant studies, showed that injections of monoclonal antibodies of certain specificities caused hippocampal neurone apoptosis, possibly via crosslinking of PrP^C. Interestingly, we never found any indication of this in mice treated for many months with large amounts of intravenously administered antibodies. Clearly, further work is needed to establish the safety and efficacy of antibodies passively transferred directly into the brain. Small molecule inhibitors of prion replication with the potential to better cross the blood–brain barrier are being developed. Some drugs in established use are under trial in various centers. Unfortunately, agents such as chlorpromazine and quinacrine, which are potent inhibitors in cell culture models, are not having a significant impact on patients, though useful information about the stages of disease will undoubtedly be gleaned from the studies in progress. Given that quinacrine does not have any significant measurable effect at suppressing disease in rodent models (53), the results in the clinic are unsurprising. Results from inhibiting murine or ovine prion replication may not translate in any case to efficacy against human prion replication and cell lines that are permissive for human prion replication are urgently needed. Several patients with CJD are being treated with intraventricular pentosan polysulphate. Pentosan is known to achieve impressive suppression of prion replication in Sc N2a cells, and to have minor effects in murine in vivo models, yet one patient with variant CJD treated with intraventricular pentosan polysulphate is the longest surviving patient with variant CJD. As time elapses the case for treating other patients in the setting of a controlled study strengthens. There is a widespread view that once clinical disease in humans is apparent, it is unlikely that treatment will be effective. However, there are experimental data, which indirectly suggest that a certain amount of reversibility could occur in the neuropathology (54). To conclude, determining what is or is not irreversible requires effective means of switching off prion replication in the CNS.

REFERENCES

1. Prusiner SB. Prions. Proc Natl Acad Sci USA 1998; 95:13363–13383.
2. Collinge J. Variant Creutzfeldt-Jakob disease. Lancet 1999; 354:317–323.
3. Collinge J. Molecular neurology of prion disease. J Neurol Neurosurg Psych 2004; 76:906–919.
4. Glatzel M, Stoeck K, Seeger H, Luhrs T, Aguzzi A. Human prion diseases. Molecular and clinical aspects. Arch Neurol 2005; 62:545–552.
5. Smith PG, Bradley R. Bovine spongiform encephalopathy (BSE) and its epidemiology. Br Med Bull 2003; 66:185–198.
6. Hunter N. Scrapie and experimental BSE in sheep. Br Med Bull 2003; 66: 171–183.
7. Alper T, Cramp WA, Haig DA, Clarke MC. Does the agent of scrapie replicate without nucleic acid? Nature 1967; 214:764–766.
8. Griffith J, Self-replication and scrapie. Nature 1967; 215:1043–1044.
9. Bolton DC, McKinley MP, Prusiner SB. Identification of a protein that purifies with the scrapie prion. Science 1982; 218:1309–1311.
10. Prusiner SB. Novel proteinaceous infectious particles cause scrapie. Science 1982; 216:136–144.
11. Bueler H, Aguzzi A, Sailer A, Greiner RA, Autenried P, Aguet M, Weissmann C. Mice devoid of PrP are resistant to scrapie. Cell 1993; 73:1339–1347.
12. Peretz D, Williamson RA, Kaneko K, Vergara J, Leclerc E, Schmitt-Ulms G, Mehlhorn IR, Legname G, Wormald MR, Rudd PM, Dwek RA, Burton DR, Prusiner SB. Antibodies inhibit prion propagation and clear cell cultures of prion infectivity. Nature 2001; 412:739–743.
13. Enari M, Flechsig E, Weissmann C. Scrapie prion protein accumulation by scrapie-infected neuroblastoma cells abrogated by exposure to a prion protein antibody. Proc Natl Acad Sci USA 2001; 98:9295–9299.
14. Beringue V, Vilette D, Mallinson G, Archer F, Kaisar M, Tayebi M, Jackson GS, Clarke AR, Laude H, Collinge J, Hawke S. PrPSc binding antibodies are potent inhibitors of prion replication in cell lines. J Biol Chem 2004; 279:39671–39676.
15. White AR, Enever P, Tayebi M, Mushens R, Linehan J, Brandner S, Anstee D, Collinge J, Hawke S. Monoclonal antibodies inhibit prion replication and delay the development of prion disease. Nature 2003; 422:80–83.
16. Castilla J, Saa P, Hetz C, Soto C. In vitro generation of infectious scrapie prions. Cell 2005; 121:195–206.
17. Beringue V, Mallinson G, Kaisar M, Tayebi M, Sattar Z, Jackson G, Anstee D, Collinge J, Hawke S. Regional heterogeneity of cellular prion protein in the mouse brain. Brain 2003; 126:2065–2073.

18. Santuccione A, Sytnyk V, Leshchyns'ka I, Schachner M. Prion protein recruits its neuronal receptor NCAM to lipid rafts to activate p59fyn and to enhance neurite outgrowth. J Cell Biol 2005; 169:341–354.
19. Zhou WQ, Gambetti P. From microbes to prions the final proof of the prion hypothesis? Cell 2005; 121:155–157.
20. Chesebro B, Trifilo M, Race R, Mead-White K, Teng C, LaCasse R, Raymond L, Favara C, Baron G, Priola S, Caughey B, Masliah E, Oldstone M. Anchorless prion protein results in infectious amyloid disease without clinical scrapie. Science 2005; 308:1435–1439.
21. Gibbs CJ, Gajdusek DC, Asher DM, Alpers MP, Beck E, Daniel PM, Matthews WB. Creutzfeldt-Jakob disease (spongiform encephalopathy): transmission to the chimpanzee. Science 1968; 161:388–389.
22. Silveira J, Raymond GJ, Hughson AG, Race RE, Sim VL, Hayes SF, Caughey B. The most infectious prion protein particles. Nature 2005; 437:257–261.
23. Lasmezas CI, Deslys JP, Robain O, Jaegly A, Beringue V, Peyrin JM, Fournier JG, Hauw JJ, Rossier J, Dormont D. Transmission of the BSE agent to mice in the absence of detectable abnormal prion protein. Science 1997; 275:402–405.
24. Hill AF, Joiner S, Linehan J, Desbruslais M, Lantos PL, Collinge J. Species-barrier-independent prion replication in apparently resistant species. Proc Natl Acad Sci USA 2000; 97:10248–10253.
25. Legname G, Baskakov IV, Nguyen HO, Riesner D, Cohen FE, DeArmond SJ, Prusiner SB. Synthetic mammalian prions. Science 2004; 305:673–676.
26. Weissmann C. Birth of a prion: spontaneous generation revisited. Cell 2005; 122:165–168.
27. Mabbott N, Turner M. Prions and the blood and immune systems Haematologica 2005; 90:542–548.
28. Borchelt DR, Scott M, Taraboulos A, Stahl N, Prusiner SB. Scrapie and cellular prion proteins differ in their kinetics of synthesis and topology in cultured cells. J Cell Biol 1990; 110:743–752.
29. Bueler H, Raeber A, Sailer A, Fischer M, Aguzzi A, Weissmann C. High prion and PrP^{Sc} levels but delayed onset of disease in scrapie-inoculated mice heterozygous for a disrupted PrP gene. Mol Med 1994; 1:19–30.
30. Will R, Ironside JW, Zeidler M, Cousens SN, Estibeiro K, Alperovitch A, Poser S, Pocchiari M, Hofman A, Smith PG. A new variant of Creutzfeldt-Jakob disease in the UK. Lancet 1996; 347:921–925.
31. Collinge J, Sidle KC, Meads J, Ironside J, Hill AF. Molecular analysis of prion strain variation and the aetiology of 'new variant' CJD. Nature 1996; 383:685–690.
32. Brown P, Preece M, Brandel J-P, Sato T, McShane L, Zerr I, Fletcher A, Will RG, Pocchiari M, Cashman NR, d'Aignaux JH, Cervenakova L, Fradkin J, Schonberger LB, Collins SJ. Iatrogenic Creutzfeldt-Jakob disease at the millennium. Neurology 2000; 55:1075–1081.
33. Collins S, Law MG, Fletcher A, Boyd A, Kaldor J, Masters CL. Surgical treatment and the risk of sporadic Creutzfeldt-Jakob disease: a case control study. Lancet 1999; 253:693–697.
34. Lloyd SE, Onwuazor ON, Beck JA, Mallinson G, Farrall M, Targonski P, Collinge J, Fisher EM. Identification of multiple quantitative trait loci linked to prion disease incubation period in mice Proc Natl Acad Sci USA 2001; 98:6279–6283.

35. Jackson GS, Hosszu LL, Power A, Hill AF, Kenney J, Saibil H, Craven CJ, Waltho JP, Clarke AR, Collinge J. Reversible conversion of monomeric human prion protein between native and fibrilogenic conformations. Science 1999; 283:1935–1937.

36. Boesenberg C, Schulz-Schaeffer WJ, Meissner B, Kallenberg K, Bartl M, Heinemann U, Krasnianski A, Stoeck K, Varges D, Windl O, Kretzschmar HA, Zerr I. Clinical course in young patients with sporadic Creutzfeldt-Jakob disease. Ann Neurol 2005; 58:533–543.

37. Hill AF, Joiner S, Wadsworth JDF, Sidle KCL, Bell JE, Budka H, Ironside JW, Collinge J. Molecular classification of sporadic Creutzfeldt disease. Brain 2003; 126:1333–1346.

38. Cooper SA, Murray KL, Heath CA, Will RG, Knight RSC. Isolated visual symptoms at onset in sporadic Creutzfeldt-Jakob disease: the clinical phenotype of the 'Heidenhain variant.' Br J Ophthalmol 2005; 89:1341–1342.

39. Shiga Y, Miyazawa K, Sato S, Fukushima R, Shibuya S, Sato Y, Konno H, Doh-ura K, Mugikura S, Tamura H, Higano S, Takahashi S, Itoyama Y. Diffusion weighted MRI abnormalities as an early diagnostic marker for Creutzfeldt-Jakob disease. Neurology 2004; 63:443–449.

40. Tschampa H, Kallenberg K, Urbach H, Meissner B, Nicolay C, Ketzschmar HA, Knauth M, Zerr I. MRI in the diagnosis of sporadic Creutzfeldt-Jakob disease: a study on inter-observer agreement. Brain 2005; 128:2026–2033.

41. Zeidler M, Sellar RJ, Collie DA, Knight R, Stewart G, Macleod MA, Ironside JW, Cousens S, Colchester AC, Hadley DM, Will RG. The pulvinar sign on magnetic resonance imaging in variant Creutzfeldt-Jakob disease. Lancet 2000; 355:1412–1418.

42. Henkel K, Zerr I, Hertel A, Gratz KF, Schroter A, Tschampa HJ, Bihl H, Bull U, Grunwald F, Drzezga A, Spitz J, Poser S. Positron emission tomography with [(18)F]FDG in the diagnosis of Creutzfeldt-Jakob disease (CJD). J Neurol 2002; 249:699–705.

43. Steinhoff BJ, Zerr I, Glatting M, Schulz-Schaeffer W, Poser S, Kretzschmar HA. Diagnostic value of periodic complexes in Creutzfeldt-Jakob disease. Ann Neurol 2004; 56:702–708.

44. Bonora S, Zanusso G, Raiteri R, Monaco S, Rossati A, Ferrari S, Boffito M, Audagnotto S, Sinicco A, Rizzuto N, Concia E, DiPerri G. Clearance of 14-3-3 protein from cerebrospinal fluid heralds the resolution of bacterial meningitis. Clin Infect Dis 2003; 36:1492–1495.

45. Zerr I, Pocchiari M, Colllins S, Brandel JP, de Pedro Cuesta J, Knight RS, Bernheimer H, Cardone F, Delasnerie-Laupretre N, Cuadrado Corrales N, Ladogana A, Bodemer M, Fletcher A, Awan T, Ruiz Bremon A, Budka H, Laplanche JL, Will RG, Poser S. Analysis of EEG and CSF 14-3-3 proteins as aids to the diagnosis of Creutzfeldt-Jakob disease. Neurology 2000; 55:811–815.

46. Palmer MS, Collinge J. Mutations and polymorphisms in the prion protein gene. Hum Mutat 1993; 2:168–173.

47. Wadsworth JD, Joiner S, Hill AF, Campbell TA, Desbruslais M, Luthert PJ, Collinge J. Tissue distribution of protease-resistant prion protein in variant Creutzfeldt-Jakob disease using a highly sensitive immunoblotting assay. Lancet 2001; 358:171–180.

48. Hill AF, Butterworth RJ, Joiner S, Jackson G, Rossor MN, Thomas DJ, Frosh A, Tolley N, Bell JE, Spencer M, King A, Al-Sarraj S, Ironside JW, Lantos PL, Collinge J. Lancet 1999; 353:183–189.
49. Castilla J, Saa P, Soto C. Detection of prions in blood. Nat Med 2005; 11:982–985.
50. Peden AH, Head MW, Ritchie DL, Bell JE, Ironside JW. Preclinical vCJD after blood transfusion in a PRNP codon 129 heterozygous patient. Lancet 2004; 364:527–529.
51. Weissmann C, Aguzzi A. Approaches to therapy of prion diseases. Ann Rev Med 2005; 56:321–344.
52. Solforosi L, Criado JR, McGavern DB, Wirz S, Sancez-Alavez M, Sugama S, DeGiorgio S, Volpe BT, Wiseman E, Abalos G, Masliah E, Gilden D, Oldstone MB, Conti B, Williamson RA. Cross-linking cellular prion protein triggers neuronal apoptosis in vivo. Science 2004; 303:1514–1516.
53. Collins S, Lewis V, Brazier M, Hill AF, Fletcher A, Masters CL. Quinacrine does not prolong survival in a murine Creutzfeldt-Jakob disease model. Ann Neurol 2002; 52:503–506.
54. Mallucci G, Dickenson A, Linehan J, Klohn PC, Brandner S, Collinge J. Depleting neuronal PrP in prion infection prevents disease and reverses spongiosis. Science 2003; 302:871–874.
55. Spencer MD, Knight RSG, Will RG. First hundred cases of variant Creutzfeldt-Jakob disease: retrospective case note review of early psychiatric and neurological features. BMJ 2002; 324:1479–1482.
56. Collinge J, Palmer MS, Dryden AJ. Genetic predisposition to iatrogenic Creutzfeldt disease. Lancet 1991; 337:1441–1442.

4

The Dementia of the Adult Hydrocephalus Syndrome

David J. Gill and Roger Kurlan

Department of Neurology, University of Rochester Medical Center, Rochester, New York, U.S.A

Normal pressure hydrocephalus (NPH) was first described as a defined syndrome by Adams and Hakim in 1965 (1,2). There are, however, case reports of patients with dementia and gait disturbance in the setting of hydrocephalus with normal cerebrospinal fluid (CSF) pressures that predate their publications (3). The syndrome described by Adams and Hakim included memory impairment, gait unsteadiness, and urinary incontinence, which improved with ventricular shunting. Since their initial description there have been many attempts to identify the pathogenesis of the disease, and develop diagnostic criteria, as well as characterize the nature of the dementia in order to predict which patients will respond to shunting. Thus far, these goals have remained elusive. There is also evidence that the intracranial pressure in many instances is not normal. Because of this, the term adult hydrocephalus syndrome (AHS) has begun to be used. In many cases, an antecedent cause for the syndrome can be found, that is, prior subarachnoid hemorrhage or head trauma, and these cases are more aptly termed as symptomatic AHS as opposed to those without a known cause, which are termed as idiopathic AHS.

EPIDEMIOLOGY

The exact rate of patients with AHS is difficult to ascertain, given the uncertainty in diagnosis. Several studies of elderly ambulatory patients have shown the rate of AHS in the general population to be less than 0.5% (4,5) Of patients with dementia, it is estimated that about 2% have AHS (6). The rate of AHS that is responsive to shunting is estimated to be in the range of 1.3–2.2 per million people per year (7).

GENERAL NEUROLOGIC CLINICAL CHARACTERISTICS

Gait disturbance is usually the first symptom in AHS (8,9), but there is no typical gait pattern. The original description of the gait disturbance was a broad-based gait with superimposed unsteadiness (1). Subsequently, the gait in AHS has been termed gait apraxia, magnetic gait, or frontal gait (10). Presently, the gait disorder in AHS is felt to begin in a subtle fashion with a wide base and mild ataxia. As the disease progresses, the gait worsens with prominent hypokinesis, short stride length, and prominent postural instability. Modern kinematic studies of the gait in AHS have found a triad of reduced stride length, reduced foot to floor clearance and a wide base (11). Along with this gait, patients also exhibit hyperreflexia, extensor plantar reflexes, and even freezing episodes akin to those seen in parkinsonism.

Frank urinary incontinence occurs late in the disease, but urinary urgency can be present much earlier. Urodynamic studies have shown hyperreflexia of the detrusor muscle. If the disease becomes severe and includes prominent dementia, the urinary incontinence may also be accompanied by a lack of concern for both urinary and fecal incontinence.

NATURE OF DEMENTIA

Many authors have described the cognitive difficulties associated with AHS, but the descriptions are varied. This is likely due to the difficulty with diagnosis and the varying methods of cognitive testing. In addition, there is overlap between AHS and other illnesses, such as Alzheimer's disease.

The cognitive deficits caused by AHS can be subtle or minor, especially at the onset (8). The profile of deficits is characterized by frontal and subcortical dysfunction, demonstrated by psychomotor slowing and poor performance on attentional tasks (2,10,12–20). These abnormalities may occur prior to the onset of observable memory difficulty (17). As the disease progresses, the patient then begins to demonstrate memory difficulty, which can be observed in verbal or non-verbal memory tests (12,13). Several authors also identified difficulty with visuospatial function on tasks of block design (12,13,15,20). At late stages, the dementia can also appear global in nature (17).

It has been thought that the dementia of AHS should not comprise any of the cortical deficits seen in dementias, such as Alzheimer's, namely aphasia, apraxia, or agnosia. If these are present, the patient may not have AHS (10). In fact, it has been proposed that in its early stages, the psychometric profile of frontosubcortical dysfunction without memory impairment or cortical deficits can help distinguish AHS from Alzheimer's dementia (12,17), while others have concluded that cognitive testing cannot distinguish between the two conditions (21). On the other hand, several authors have suggested that Alzheimer's pathology may co-exist with an AHS state, and that the rate seems to increase in those patients with more severe dementia (22).

Another condition in the differential of AHS is vascular dementia. One study looked at the psychometric profiles of patients with Binswanger's syndrome and AHS, finding that overall they are remarkably similar, except that patients with AHS perform significantly worse on the phrase construction, long-term memory, and spatial span portions of the mental deterioration battery (17). Again, it is not clear if these differences would be able to distinguish the two conditions from each other. Several authors have also noted prominent confabulation in patients with AHS similar to that seen Korsakovian dementias (12,13), as well as an association with depression (23).

PATHOGENESIS

A distinction should be made between idiopathic and symptomatic AHS. In about 50–70% of the cases, an identifiable cause can be found (24,25). The causes are often due to processes that impair the ability to reabsorb CSF. These include prior subarachnoid hemorrhage, meningitis, head injury, brain surgery, or current carcinomatous meningitis. Less often, symptomatic AHS is associated with conditions that cause a non-communicating hydrocephalus, such as a mass lesion. With idiopathic AHS, it is thought that an unknown process increases CSF outflow resistance. One current theory is that this is caused by increased transvenular resistance around the superior sagittal sinus (26).

The elevated CSF outflow resistance is thought to cause a transient elevation of CSF pressure and subsequent ventricular enlargement. As the ventricles enlarge, equilibrium is reached between the raised CSF pressure and the dilated ventricles that allows normalization of the CSF pressures according to Pascal's law (10). In pathologic studies the leptomeninges have not shown a direct associated fibrosis in patients with AHS, suggesting that the problem may not be at the arachnoid granulations (27,28). Data from continuous CSF pressure monitoring have shown that patients diagnosed with AHS have episodic elevations of their CSF pressure, the Lundberg B-waves (24,25). These are oscillations of CSF pressure at the rate of 0.5–2/min. The fact that patients with AHS actually have transient elevations of their CSF pressure lends credence to the nomenclature of "adult hydrocephalus syndrome" as opposed to NPH.

Along with the dilated ventricles, the white matter surrounding the ventricles displays decreased cerebral blood flow as demonstrated by functional imaging (29). The mechanism for this has not been established, but subcortical dysfunction secondary to the reduced blood flow is consistent with the nature of the dementia of AHS. The mechanism of the gait disturbance and bladder incontinence felt is explained by involvement of the subcortical areas of the frontal horns, as these are the general locations of fibers supplying the legs as well as the bladder sphincter (10).

There is evidence that vascular risk factors, especially hypertension, are significantly associated with AHS (30), but it is not clear at this point if hypertension plays a primary role in the pathogenesis of this condition.

EVALUATION

Adult hydrocephalus syndrome is suspected in cases of cognitive impairment with associated gait disturbance and urinary incontinence. The triad of symptoms is seen in the majority of patients (31). The history-taker should evaluate for the secondary causes mentioned earlier. The examiner should also identify the time course of the gait disturbance versus any cognitive impairment. The psychometric profile is not specific enough to enable a diagnosis merely on the basis of a neuropsychologic assessment. The common occurrence of a frontosubcortical dementia can be detected by the use of frontal-specific tests, such as the Trail-Making tests B and C and the Stroop test (32). In addition, the head circumference should be measured, looking for evidence of long-standing hydrocephalus as opposed to an acquired disorder.

CT

With regard to neuroimaging, the classic appearance is ventricular enlargement out of proportion to cortical atrophy as seen on CT scan. The proportion of cortical atrophy to ventricular size can be calculated by the frontal horn ratio, also referred to as the Evans Index (33). In this calculation, the maximum width of the frontal horns is divided by the width of the inner cranium at the same level. It has been suggested that a ratio of 0.32 or more is required for AHS, but other studies have shown that there is a wide variability in the Evans Index in patients with AHS (25). There is often evidence of periventricular lucencies on CT.

MRI

Because of the great anatomic detail that MRI provides, it is considered as the best neuroimaging technique for patients undergoing evaluation for AHS. MRI will show the ventricular enlargement out of proportion to cortical atrophy, but also can provide for volumetric measurements of the hippocampus, which is typically atrophied in Alzheimer's disease. A large amount of hippocampal atrophy and associated enlargement of the perihipppocampal fissure suggests Alzheimer's disease as opposed to AHS (34,35). On T2-weighted sequences, there can be decreased signal in the cerebral aqueduct that is felt to be due to increased velocity of CSF and is described as a "CSF flow-voiding sign" (36). Recent studies have shown that the CSF flow-voiding sign does not help predict response to shunting (37) and the significance of this sign is unclear.

The velocity of CSF flow through the cerebral aqueduct can also be measured by MRI and may be able to predict outcome to shunting, but is technically difficult to perform (38). Compared to CT, MRI is better able to detect periventricular lucencies, which are felt to represent transependymal edema from the intermittently elevated CSF pressure that causes the ventricular enlargement. It is not uncommon in this aged population to see white matter ischemic lesions, and distinguishing between these and periventricular lucencies can be difficult. The newer techniques of diffusion tensor imaging may provide some information in this area, but their value has not been established.

Functional Imaging

Postitron emission tomography (PET) scanning has demonstrated generalized decreased glucose metabolism most prominent in the frontal lobes (10). PET scanning may be able to differentiate patients with AHS from normal patients, but it has not been able to predict response to shunting (39).

CSF Removal

The CSF "tap test," where a large volume of CSF is removed (usually over 30 mL) to see if the cognitive and gait functions improve, has long been a standard of diagnosis of AHS. It has also been used to suggest whether a patient will respond to shunting. Recently, however, several authors have found that the CSF tap test does not allow prediction of successful shunting (40) and continuous external lumbar drainage provides better predictive information (41). The continuous external lumbar drainage involves drainage of 100–200 mL of CSF per day for 3–6 days. A standardized measure of gait and cognition is assessed prior to and after removal of CSF. Overall, if a patient improves, it is felt to be a good predictor of response to shunting, but the lack of improvement after CSF removal does not preclude a good outcome (41). The risks of this procedure include meningitis, subdural hematoma, and radiculitis.

CSF Dynamics

Continuous intracranial pressure monitoring has demonstrated the presence of Lundberg B-waves in AHS patients and if these are a frequent occurrence (>50%). On continuous monitoring this is predictive of a good response to shunting and the absence of B-waves predicts a poor response (24). As this technique requires placement of an intraventricular pressure monitor, this is not performed frequently. More commonly used measures of CSF dynamics are the lumbar CSF infusion and conductance tests. In the former, the resistance of CSF outflow is measured after installation of saline or artificial CSF. The ability of this test to predict response to shunting is variable, but it seems that if the resistance is above 18 mm Hg/mL, this is suggestive that a patient will respond to shunting (42). As in the case of CSF removal tests, however, a normal resistance does not preclude improvement (43). A recent study found that the lumbar CSF infusion test is more reliably predictive of clinical response to shunting than the CSF tap test (44).

The lumbar CSF conductance (the reciprocal of CSF resistance) can also be obtained by measuring CSF reabsorption either in the lumbar region or directly via a ventriculostomy. However, there is some variability in this test's ability to diagnose AHS as well as predict response to shunting. Considering its invasiveness, measurement of CSF conductance is not often done (32).

Other Tests

Radionuclide cisternography has frequently been used in the past to help diagnose AHS and predict response to shunting. Neither the positive or negative predictive values of this test are significant, however, and this test does not add much to the work-up of AHS. Cerebral blood flow studies have demonstrated reduced flow around the ventricles, but these findings do not discriminate AHS from non-AHS-caused dementias and do not predict which patients will respond to shunting (45). Finally, small molecules such as tau, neurofilament triplet protein, and galanin are being investigated as aides to diagnosis.

TREATMENT

Ventricular shunting is the recommended treatment for patients with AHS. As discussed, however, the diagnosis of AHS can prove difficult, and there is no agreement upon criteria for diagnosis (46). Because of this, outcomes with shunting vary based on the definition of the patients with the disease. There are, however, clinical characteristics that are associated with a good response to CSF diversion, as shown in Table 1.

Unfortunately, the absence of these positive predictors does not exclude the possibility of a good response. The most consistent finding suggestive of poor response to shunting is early and/or severe cognitive impairment (32), which is thought to suggest a co-morbid or alternative cause of dementia, such as

Table 1   Factors Predictive of a Good Response to Shunting

1. Secondary cause of hydrocephalus (symptomatic AHS)
2. Short (<36 months) duration of illness, especially the dementia (47)
3. Gait disorder preceding other symptoms (39,41,42)
4. Mild dementia symptoms
5. Enlarged frontal horn index/hydrocephalus out of proportion to atrophy (41,42)
6. Significant improvement after CSF removal via lumbar puncture or lumbar CSF drainage (39)
7. CSF resistance >18 mm Hg/mL (42)
8. B-waves for more than 50% of ICP recording (18)

vascular dementia or Alzheimer's disease. The presence of cerebrovascular disease has been associated with poor outcomes after shunting in some studies (48), but not in others (49). With regard to Alzheimer's disease, the presence of Alzheimer's disease in patients undergoing work-up for AHS has been shown to be between 18% and 75% (50,51). Outcomes after shunting for AHS were similar with or without co-morbid Alzheimer's disease (51). One author suggested that this is because the primary pathogenesis of both Alzheimer's disease and AHS is poor CSF turnover, and increasing CSF circulation can improve either condition (52).

It is known that of the components of the clinical triad of AHS, dementia is the least likely to respond (21,31). Because of this, it may be useful to think of AHS as a reversible cause of gait disturbance and not of dementia.

While up to 60% of the patients can demonstrate improvement with shunting (39), it is important to note that the complication rate of shunt placement is high. On average, 40% of the patients have a complication, with 6% having a serious complication, such as subdural hematoma, stroke, or infection. It is interesting to note that the most recent Cochrane review concluded that: "There is no evidence to indicate whether placement of a shunt is effective in the management of NPH" (53), citing the lack of any placebo-controlled randomized trials.

CONCLUSIONS

AHS is an uncommon cause of cognitive impairment, gait troubles, and urinary incontinence. There is still much uncertainty about its pathogenesis, diagnosis, and treatment. The dementia of AHS is usually frontosubcortical, but the psychometric profile does not appear distinct from other disorders of cognitive function. Ventricular shunting does not provide a major improvement in the cognition of patients, but may significantly improve gait. The substantial complication rate of shunting must be balanced against this potential benefit.

REFERENCES

1. Hakim S, Adams R. The special clinical problem of symptomatic hydrocephalus with normal cerebrospinal fluid pressure. J Neurol Sci 1965; 2:307–327.
2. Adams RD, Fisher CM, Hakim S, Ojemann RG, Sweet, WH. Symptomatic occult hydrocephalus with "normal" cerebrospinal-fluid pressure. N Engl J Med 1965; 272:117–126.
3. Foltz EL, Ward AA. Communicating hydrocephalus from subarachnoid bleeding. J Neurosurg 1956; 13:546–566.
4. Larson EB, Reifler BV, Featherstone HJ, English DR. Dementia in elderly outpatients: Prospective study. Ann Intern Med 1984; 100:417–423.
5. Trenkwalder C, Schwarz J, Gebhard J, Ruland D, Tenkwalder P, Hense H, Oertel WH. Starnberg trial on epidemiology of parkinsonism and hypertension in the elderly. Arch Neurol 1995; 52:1017–1022.
6. Clarfield AM. The reversible dementias: do they reverse? Ann Intern Med 1988; 109:476–486.

7. Vanneste J, Augustijn P, Dirven C, Tan WF, Goedhart ZD. Shunting normal-pressure hydrocephalus: do the benefits outweigh the risks? Neurology 1992; 42: 54–59.
8. Fisher CM. Hydrocephalus as a cause of disturbances of gait in the elderly. Neurology 1982; 32:1358–1363.
9. Graff-Radford NR, Godersky JC. Normal-Pressure hydrocephalus. Arch Neurol 1988; 43:940–942.
10. Mendez MF, Cummings JL. Miscellaneous dementia syndromes. Dementia: A Clinical Approach. 3rd ed. Boston: Butterworth Heinemann, 2003:503–558.
11. Stolze H, Kuhtz-Bushbeck JP, Drücke H, Jöhnk K, Diercks C, Palmié, Mehdorn HM, Illert M, Deutchl G. Gait analysis in idiopathic normal pressure hydrocephalus— which parameters respond to the CSF tap test? Clin Neurophysiol 2000; 111: 1678–1686.
12. Gustafson L, Hagberg B. Recovery in hydrocephalic dementia after shunt operation. J Neurol Neurosurg Psych 1978; 41:940–947.
13. Berglund M, Gustafson L, Hagberg B. Amnestic-confabulatory syndrome in hydrocephalic dementia and Korsakoff's psychosis in alcoholism. Acta Psychiat Scand 1979; 60:323–333.
14. Caltagirone C, Gainotti G, Masullo C, Villa G. Neurophysiologic study of normal pressure hydrocephalus. Acta Psychit Scand 1982; 65:93–100.
15. Thomsen AM, Børgesen SE, Bruhn P, Gjerris F. Prognosis of dementia in normal-pressure hydrocephalus after a shunt operation. Ann Neurol 1986; 20:304–310.
16. Stambrook M, Cardoso E, Hawryluck GA, Eirikson P, Piatek D, Sicz George. Neuropsychological changes following neurosurgical treatment of normal pressure hydrocephalus. Arch Clin Neuropsychol 1988; 3:323–330.
17. Gallassi R, Morreale A, Montagna P, Sacquegna T, Di Sarro R, Lugaresi E. Binswanger's disease and normal-pressure hydrocephalus. Arch Neurol 1991; 48: 1156–1159.
18. Raftopoulos C, Deleval J, Chaskis C, Leonard A, Cantraine F, Desmyttere F, Clarysse S, Brotchi J. Cognitive recovery in idiopathic normal pressure hydrocephalus: A prospective study. Neurosurgery 1994; 35:397–405.
19. Iddon JL, Pickard JD, Cross JJL, Friffiths PD, Czosnyka M, Sahakian BJ. Specific patterns of cognitive impairment with idiopathic normal pressure hydrocephalus and Alzheimer's disease: a pilot study. J Neurol Neurosurg Psych 1999; 67:723–732.
20. Mataró M, Poca MA, del mar Matarín M, Catalan R, Sahuquillo J, Galard R. CSF galanin and cognition after shunt surgery in normal pressure hydrocephalus. J Neurol Neurosurg Psych 2003; 74:1272–1277.
21. Savolainen S, Hurskainen H, Paljärvi, Alafuzoff I, Vapalahti M. Five-year outcome of normal pressure hydrocephalus with or without a shunt: Predictive value of the clinical signs, neuropsychological evaluation and infusion test. Acta Neurochir (Wien) 2002; 144:515–523.
22. Golomb J, Wisoff J, Miller DC, Boksay I, Kluger A, Weiner H, Salton J, Graves W. Alzheimer's disease comorbidity in normal pressure hydrocephalus: Prevalance and shunt response. J Neurol Neurosurg Psych 2000; 68:778–781.
23. Rosen H, Swigar M. Depression and normal pressure hydrocephalus. J Nerv Ment Dis 1976; 163(1):35–40.

24. Børgesen SE, Flemming G. The predictive value of conductance to outflow of CSF in normal pressure hydrocephalus. Brain 1982; 105:65–86.
25. Sahuquillo J, Rubio, E, Codina, A Molins A, Guitart JM, Poca MA, Chasampi A. Reappraisal of the intracranial pressure and cerebrospinal fluid dynamics in patients with the so-called "normal pressure hydrocephalus" syndrome. Acta Neurochir (Wien) 1991; 112:50–61.
26. Bateman GA. Vascular compliance in normal pressure hydrocephalus. AJNR 2000; 21:1574–1585.
27. Bech RA, Juhler M, Waldemar G, Klinkin L, Gjerris F. Frontal brain and leptomeningeal biopsy specimens correlated with cerebrospinal fluid outflow resistance and B-wave activity in patients suspected of normal-presssure hydrocephalus. Neurosurgery 1997; 40:497–502.
28. Bradley WG. Normal pressure hydrocephalus: New concepts in etiology and diagnosis. AJNR 2000; 21:1586–1590.
29. Momjian S, Owler B, Czosnyka Z, Czosnyka M, Pena A, Pickard JD. Pattern of white matter regional cerebral blood flow and autoregulation in normal pressure hydrocephalus. Brain 2004; 127:965–972.
30. Krauss JK, Regel JP, Vach W, Droste DW, Borremans JJ, Mergner T. Vascular risk factors and arteriosclerotic disease in idiopathic normal-pressure hydrocephalus of the elderly. Stroke 1996; 27:24–29.
31. Poca MA, Mataró M, Del Mar Matarín M, Arikan F, Junqué C, Sahuquillo J. Is the placement of shunts in patients with idiopathic normal-pressure hydrocephalus worth the risk? Results of a study based on continuous monitoring of intracranial pressure. J Neurosurg 2004; 100:855–866.
32. Vanneste JAL. Diagnosis and management of normal-pressure hydrocephalus. J Neurol 2000; 247:5–14.
33. Evans WA. An encephalographic ratio for estimating ventricular enlargement and cerebral atrophy. Arch Neurol Psychiatry 1942; 47:931–937.
34. Savolainen S, Laakso MP Paljärvi L, Alafuzoff I, Hurskainen H, Partanen K, Soininen H, Vapalahti. MR imaging of the hippocampus in normal pressure hydrocephalus: Correlations with cortical Alzheimer's disease confirmed by pathologic diagnosis. AJNR 2000; 21:409–414.
35. Holodny AI, Waxman R, George AE, Rusinek H, Kalnin AJ, de Leon M. MR Differential diagnosis of normal-pressure hydrocephalus and Alzheimer disease: Significance of perihippocampal fissures. AJNR 1998; 19:813–819.
36. Bradley WG, Whittemore AR, Kortman KE, Watanabe AS, Homyak M, Teresi LM, Davis SJ. Marked cerebrospinal fluid void: Indicator of successful shunt in patients with suspected normal-pressure hydrocephalus. Radiology 1991; 178: 459–466.
37. Krauss JK, Regel JP, Vach W, Jüngling FD, Droste DW, Wakhloo AK. Flow void of cerebrospinal fluid in idiopathic normal pressure hydrocephalus of the elderly: Can it predict outcome after shunting? Neurosurgery 1997; 40:67–74.
38. Bradley WG, Scalzo D, Queralt J, Nitz WM, Atkinson DJ, Wong P. Normal-pressure hydrocephalus: Evaluation with cerebrospinal fluid flow measurements at MR imaging. Radiology 1996; 198:523–529.
39. Hebb AO, Cusimano MD. Idiopathic normal pressure hydrocephalus: A systematic review of diagnosis and outcome. Neurosurgery 2001; 49:1166–1186.

40. Malm I, Kristensen B, Karlsson T, Fagerlund M, Elfverson J, Ekstedt J. The predictive value of cerebrospinal fluid dynamic tests in patients with the idiopathic adult hydrocephalus syndrome. Arch Neurol 1995; 52:783–789.

41. Walchenbach R, Geiger E, Thomeer RTWM, Vanneste JAL. The value of temporary external lumbar CSF drainage in predicting the outcome of shunting on normal pressure hydrocephalus. J Neurol Neurosurg Psych 2002; 72:503–506.

42. Boon AJ, Tans JTJ, Delwel EF, Egeler-Peerdeman, Hanlo PW. The Dutch normal-pressure hydrocephalus study: How the select patients for shunting? An analysis of four diagnostic criteria. Sug Neurol 2000; 53:201–207.

43. Boon AJ, Tans JTJ, Delwel EJ, Egeler-Peerdeman SM, Hanlo PW, Wurzer HAL, Avezaat CJJ, deJong DA, Gooskens RHJM, Hermans J. Dutch normal-pressure hydrocephalus study: Prediction of outcome after shunting by resistance to outflow of cerebrospinal fluid. J Neurosurg 1997; 87:687–693.

44. Kahlon B, Sundbarg G, Rehncrona S. Comparison between the lumbar infusion and CSF tap tests to predict outcome after shunt surgery in suspected normal pressure hydrocephalus. J Neurol Neurosurg Psych 2002; 73:721–726.

45. Hebb AO, Cusimano MD. Idiopathic normal pressure hydrocephalus: A systematic review of diagnosis and outcome. Neurosurgery 2001; 49:1166–1186.

46. Kreft TA, Graff-Radford NR. Normal pressure hydrocephalus. Behavioral Neurology and Neuropsychology, 2nd ed. McGraw-Hill, 2003:659–673.

47. Meier U, Zeilinger FS, Kintzel D. Signs, symptoms and course of normal pressure hydrocephalus in comparison with cerebral atrophy. Acta Neurochir (Wien) 1999; 141:1039–1048.

48. Boon AJW, Tans JTJ, Delwel EJ, Egeler-Peerdeman SM, Hanlo PW, Wurzer HAL, Hermans J. Dutch normal-pressure hydrocephalus: The role of cerebrovascular disease. J Neurosurg 1999; 90:221–226.

49. Tullberg M, Jensen C, Ekholm S, Wikkelsø C. Normal pressure hydrocephalus: Vascular white matter changes on MR images must not exclude patients from shunt surgery. AJNR 2001; 22:1665–1673.

50. Savolainen S, Paljärvi L, Vapalahti M. Prevalence of Alzheimer's disease in patient investigated for presumed normal pressure hydrocephalus: A clinical and neuropathological study. Acta Neurochir (Wien) 1999; 141:849–853.

51. Golomb J, Wisoff J, Miller DC, Boksay I, Kluger A, Wiener H, Salton J, Graves W. Alzheimer's disease comorbidity in normal pressure hydrocephalus: Prevalence and shunt response. J Neurol Neurosurg Psych 2000; 68:778–781.

52. Silverberg GD, Mayo M, Saul T, Rubenstein E, McGuire D. Alzheimer's disease, normal-pressure hydrocephalus and senescent changes in CSF circulatory physiology: A hypothesis. Lancet Neurol 2003; 2:506–511.

53. Esmonde T, Cooke S. Shunting for normal pressure hydrocephalus. Cochrane Database of Systematic Reviews. 2004; 3.

5

Traumatic Brain Injury

Denise Burton and Mindy Aisen

*Veteran's Health Administration, Rehabilitation Research and
Development Service, Washington, D.C., U.S.A.*

INTRODUCTION

Traumatic brain injury (TBI) can be mild to severe, resulting in a range of deficits
from mild and temporary to disabling and permanent impairment. TBI can occur
in the setting of motor vehicle accidents, falls, violence, and sports. Moderate to
severe injuries result in widespread, diffuse damage to the brain because the brain
"ricochets" within the skull; there is commonly diffuse axonal injury and multifocal damage. The brain stem, frontal lobe, and temporal lobe are particularly
vulnerable to this because of their location near bony protrusions.

TBI is a broad category that encompasses closed head injury, open head
injury, and penetrating head injury. A closed head injury occurs when the head
suddenly and violently strikes an immovable object, but there is no skull fracture
and the dura remains intact. An open head injury implies that skull and dural
integrity are compromised. When an object pierces the dura and enters the
brain (stab wounds and missile wounds are most often the cause), a penetrating
head injury results. Closed, open, and penetrating brain injuries lead to combinations of focal and diffuse brain damage. There are varying degrees of closed
brain/head injury that range from mild to moderate to severe. The Glasgow
Coma Scale (GCS) is an internationally accepted standardized quantitative
descriptive scale used to establish functional severity of acute neurological
damage in TBI.

Several types of trauma can affect the head and brain: concussion,
depressed skull fracture, contusion, contre-coup, shaken baby syndrome, epidural

hematoma, subdural hematoma, anoxia, and hypoxia. In a depressed skull fracture, broken skull pieces press into the tissue of the brain. This can cause contusion with edema and disruption of blood vessels. A penetrating skull fracture occurs when an object pierces the skull, such as a bullet, resulting in a focal injury to the brain tissue. A contusion can also occur in closed injury when there is shaking of the head back and forth with sufficient force that the brain impacts the skull. Shaken baby syndrome is a severe form that occurs when a baby is shaken forcibly enough to cause contusion and, if blood vessel integrity is impaired, intraparenchymal hematoma. Brain damage can be caused by blood compressing the brain, bleeding into the tissue of the brain, or inadequate blood flow to regions of the brain. Bleeding into the area between the dura and skull, generally brisk and of arterial origin is known as an epidural hematoma. With a subdural hematoma, the bleeding is confined to the area between the dura and the arachnoid membrane. Bleeding within the brain itself is known as intraparenchymal hematoma.

Other types of brain injury include those caused by insufficient oxygen to tissues, anoxia, and hypoxia. These types of injuries are often experienced by near-drowning victims and individuals who experience cardiac arrest. Diffuse hypoxic ischemic damage leads to neurogenic edema—unresponsive to steroid therapy—and increased intracranial pressure. Neurosurgical intervention is often needed to monitor and manage intracranial pressure, just as it is necessary to evacuate epidural and large subdural hematomas.

The severity of TBI can range from mild to the extremes of irreversible coma or even death. The most common type of TBI and the most minor is *concussion*, in which there is a closed head injury and brief loss of consciousness. In many MTBI cases, the person shows no obvious residual deficits, yet continues to endure chronic functional problems. Some people suffer long-term effects of MTBI, known as post-concussive syndrome (PCS). PCS can be associated with changes in cognition and personality.

One or more of the following symptoms defines mild TBI: a brief loss of consciousness, loss of memory immediately before or after the injury, any alteration in mental state at the time of the accident, or focal neurological deficits. The GCS score can range from 13 to 15 at the lowest functional point. Moderate TBI is defined by a GCS score of 9–12, and a GCS score of eight or lower defines severe TBI.

After the patient is stabilized medically, neurosurgeons evaluate the severity of injury to the nervous system. The GCS is used to categorize functional severity of acute neurological damage in TBI in most centers. The GCS provides a quantitative assessment of clinical status. Next, clinical exam and neuroimaging are used to identify the type(s) and location(s) of the brain injury. The areas most sensitive to mechanical trauma are the brainstem/midbrain (shearing forces), anterior temporal lobes and frontal lobes (due to impact against the skull). The area most sensitive to hypoxia/ischemia is the hippocampus region of the temporal lobe.

The brain stem is located at the base of the brain, and regulates basic arousal, autonomic functions, and cranial nerve functions. The midbrain, meso-temporal, and temporal lobe regions are involved in attention and short-term memory, and regulate emotions. Trauma to this area can lead to disorientation, frustration, and anger. In addition to memory and emotional functions, the tem-poral lobes are critical in language comprehension and visual pathways. The frontal lobe is almost always injured due to its large size and location near the front of the cranium. Damage to this area can impair judgment, increase impul-sitivity and can cause apathy. Since the brain is complex, every brain injury is different. Some symptoms may appear right away. Other symptoms may not show up for days or weeks. Sometimes the injury makes it difficult for the person with TBI to recognize his or her own deficits.

Mild TBI, concussion, is the most common type of TBI. The individual may have no residual symptoms, or may experience persistent headaches or neck pains that do not dissipate, tinnitus, mild diplopia, loss of sense of smell or taste, nausea, feeling "easily confused," slowness in thinking, speaking, acting, or reading. Children with TBI have the same symptoms as adults; however, because of their communication skills may not be as refined as an adult, the signs and symptoms manifest as: tiredness or listlessness, changes in eating, sleeping patterns, playing habits, loss of balance and of new skills such as toilet training, and vomiting.

Moderate to severe TBI results in persistent deficits in cognition, memory, language function, articulation, paralysis, sensory impairments, ataxia, and tremor. Clinical management of the moderate to severe TBI patient will be covered in subsequent sections of this chapter.

EPIDEMIOLOGY

The overall incidence of TBI in the United States is 1.5–2 million. Prevalence estimates indicate that there are 5.3 million living Americans who have sustained a TBI. It is estimated that more than $48 billion dollars a year is being spent for TBI healthcare, and related expenses. The risk for TBI is especially high among adolescents and young adults (ages 15–24). Young children (under the age of five years) and the elderly (over the age of 75 years) are also at high risk. For persons of all ages, the risk of TBI among males is twice the risk among females.

According to the CDC, 270,000 people experience a moderate or severe TBI annually. The annual mortality rate is 70,000. Over a million people are treated and released from hospital emergency departments each year, and an esti-mated 230,000 Americans survive a hospitalization for TBI; approximately 80,000 of these Americans are discharged with significant TBI-related disabil-ities. According to the CDC, there are various types of impairments that may occur as a result of TBI: (i) cognition-concentration, memory, judgment, and mood, (ii) mobility-strength, coordination, and balance, (iii) sensation-tactile sensation and special senses, such as vision, and (iv) sometimes seizure disorders (epilepsy). Approximately, 60,000 new cases of epilepsy occur as a result of head trauma and about 1% of persons with severe TBI survive in a state of persisting unconsciousness.

The leading causes of TBI vary by age: falls are the leading cause of TBI among persons aged 65 years or older, whereas transportation leads to TBI among persons aged 5–64 years and involves motorcycles, bicycles, and pedestrians. The outcome of these injuries varies greatly depending on the cause: 91% of firearm-related TBIs resulted in death, but only 11% of fall-related TBIs are fatal. Each year, the incidence and prevalence of TBI-related disability is increasing.

There are several published epidemiological studies of TBI-related hospitalizations and deaths in the United States. Recent data suggest a decline in rates of hospitalization for less severe TBI, possibly due to changes in hospital admission criteria. The lower incidence rate seen today may be due in part to a real decline in brain injuries but also appears to be an artifact of counting methods, which capture only hospitalized and fatal cases.

There was a 22% decline in the TBI-related death rate from 24.6/100,000 U.S. residents in 1979 to 19.3/100,000 in 1992. Firearm-related rates increased 13% from 1984 through 1992, undermining a 25% decline in motor-vehicle-related rates for the same period. Firearms surpassed motor vehicles as the largest single cause of death associated with TBI in the United States in 1990. These data highlight the success of efforts to prevent TBI due to motor vehicles and failure to prevent such injuries due to firearms. Nearly two-thirds of firearm-related TBIs are classified as suicidal in intent. The increasing importance of penetrating injury has important implications for research, treatment, and prevention of TBI in the United States.

The cost of TBI to those who are injured, as well as their caregivers, is immeasurable. The social as well as psychological upheaval is devastating, and subsequently, only a few analyses of the monetary costs of these injuries are available, including the following estimate from the CDC (lifetime cost of all brain injuries occurring in the United States): direct annual expenditures, 10.5 billion; indirect annual costs, 38.3 billion; total costs, 48 billion dollars.

IMMEDIATE, SUBACUTE CHRONIC IMPACTS OF HEAD INJURY AT THE MOLECULAR AND CELLULAR LEVEL

Despite preventive measures to reduce the number and risk of TBI cases that occur in the United States each year, the number of TBI patients seeking hospital services has increased. This is due in part to improved acute care, which has improved the survival rates of TBI patients. Continued advancements in the clinical arena are dependent upon the elucidation of the cellular and molecular mechanisms of TBI. Understanding the molecular and cellular mechanisms underlying the pathophysiology in immediate, subacute severe head trauma will be vital to the development of novel pharmaceutical and gene-based therapies to restore physical, cognitive, behavioral, and emotional function to patients who sustain a TBI.

The pathophysiology of TBI can be categorized as primary or secondary injury. Initial neurochemical damage, which occurs at the time of initial contact, is known as primary injury and a secondary injury is the progressive, degradative cascade of cellular damage that is set at the time of primary insult (1,2). The pathophysiological process—the molecular mechanism underlying secondary or delayed cell death that is evoked following TBI—is highly complex and poorly understood. However, recent scientific advancements have provided some insight into the cascade of cellular events, the secondary process of cell death that the brain initiates after primary physical assault and injury.

In experimental and clinical TBI, the first couple of hours post-injury is critical because the nerve cell's axon is extremely damaged due to shearing, which is termed diffuse axonal injury. Events such as axonal swelling, disconnection from the cell body of the neuron, degeneration of communicating junctions, and the release of toxic levels of neurotransmitters into the synapse, damages nearby neurons through a secondary neuroexcitatory cascade. This process is the mechanism by which neurons that were undamaged during the primary trauma suffer damage in this secondary assault. Vulnerable regions of the brain, such as the cerebral cortex, hippocampus, thalamus and substantia nigra, and subcortical nigra (3), are selectively affected because of the diffuse and widespread neuronal damage and apoptosis that occur. Spanning from hours to days, the acute phase of neurological damage is followed by recovery (hours to months), then the chronic/plateau phase of neurodegeneration that can last months to years. The acute phase is followed by the chronic phase of neurodegeneration that can last several years post-injury (4,5). Many of the molecular and cellular sequelae are neuroprotective in nature and involve the release of signals from neurons and glia designed to prevent further injury. Expression of neurotrophic factors, activation of cell death genes (apoptosis), the activation of reactive oxygen species (ROS), alterations in calcium homeostasis, and activation of intracellular proteases (calpains) are thought to be pivotal in the process of mediating delayed cell death in TBI. The final target of all of these cascades of events is thought to be the mitochondria via alteration in the mitochondrial permeability transition pore. The inflammatory response is also believed to be involved in exacerbating the secondary damage.

The role of neurotroprotective factors (NPFs) has been well documented in TBI. A large number of NPFs, whose expression increases in response to brain injury, have been identified and include the neurotrophins (NGF, NT-3, NT-5, and BDNF), bFGF, IGFs, TGFs, TNFs and secreted forms of the beta-amyloid precursor protein. It has been postulated that perhaps this alteration following brain injury may be a response to promote neuronal survival and repair and induce sprouting of neuritis in order to re-establish functional connections in an injured brain (neuronal plasticity) (3). Animal and cell culture studies have shown that NPFs can attenuate neuronal injury initiated by insults believed to be relevant to the pathophysiology of TBI, including exocitoxins, ischemia, and free radicals. Intraparenchymal administration of NGF can attenuate cognitive but not neurobehavioral motor deficits or hippocampal cell loss following lateral FP brain injury (3,6,7). Studies of the mechanism of action of these NPFs indicate that they enhance cellular systems involved in the maintenance of Ca^{2+} homeostasis and free radical metabolism.

Ca^{2+} homeostasis research shows promising potential in understanding TBI. Numerous studies have shown that brain Ca^{2+} homeostasis and membrane receptors/channels associated with Ca^{2+} -ion influx into the damaged neuron causes delayed cell death, vasospasm, and regional cerebral edema (3,8,9). Voltage-sensitive Ca^{2+} channels are intimately involved in mediating cellular dysfunction via voltage-sensitive Ca^{2+} channels (VSCC) antagonists, such as S-emopamil, which has Ca^{2+} channel and 5-HT2 and antagonist effects (10). In rat model systems, Okiyama et al. (11) demonstrated that a reduction in regional cerebral edema, attenuation of neurological motor and cognitive dysfunction, and improved cerebral blood flow to critically injured brain regions, could be accomplished.

Lipid metabolism has also been implicated in the pathogenesis of TBI via the activation of Ca^{2+}-dependent phospholipases in response to post-traumatic increases in intracellular calcium. Trauma-induced increases in intracellular Ca^{2+} cause an attack on the cellular membrane, mediated by phospholipases A2 (PLA2) and C (PLC), that results in release of fatty acids (FFAs) and diacylglycerol (DAGs). Cerebral edema has been shown to be associated with brain-induced DAG formation (12), and to activate protein kinase C (PKC), which may in turn modulate other signal transduction pathways. Sun and Faden (13) demonstrated in rat models that after FP brain injury, PKC increases over time in the cortex and hippocampus.

Following brain trauma, ROS such as free radicals have been shown to be associated with alterations in regional cerebral blood flow, production of intracellular arachidonic acid, acid cascade metabolites, and specifically with increased intracellular Ca^{2+}, which can induce ROS release from mitochrondria or via cytoplasmic generation (3,14). Moreover, glutamate, and EAA can also induce formation of ROS in high levels, which in turn can cause peroxidative destruction of the cell membrane and attack the cerebrovasculature. Hydrogen peroxide induces the expression of IEGs, c-fos and c-jun (15), and calmodulin-regulated gene transcription and intracellular transduction cascades are disrupted via oxidative damage (16). In a weight drop model of brain injury, rat model studies have demonstrated ROS formation (17).

Calpains, a family of non-lysosomal cysteine proteases, break down proteins that maintain the structure of the axon. Calpain, has been localized to both neurons and glia (18) and appears to be involved in post-traumatic cytotoxicity associated with increases in intracellular Ca^{2+}. The activation of calpain, which is irreversibly activated when free intracellular Ca^{2+} increases above threshold, causes cytoskeletal proteolysis. Moreover, when calpain activation is unregulated and prolonged, irreversible structural and functional alterations occur and have been implicated in neuronal toxicity (3,19). In regions that sustain neuronal loss and axonal injury following lateral CCI brain injury in rats, Kamplf et al. (20) demonstrated that as early as 15–30 min post-TBI, calpain activation occurs and continues for at least 24 hours. TBI has been shown to produce structural disruptions, altered distribution, and even degradation of neurofilaments and microtubules in several species, including rodents, cats, and pigs (21). Through the absorbance of excess Ca^{2+}, the mitochondria swell and cease functioning. If enough mitochondria are damaged, the nerve cell degenerates. Ca^{2+} also damages the cell by activating caspases that serve to damage the DNA and trigger programmed cell death.

In both clinical and experimental TBI, apoptosis and programmed cell death, necrosis, have been documented extensively in the acute (first 24-hours) period (3). It has been hypothesized that the diffuse and progressive cell death observed following brain trauma may be related to the induction of programmed cell death (PCD) which, unlike necrosis, involves the initiation and active expression of transcription- and translation-dependent pathways (3). A study by Conti et al. (22) reported that following brain assault, specific temporal and regional patterns of progressive apoptotic cell death are initiated. With the temporal span of 24–72 hours, maximal apoptotic cell death occurred in the injured cortex, which resolved by two months post-injury. Associated with the process of trauma-induced apoptosis is altered gene expression in the Bcl-2 and the caspase gene family. The Bcl-2 family of proteins are made up of proteins that serve to promote (Bax, Bad, Bcl-xs, Bak, Bik, Bid, Krk) or inhibit (Bcl-2, bcl-xl, Bfl-1, Brag-1, Ced-9, Mcl-1, A1) apoptosis. In trauma-induced cell death in the brain, alterations in Bcl-2 gene family appears to be an important factor in mediating such an event. Clark et al. (23) reported that following CCI brain injury in rats in which cells appear to be protected from apoptotic cell death, bcl-2 mRNA is induced in the injured cortex, hippocampus, and dentate gyrus between eight and 168 hours.

The role of caspases in the final step of the process of apoptosis is well established. In injured cortex fivefold increased expression of caspase-3 mRNA was reported by Yakolev et al. and twofold increased expression in the hippocampus at 24 hours after lateral FP brain injury in rats. The administration of a specific tetrapeptide inhibitor of caspase-3, Z-DEVD-FMK, prior to and following injury markedly reduced post-traumatic apoptosis and significantly improved neurological function. Such studies reveal that caspase-3-like proteases and PCD are pivotal in cell death pathways that result from brain injury.

Currently, inflammation and the role of cytokines in head injury is an area that is being thoroughly researched. Studies have shown that specific cytokines, tumour necrosis factor (TNF), and interleukin (IL) family of peptides, are involved in post-traumatic neuropathological damage. Regional concentrations of IL-1, IL-6, and TNF peptides have been shown to markedly increase in the acute post-traumatic period following experimental brain trauma in the rat, while circulating TNF and IL-6 have been shown to be increased in head injury (3).

CLINICAL MANAGEMENT: INTRODUCTION

This section will introduce traditional rehabilitation approaches in common practice for TBI and the roles of the members of the multidisciplinary rehabilitation team.

Effective management of the TBI patient requires accurate diagnosis of the etiology underlying behavioral/cognitive abnormalities. Abnormal behaviors, such as irritability, flattened affect, attention deficit, forgetfulness, and agitation may be seen as the result of psychogenic or structural brain disorders, and although the signs may be almost clinically indistinguishable, successful clinical management requires correct diagnosis. Reactive depression and post-traumatic stress disorder require very different intervention than do apathy or irritability and agitation from frontal lobe damage.

Rehabilitation focuses on optimizing physical, cognitive, and psychosocial function by finding compensatory strategies for various linguistic, cognitive, perceptual, behavioral, motor, and sensory deficits that result from damage to the nervous system. Initial evaluation must establish the nature and origin of the deficits the TBI patient has: primary (direct consequences of nervous system damage: motor, sensory, cognitive, autonomic), secondary (the medical consequences, such as falls due to gait impairment, visual field impairments, and impulsivity), and tertiary (psychosocial).

The goal of rehabilitation is to optimize quality of life and personal autonomy. A critical element of success is active comprehension of the family about the nature and extent of each of these challenges and involving them in treatment strategies. Inpatient rehabilitation requires an all-enveloping, around-the-clock consistent program incorporating the entire rehabilitation team's efforts. Important elements of such a program include compensatory training and assistive devices to improve communication skills, cognitive performance, behavior, strength and range of motion, and self-care activities. Other deficits requiring evaluation and treatment include sexual and reproductive dysfunction, psychiatric complications, and loss of job skills.

Experience has shown that a coordinated team effort leads to effective utilization of time and facilities. Outcomes are enhanced when there is integrated patient and family participation and true interdisciplinary cooperation (24). Data suggest that the organization of therapeutic programs may be more important than the type of hospital providing care (25,26).

The core rehabilitation team generally has physicians (primary care and consultants), nurses (skilled in rehabilitation techniques), discharge planners, physical therapists, occupational therapists, speech pathologists, psychologists, and social workers. Often the expertise of dietitians, neuropsychologists, audiologists, optometrists, podiatrists, dentists, orthotists, recreational therapists, and vocational counselors is required. Active involvement from clergy, homecare agencies, liaison representatives from long-term care facilities, and representatives from self-help groups may be important at different points in the rehabilitation process and, from time to time, the "care group" may change. Traditionally, the team leader is the physician in charge of the patient's principal care. For patients with persistent disabilities caused by injury to the nervous system, physicians with substantial training in neurology and rehabilitation are best suited for this responsibility. It is critical for the physician to understand the neurobiology of recovery and mechanisms underlying neurological deficits, and to be able to track changes in the neurological examination that may signal new or worsening underlying disease. Experience has shown that an interdisciplinary rehabilitation team works most effectively in TBI if the team members are permanently assigned to work with TBI patients.

In the following sections, strategies, underlying philosophies, and vernacular used by rehabilitation therapists will be reviewed. The neurological impairments caused by TBI and dealt with in the rehabilitation setting are cognitive (including dysphasia, apraxias, neglect, agnosia, apathy, abulia, memory impairment, and impulsivity), motor (weakness and spasticity, ataxia, and tremor), and sensory (visual/perceptual, and tactile). In TBI, brain pathology is usually multifocal. Severity of deficit is proportional to the size of the brain lesions and the nature of the deficit is directly related to the location of the lesions (anterior versus posterior circulation, right versus left hemisphere). A well-defined baseline neurological examination and lesion definition by imaging is important to anticipate the needs of the patient during rehabilitation.

Physical medicine and neurological rehabilitation for TBI has always focused foremost on safety of the patient and caregivers, and adaptation to newly acquired cognitive and behavioral dysfunction. It is also important to consider the potential for rehabilitation as a restorative therapy. For this reason, this chapter will also review selected "experimental" motor therapies, such as body weight-supported treadmill training (BWSTT), constraint-induced therapy (CIT), and other forms of "mass practice" motor learning therapy. The neurobiological hypotheses underlying rehabilitation will also be described.

The Evolving Philosophy of Rehabilitative Clinical Care

The first systematized attempt to rehabilitate people surviving traumatic injuries occurred during World War I, when "reconstruction aides," the forerunners of modern physical and occupational therapists, began treating soldiers with orthopedic injuries (27). Patients with brain injuries generally did not survive. Those with TBI who did survive were managed with months of bed rest, massage, passive range of motion, and heat.

During the poliomyelitis epidemic, Sister Kenny introduced a new theory—the muscle re-education model—suggesting that patients would benefit more from activity than from rest, and encouraging patients to actively participate in their own recovery. The goal was to enhance the strength of the remaining motor units (Sister Kenny 1943). Kenny's approach was based on muscular strengthening, and her polio patients reportedly fared better than did those treated conventionally. Her insistence upon physical activity as the cornerstone of a rehabilitation program, then considered revolutionary, was soon commonly accepted. Motor rehabilitation care began to emphasize compensatory use of unimpaired limbs to perform activities of daily living, and the patient's active engagement in self-care. Technologic and medical advances resulted in the greatly improved survival rate of soldiers wounded in World War II. During his military service, Dr. Howard Rusk developed a comprehensive treatment philosophy that combined supportive care and rehabilitation for traumatic-deployment-related conditions, and a new medical specialty, Physical Medicine, was born (27).

In the following decades, leading rehabilitation professionals began to focus on the neuroanatomy of brain dysfunction and the structural–functional relationships between brain lesion and motor changes. Kabat, Knott, Voss, Rood, Brunnstrom and Bobath were among the key figures in developing a new, theoretically-based approach to rehabilitation exercises for treating brain injury (28–34). A unifying concern was that exclusive focus on residual function would lead to fixed deformity and suboptimal recovery; however, the approaches often were based on nearly diametrically opposed theories of recovery. The neurofacilitation approach, espoused by Bobath, Kabat, Brunnstrom and Rood, represented the first attempts to use movement to treat central nervous system disorders. These approaches were based on the reflex model (35), which held that movements were composed of a series of reflexes. Therapists therefore attempted to facilitate "good" reflexes, and inhibit "bad" reflexes.

The Hierarchical model, first espoused by Hughlings Jackson (36), stated that the nervous system was organized hierarchically, with higher centers controlling lower ones. Believing that damage to a higher center would cause the "release" of pathologic movement from lower centers, therapists focused on blocking pathologic movement, believing this was necessary before normal movement could occur.

In some cases, the different schools of thought promoted contradictory clinical approaches. The Neurodevelopmental Treatment (NDT) School of Bobath espoused the view that recovery from central nervous system deficit recapitulated normal infant development, and therefore patients were taught to crawl and kneel prior to ambulating (37). The shortcomings of these models became apparent when it was observed that blocking abnormal movement did not necessarily produce normal movement. Furthermore, patients who were able to successfully perform functional tasks using abnormal movement were unable to perform the same tasks if the abnormal movement was inhibited.

The prevailing belief in the neurological clinical community during the 1970s and 1980s was that rehabilitation had very little impact on restoration of neurological function. Rehabilitation efforts mirrored these beliefs and focused on treating the medical, surgical, and psychosocial consequences of chronic illness, using assistive technologies to help compensate for disability. Physical, occupational, and speech therapies also were seen as means to prevent orthopedic complications (such as contracture), strengthen residual muscle function, and train patients to use compensatory strategies to promote independence in performing activities of daily living. The prevailing belief in the medical community was that rehabilitation therapies did not contribute in a meaningful way to neural restoration.

The motor learning approach grew out of Bernstein's ideas and the study of how movement was learned in normals (38). This approach fosters the immediate acquisition of motor skills. The different roles of acquisition, retention, and generalization of motor skills are key in motor learning. A major principle of motor learning is that of whole practice, meaning that tasks to be relearned must be practiced in their entirety rather than as isolated movements (39). Motor learning theory advocates blending an approach in which new motor skills are learned in a random manner rather than in a blocked repetitive fashion. This approach purportedly enhances retention while making acquisition more difficult. Conversely, learning skills in a repetitive manner enhances acquisition but decreases retention, perhaps because learning and retaining a skill is best accomplished by engaging in active problem-solving (40).

In the meantime, clinical approaches to neurological rehabilitation were based on empirical observations in small and disparate subject samples and untested hypotheses. Objective efficacy studies and comparative studies were not done. Neurological rehabilitation treatment was based on the training and intuitive beliefs of the treating therapist. Neurologists and physiatrists remained convinced that rehabilitation therapies were important to prevent complications, enhance residual functions, and help the patient reintegrate into society.

Rehabilitation as Restorative Therapy: Progress in Regeneration and Plasticity

Neuroscience compelled clinicians to re-examine traditional approaches to rehabilitation. Basic investigation into molecular and cellular responses to neural injury identified mechanisms of lost regenerative capability in adult animals. Therapies (pharmacologic and physical) which promote neuronal survival and exploit the CNS's innate capacity for regeneration and plasticity are now on the horizon.

Many questions still require investigation, including the functional impact of this approach in improving outcome after TBI, issues of timing (e.g., is there any effect of interventions long after injury?), long-term consequences, and alternative modes of delivering therapy. Ultimately this approach may have important clinical implications, such as restoration of motor, sensory, and cognitive function after TBI. The more that is learned about the mechanisms of injury and early and late cell death, the more opportunities for therapeutic interventions.

Plasticity and Learning

Optimizing appropriate dendritic connections is almost certainly dependent on environmental stimulation and physical experience. Transplantation and other therapies may have impact on the chronic "stable" patient, so the window of opportunity for effective rehabilitation may be greater than imagined.

Plasticity can be defined as "an adaptive mechanism by which the nervous system restores itself towards normal levels of functioning after injury. . . . Neural plasticity is the series of steps by which specific injured central circuits attempt to repair themselves after injury and to restore function directly by the repair of the damaged circuits" (41).

Neuroplasticity can also be defined across several domains. Anatomically, it refers to changes in nerve morphology, such as increased terminal sprouting and regeneration of damaged axons. Physiologically, it refers to a lower firing threshold, increased conduction velocity, improved synaptic efficiency, disinhibition, and activation of latent or redundant pathways. Behaviorally, it can refer to improved recovery of function or improved learning or relearning of functional skills (42).

Complex motor actions can rarely be performed accurately on "first try" in the neurologically intact individual. Motor learning occurs on the basis of practice: executing an action, detecting errors (through visual, proprioceptive, auditory, and other sensory feedback), performing corrections, and repeating the process. This learning process also forms the basis for some approaches to motor training in individuals with central nervous system deficits. The extent to which improvement in motor function during neurorehabilitation involves brain plasticity versus adaptation remains uncertain.

If therapy can capitalize on the innate plasticity of the nervous system, the rehabilitation environment can play a role in restoration. Positron emission tomography studies have shown an increase in relative oxygen metabolism in the cortex of the nondiseased, ipsilateral cortical hemisphere coincident with motor recovery in some hemiplegic stroke patients (43). A study of ten patients with motor recovery following striatocapsular infarction showed activation of bilateral motor pathways; increased activation of posterior cingulate and prefrontal cortices was also evident, which the authors interpreted to indicate intentional and attentional mechanisms in the recovery process (44). Clinico-pathologic observations similarly have invoked ipsilateral corticospinal involvement in the motor recovery process (45). Experiments have shown that an enriched environment can significantly improve outcome in laboratory animals after brain infarction (46). Animal models also suggest that increased functional demand on an impaired limb increases the plastic response (47). It is now critical to identify the appropriate physical therapies to promote optimal adaptive reorganization in the adult human nervous system.

The discovery that cats with complete paraplegia retain rudimentary ambulatory ability when suspended over a moving treadmill led to the description of central pattern generators (CPGs), dedicated local circuits within the spinal cord which produce complex, sequential motor actions (48,49). The afferent stimulation of the hind limbs produced by partial weight bearing and the moving treadmill produce reflexive walking. Experiments showed that early and intensive treadmill training leads to improved hindlimb function and ambulation. Later, Barbeau et al. demonstrated the same mechanisms in normal humans, using different degrees of body weight support, electromyography, and kinesiology techniques (50).

In BWSTT, the patient is suspended upright over a treadmill. The minimum required support is provided to allow the patient to stand. A physical therapist stands behind the patient to monitor and correct posture, while one or two therapists assist with leg advancement and foot placement.

Carr and Shepherd (51) summarize the benefits of BWSTT as follows:

- Walking is accomplished without danger or fear of falls.
- Ambulation can be practiced early in the subacute period, before the patient is capable of fully supporting body weight. Locomotor training can occur as a whole rather than in its component parts.
- The upper extremities are no longer required to make adaptive movements or use assistive devices.
- Treadmill speed can be varied.
- As a result of the stretch facilitation of the hip flexors, BWSTT "forces" initiation of swing. Similarly, the movement of the treadmill itself facilitates movement of the leg through stance.
- It allows for appropriate loading of the limb so that stepping can occur without stimulating a hyperactive stretch reflex.
- It increases aerobic demands for patients who would otherwise be unable to exercise.

BWSTT is being studied in patients with stroke, spinal cord injury, and Parkinson's disease; its clinical application is becoming widespread, although its therapeutic efficacy has not yet been established.

BWSTT

Hesse et al. (52) compared BWSTT with "standard physical therapy" in seven nonambulatory stroke patients using an A-B-A design. The patients only improved during the BWSTT phase. However, the "standard physical therapy" component of the trial specified the use of isolated elements of gait rather than the task of gait itself.

Pursuing these findings, Kosak and Reding (53) compared BWSTT with aggressive brace-assisted walking in 56 acute stroke patients and found no difference between groups. However, a subgroup of more severely involved stroke patients (defined by the presence of hemiparesis, hemianopsia, and hemihypesthesia) who received BWSTT performed better than the brace-assisted group in endurance and speed measures.

Treadmill training requires rigorous efficacy studies. It is extremely labor-intensive. The evidence is scant in that it is actually superior to traditional physical therapy, as most studies to date have included patients who may not yet have stabilized neurologically, or compared the BWSTT to an intervention, which included little ambulation. A skilled therapist can also support the body weight of a patient, and has the advantage of being able to alter the amount of weight supported throughout the gait cycle, depending on the needs of the patient. BWSTT is not tantamount to true ambulation as it occurs in an artificial environment, and therefore its ability to generalize to functional ambulation is questionable.

Mass Practice

In CIT the stronger arm in the person with hemiplegia is constrained from use to force the use of the involved extremity. Knapp (54) was the first to note that monkeys with deafferented forelimbs were able to regain the use of that limb if the intact limb was restricted. Later researchers restrained the use of the intact arm, using slings and mitts, in 25 hemiplegic patients with stroke or TBI (55). The arm was restrained for all waking hours for 14 days. Speed of task execution for functional tasks improved in all patients, with these gains being maintained at one year.

Taub (56) compared outcomes in chronic stroke patients receiving CIT with a control group who were instructed to "pay attention" to their involved arm. Inclusion in the study required sufficient motor strength to perform 20° of wrist extension and 10° of digit extension against gravity. The CIT group practiced six hours a day. Functional tasks performed by the affected limb included eating, throwing a ball, and peg manipulation. Results showed significant improvement in ADL skills for the constraint group compared with the control group, and these skills were sustained for two years post-intervention.

Taub's hypotheses for the mechanisms underlying CIT are twofold. First, following a stroke the patient goes through a period of cortical shock, or diaschisis, during which many of the neurons surrounding the area of the lesion are viable, but not functioning. During this time the patient attempts to use the involved extremity but fails, thus receiving negative reinforcement. Attempts to compensate with the intact extremity are successful, and therefore are positively reinforced. Over the time, the cortical shock fades, but the patient has developed "learned disuse" of the involved extremity, and although capable of using the extremity to some extent, does not.

Second, motor improvement may be the result of the intensive practice that these patients receive during the time that their intact extremity is restrained. This learning may be the result of recruiting neurons as the period of diaschisis resolves. Liepert (57), using transcranial magnetic stimulation, reported enlarged contralateral cortical representations and increased levels of neuronal excitability in 13 chronic stroke patients following a 12-day period of CIT.

However, animal studies by Kozlowski et al. (58) suggested that if constraint and mass practice is initiated too early following the initial injury, greater damage may result. As with BWSTT, CIT requires further study to determine optimal dose and timing strategies.

The 1990s witnessed the dawning of a new age in neurorehabilitation. Political and economic pressures drove clinicians to practice "evidence-based" rehabilitation medicine. Tradition and compassion were not adequate justification for rehabilitation; outcome data were necessary to show efficacy. This converged with advances in neuroscience: in the animal model it was possible to manipulate innate plasticity to improve outcome and restore function after injury to the central nervous system. Translational research was needed to test these strategies in humans, creating collaborations between the neuroscience and neurorehabilitation communities.

Neurorehabilitation became field-focused not only on compensation, but also on restoration. Advances in neuroimaging and rigorous study of the impact of intensive physical therapies on clinical function compelled the neurologic community to realize the capacity for plasticity in the adult human brain as a function of physical and cognitive activities. Today the neurologic rehabilitation community actively pursues opportunities for combinations of these therapies leading to restoration of neurologic function.

Functional Electrical Stimulation

Functional electrical stimulation (FES) bypasses the CNS to directly stimulate peripheral nerve and cause muscle contraction, and can be used anywhere in the body (59,60). Sequential stimulation of peripheral nerves has been used to improve ambulation and hand function. FES increases muscle mass, oxygen consumption, insulin-stimulated glucose use, and bone mineral content. FES in combination with BWSTT is undergoing investigation, with the underlying premise that FES can provide more powerful afferent stimulation to the spinal cord CPGs than can passive movements.

Robotics

CIT is based on the premise that time and labor-intensive repeated goal-directed therapy can enhance recovery. Robotics represent a technology, that can be designed to provide quantifiable and reproducible physical activity (61,62). Computerized robotic devices can precisely standardize the therapy delivered, providing a graded exercise program, which adjusts to patient response on a continuous basis. Robots can be made to not only administer a therapeutic exercise regimen, but also to provide on-line patient assessment and analysis. A robot is capable of delivering a precise regimen of active and passive physical therapy coupled with multisensory (visual, tactile, and auditory) feedback. Such a device lacks the compassionate human aspect of physical and occupational therapy, the effects of which cannot be discounted. However, it has certain potential advantages over traditional physical therapy. Computerized robotic devices promise a cost-effective adjunct to rehabilitation therapy.

The Rehabilitation Team

Physicians

The neurologist may provide principal care or serve as a consultant to the physiatrist—more often the medical doctor who provides leadership to the team providing rehabilitation care. After meticulous neurological evaluation to ascertain severity and location of neurologic disease, the neurologist can develop a comprehensive rehabilitation program, helping other staff members understand and define the patient's neurologic findings, medical limitations, and the rationale for prescribed pharmacologic interventions, including post-traumatic epilepsy prophylaxis, treatment, and tapering of anticonvulsants as appropriate. The physician's assessment of the patient's medical condition and prognosis plays a pivotal role in planning long-term care needs.

Rehabilitation Nurse

The primary care nurse coordinates all daily activities of the patient, is actively involved in detecting and treating the medical complications of the patients, acts as liaison between the patient, family, and others on the team, provides skilled rehabilitation treatment, and provides routine nursing care (24,63). Nursing staff spend more time with patients than any other members of the team and frequently know the most about the patient's emotional state, adjustment, and everyday concerns (64).

Incontinence and bowel and bladder retraining: Many patients who have suffered a major TBI develop urinary retention or incontinence. Using the approach outlined, most patients regain bladder control (63). Guidelines for the management of urinary retention or incontinence are as follows:

1. Measure residual urine. If residual is more than 100–150 cc, assess the reason for retention (which may or may not be associated with incontinence). Common causes of retention and overflow incontinence include: functional bladder outlet obstruction, bladder spasticity, absence of conscious desire to void, and infection.
2. Begin intermittent catheterizations every six hours (more often if necessary). During this time, monitor input and output, offer the patient the toilet/commode/urinal every two hours while awake, awaken patient two or three times a night to offer the toilet/commode/ urinal. If this is successful, gradually decrease the number of and frequency of catheterizations and increase the time between voiding trials. If unsuccessful, an indwelling catheter may be necessary.

3. For patients requiring long-term in-dwelling catheters, change catheter every two weeks. Catheter removal should be attempted on a regular basis if the patient is not severely confused or perceptually impaired and if there are no medical contraindications (64).

Whether because of immobility, medications, or hospital diet, many TBI patients also develop constipation. This can be avoided by a proper diet, adequate hydration, and a bowel regimen of stool softeners and mild cathartics. Enemas are then rarely needed. Fecal incontinence usually occurs in severely confused, perceptually unaware patients who do not know that they have moved their bowels. Patients will frequently become impacted. This almost always presents with diarrhea or incontinence because only loose stool can pass through the partially obstructed bowel. Treatment of incontinence and impaction depends on the underlying cause. For confused, perceptually unaware patients, a timed voiding schedule similar to the bladder routine just described may stop fecal incontinence. The nurses and nursing aides are most directly involved with bowel and bladder retraining and provide invaluable input in establishing optimal medical and physical routines.

Neuropsychologist

This team member identifies, quantifies, and helps predict the impact of deficits of a cognitive or perceptual nature. These data are useful in the planning of specific treatment and the monitoring of recovery. The neuropsychologist can help distinguish affective from organic brain disease and design behavioral and pharmacologic interventions with the physician and other team members. Neuropsychologists help the therapeutic team, patient, and family understand the nature and severity of deficits and help predict prognosis.

Common neurobehavioral issues: Confused and perceptually unaware patients may have "bizarre" behavior. Confused patients forget, wander, confabulate, and they may get agitated when they become frightened. Mild sedation with small doses of Benadryl or meprobamate sometimes calms the anxiety and makes it easier for confused patients to cope with stress. However, major tranquilizers and their derivatives frequently produce extrapyramidal dysfunction in (especially in) elderly patients with brain injury and should be avoided. Short-acting benzodiazapines, in very small doses, are sometimes effective, but more of such treatment causes sedation (aggravating confusion) before it calms anxiety.

Patients with neglect often show surprising and unusual behaviors. They may dress only half of the body, and fail to notice this even when looking at themselves in the mirror. They may tell you that an arm is missing or that they have several legs around with spares in the closet, at home, and an extra in the bed. They may say that an arm or leg is not part of their body, but is instead a club, a salami, a tennis racket, and so forth. Yet these patients may not be confused per se, and they may perform quite well on formal psychometric testing. They have an altered concept of the way in which the world is organized and this causes them to do things that look peculiar, but that may be very reasonable within the context of their own distorted world.

Apraxic patients also show abnormal behavior. Thus, they cannot use utensils correctly, they may eat with their razor and write with a comb, yet they may have good memory and be able to calculate, reason, and abstract. Apraxic patients and patients with neglect frequently get frustrated and agitated because they operate in a distorted world that does not reflect the real world adequately. Goal-oriented behavior often ends in dismal failure. Tranquilizers and sedatives almost always make the undesirable behavior worse because these people are frequently tottering on the brink of the real and the surreal. By dulling their sensibilities with drugs, the "thin edge of reality" is often removed, making the abnormal behavior even worse.

Sleep–wake cycle disruption commonly complicates stroke. Sleep deprivation contributes to behavioral complications. Patients try to get up at night and dress to prepare for the day's activities. When put back to bed, they may awaken again and again to restart the ritual. Others may fall asleep in the middle of an interview, in the middle of a sentence, while scratching their knees, or while wheeling their wheelchairs. Some types of behavioral abnormalities regularly follow stroke and are unrelated to the behavioral abnormalities caused by cognitive or perceptual dysfunction. Unprovoked and often paroxysmal laughing and crying frequently occur. However, they are not associated with underlying happiness or sadness (pseudobulbar affect). Depression, anger, hostility, and the many expressions of these emotions occur frequently and are best treated with understanding, patience, and environmental manipulation. Psychiatric intervention is also sometimes needed.

Traditionally, neuropsychologists, occupational therapists (OT), psychologists, psychiatrists, nurses, and social workers have been most involved in delineating and treating these deficits. However, with the establishment of behavioral neurology sections at several major universities, neurologists may again be drawn toward the intriguing interactions of mind and brain. The traditional neurologic examination should thus be expanded to include the evaluation and description of the various cognitive, perceptual, and behavioral deficits that follow stroke (65). The fields of liaison psychiatry and geriatric psychiatry provide experts specially trained in treating patients with medical illness who also have behavioral abnormalities.

By evaluating the various cognitive, perceptual, and behavioral problems when patients return for follow-up, it may be possible to limit the use of unnecessary psychoactive drugs. It can also help the patient and families to continue to adjust and avoid unnecessary and premature nursing home placement. Studies suggest that depression (as measured by standardized depression indices) is common, but results of other studies indicate that clinically significant depression (depression that impairs function) is uncommon (63,66). Depression is more common with left hemispheric disease, but longitudinal follow-up of patients overcoming major right hemispheric infarctions showed that many of these patients developed signs of depression when they overcame their perceptual problems just enough to realize the extent of their physical disabilities (66).

Cognitive, perceptual, and behavioral issues: Confusion (cognitive dysfunction, dementia) has been classically defined as "an impairment in higher intellectual functioning" that can appear as:

1. Difficulty with orientation as to time, place, or person.
2. Diminished recall or memory (immediate more than remote).
3. A decreased fund of general information.
4. Difficulty in performing such tasks of abstract reasoning as calculations, similarities and differences, and proverbs.
5. Grossly impaired judgment.
6. Inappropriate affect or confabulation.

Perception is the way in which we interpret (or integrate) all of the complex information that constantly bombards the central nervous system. It is, in essence, the way in which we see and experience the world around us. At least 15 different perceptual abnormalities are described in patients who have suffered from stroke. They include apraxia, agnosia, denial, neglect, disordered concepts of body image and scheme, right–left disorientation, figure-ground difficulties, disordered concepts of verticality, visual-spatial distortion, disordered concepts of sequencing, disordered concepts of time, disordered sleep–wake cycles, perseveration, extinction (and cross-modal extinction), auditory mislocalization, and difficulty reading.

Such perceptual abnormalities almost always interfere with functional recovery. Perceptual deficits may be present in patients who are confused, but they may also exist as isolated phenomena in patients with no cognitive deficits. They may exist in patients with dominant or nondominant hemispheric lesions, and are sometimes seen with infratentorial lesions.

The success of programs to detect and treat cognitive and perceptual problems is predicated upon the patient's ability to remember compensatory strategies. Therapy for cognitive and perceptual dysfunction varies widely. In general, specific deficits must first be clearly labeled by using formal testing and by incorporating data gathered by observing the stroke patient in the patient's own environment. Individual programs are then devised to make the patient aware of the problems and to teach the patient to compensate for these problems. Families are often asked to participate in the treatment program because they can greatly extend the number of hours of formal treatment while they are developing the necessary expertise to carry through with these programs when the patient is discharged.

For confused patients, it is important to keep the environment simple, uncluttered, and constant. Do not change rooms or roommates frequently. Set up a strict daily schedule and post it on the wall above the bed and on the activity cards. Constantly remind patients about where they are, what day it is, the date and year, and significant current events. Calendars and clocks should be prominently displayed, and the names of each of the patients should be posted on the doors to their rooms. Sometimes other cues are needed, such as pictures of the patient or of the spouse and family.

Therapy for patients with perceptual dysfunction is deficit-specific. Constant cuing and repetition in a very structured environment is a cornerstone of remediation. The program should include frequent and consistent cuing and repetition in a very structured environment. As the patient improves, the therapist gives fewer cues, less repetitive, and may require the patient to perform in less structured environments in which it is necessary to "tune out the noise" to perform successfully.

Depression: Early initiation of rehabilitation, frequent counseling sessions for patients and their families, and continuing evaluation and discussion of staff, patient, and family expectations and limitations also help to diminish depression during the first year after TBI. Depression may sometimes be aggravated by medications used to treat underlying medical problems. Antihypertensives and corticosteroids are notable examples. Psychiatric consultation and prescription of antidepressants are indicated when patients do not respond to these measures.

Sexuality: Sexual function is a natural part of everyone's life, including the lives of people with disabilities. An evaluation and treatment program of sexual dysfunction should be included in all rehabilitation programs. In TBI, sexual dysfunction may have organic and behavioral components. Brain injury can cause a lowered or disinhibited sex drive. For most patients with unilateral hemispheric infarctions or hemorrhages, there is no physiologic impairment of erection, ejaculation, orgasm, lubrication, or ovulation after the acute stage of illness. Most people recovering from stroke can resume sexual activity but they may have to modify their emotional approach and physical techniques. Couples must work out practical techniques for overcoming their motor and sensory impairments and resulting lack of agility. Examples include use of a bedside rail, trapeze, footboard, or headboard with grab bars to assist in position changes, pillows for positioning, or alternative positions for intercourse (partner on top, side-lying). Vaginal lubricants or lubricated condoms may be helpful.

Although TBI may not alter the ability to perform sex acts, the medications used to treat concommitant medical problems, or the medical problems themselves, may impair sexual activity. Medications include major tranquilizers, minor tranquilizers, anticholinergic agents, and sedative hypnotics. It is obviously important to obtain a complete medical history prior to counseling, and referral to a urologist or gynecologist with special interest in sexual functioning may help to define any existing physiologic problems that could interfere with the sex act. Sexuality is more than the act of sexual intercourse. It involves the essence of relating to another person—the tenderness, the desire to give as well as take, the compliments, casual caresses, reciprocal concerns, tolerance, the forms of communication that both include and go beyond words: "sexuality includes a range of behaviors: from smiling—through orgasm; it is not just what happens between two people in bed" (67).

When patients return for follow-up, it is important to ask questions about sex drive, sex acts, and sexuality. This topic may be approached directly or indirectly. By inquiring, the physician may elicit important concerns or uncover unsolved medical problems. Asking the question may implicitly give the patient permission to discuss a topic the patient might be embarrassed to broach. This is another opportunity to enhance the quality of life for the patient and partner.

Social Worker

The social worker who is knowledgeable about neurologic impairment and disability counsels the individual and family during all phases of patient care. Commonly, patients have reactive depression, altered self-image, and fears of abandonment. For intensive counseling, the services of a clinical psychologist or psychiatrist are often a necessary supplement to the social worker's program of care. The social worker assesses resources of the patient and family, plays a major role in discharge planning, and assists in obtaining community support and outpatient care. In the outpatient setting, the social worker can help the patient and caregiver to coordinate efforts among healthcare providers, third-party carriers, and state and federal agencies. Continued availability of the social worker may help prevent premature institutionalization or retirement.

Occupational, Physical, and Speech Therapists

Physical therapists (PT) supervise rehabilitation exercise programs. Physical therapists and OTs use passive and active range of motion activities and strengthening exercises. Generally the physical therapist focuses on fitness, balance, lower extremity function, and ambulation. The OT provides upper extremity exercise, evaluates and prescribes adaptive equipment, and joins the PT in training the patient to safely transfer. OTs conduct elements of cognitive and perceptual rehabilitation, in conjunction with the neuropsychologist.

OT: OTs monitor motor reaction times and train their patients to practice fine motor skills and reduce impulsive behaviors. They provide memory strategies and work with the patient to develop problem-solving skills. The OT coordinates with the PT's hands-on tactile motor program and with the speech language pathologist's intensive cognitive and communication-focused therapy program.

OTs are most frequently involved with upper extremity retraining activities, but the nursing staff and family can offer invaluable assistance in carrying out therapeutic activities, even during the acute phases of stroke care. There are no statistics which accurately predict eventual functional outcome for patients with persistent upper extremity weakness. Although it is possible to brace a weak leg and foot, there is no simple device to increase function in a weak upper extremity. Recovery of power and function is often slow and incomplete and skilled hand movement rarely returns. Many patients slowly recover function over a period of years following TBI. Slings are useful only to prevent a flaccid arm from banging into things during ambulation. By "packaging" the arm, the sling often seems to promote sustained neglect and interfere with recovery.

Hand edema is almost always relieved by elevation of the hand, using an elevated arm rest support while seated. Recent data suggest that hybrid orthoses allowing proper positioning, supplemented by FES, can lead to more rapid resolution of edema and pain, and perhaps enhance motor recovery.

Following TBI, the hand flexors usually predominate, causing flexion contractures of the hand and wrist. Exercises aimed at increasing power in the flexors may hasten this unless there is a concomitant increase in power of the extensors. When spasticity threatens to cause joint deformity, various splinting devices may be used. Medications are rarely beneficial in controlling upper extremity spasticity. Frequent range of motion is still the treatment of choice. If these exercises are done several times each waking hour and combined with other therapeutic exercises, spasticity and joint contracture may be minimized.

As a result of weakness and other associated neurologic deficits following stroke, patients often need assistance with feeding, dressing, hygiene, and bowel and bladder routines. Institutes specify programs to teach these skills as soon as the patient is medically stable; this improves eventual outcome and prevents patients from becoming overly dependent. The nurses and nursing aides, because they're most involved with morning care, should be directly involved with these programs and should work closely with the OTs in planning individual programs.

Installation of rails on the stairs, grab bars in the bathroom, arm rails on the toilet, and a tub bench may make it easier to manage patients at home. Some benefit from using a commode placed near their bed. OTs may make further suggestions about clothing (e.g., Velcro closures, pullover shirts without buttons, front-closure brassieres, elastic shoe laces), kitchen (e.g., special utensils, cutting boards), dishwashing devices, and home adaptations (e.g., widening doorways, ramping, redesigning kitchen, bathroom, bedroom, and working facilities). They may suggest special adaptive equipment for the car or work environment. OTs may also recommend the most appropriate type of mobility devices.

Although it is easier to help than it is to supervise while a TBI patient spends untold minutes struggling to accomplish simple tasks, it is ultimately more therapeutic to engage and challenge the patient. Up to 56% of the patients can be expected to achieve full independence in ADL (63). When patients do not succeed, it is important to search for the underlying cause so that deficit-specific programs can be developed and initiated.

Physical therapy: PTs begin ambulation training by emphasizing activities aimed at improving sitting and standing balance. Balance activities can be started before the patient is able to stand. Later, weight-shifting techniques become important, and are termed "pre-ambulation activities." Weight-shifting techniques teach patients to put more weight on their weak leg, walk with a heel-toe gait, and discourage shoulder and hip retraction. Therapists use a variety of tactile techniques to combat scissoring, toe curl, and foot inversion.

For the patient with ataxia, balance activities should be started early in the rehabilitation process, and can be used for the patient who is not yet able to tolerate being out of bed. Later, patients are taught to balance at the hemibars (an adjustable-height, elliptic handrail), first with assistance, then independently. Patients with neglect (hemi-inattention) or with disordered perceptions of verticality frequently have difficulty with this task and must be reminded (cued) to stand straight and to distribute weight appropriately. When sitting and standing balance improves, patients are encouraged to take a few steps while still at the hemibar. When they are able to walk around the hemibar reasonably well, they are taught to walk with a four-legged cane (quad cane), a standard cane, and eventually progress to no cane at all.

Lower extremtiy braces are used to correct position, protect joints, and enhance function. The ankle foot orthosis (AFO) is used to correct ankle positioning and prevent toe drag. A lightweight polypropylene brace that slips into the shoe and extends about halfway up the calf provides dorsiflexion assistance, prevents inversion, and can help to stabilize the knee.

When patients cannot learn to walk, it is often related to:

1. Cognitive and perceptual problems, such as denial, neglect, apraxia, difficulty with sequencing (e.g., the patient literally carries the cane instead of using it for support), and difficulty with concepts of verticality.
2. Severe spasticity of the hip rotators and adductors (causing scissoring), quadriceps (causing knee hyper-extension), hamstrings (causing knee flexion), or gastrocs (causing heel cord foreshortening).
3. Ataxia resulting in inability to shift weight properly.

Careful analysis of the gait pattern and awareness of concomitant deficits is necessary for an effective retraining program. Patients can improve their gait patterns, ambulation tolerance, and even shed adaptive devices (braces, canes) years after their initial stroke. Periodic neurologic evaluation with review of all problems, progress, and programs help to coordinate the team, set goals and priorities, detect potentially correctable neurologic, medical, and functional problems, support the family structure, and provide useful consultative services to the primary care physician.

Transfer training: When patients cannot walk, they must learn to move (transfer) from the bed to a chair, from the chair to the toilet, into and out of a bathtub or shower, and into and out of a car. Patients cannot receive adequate care if the staff cannot move them easily or if it takes two staff members and a Hoyer lift to accomplish simple transfers. There are special techniques for performing these transfers, and all staff members should be trained in these techniques. Early institution of transfer training also helps to free patients of the bedpan and urinal and makes it possible for them to be out of bed much of the day, either in therapy or visiting with others. Families should be taught these transfer techniques as soon as it is safe for them to transfer their affected family members. PTs, OTs, and nurses are all involved in teaching transfer techniques.

Speech therapy: Speech language therapists evaluate and treat patients with cognitive impairments, principally with language comprehension and production difficulties. The patient with TBI often has elements of language dysfunction. In addition, they have cognitive deficits associated with short-term memory, poor attention, impulsivity, and abstract reasoning. Cognitive and perceptual testing by the speech pathologist complements the work of the neuropsychologist, and directs therapeutic linguistic programs. Speech pathologists also evaluate another set of pathological conditions resulting from TBI: buccal-lingual dysfunction, which may be associated with dysarthria, dysphagia, and aspiration.

Speech, language, and swallowing deficits: TBI can result in deficits that interfere with communication, speech (comprehension, production), language (phonemic, phonetic, lexical, syntactical), reading, writing, spelling, gesturing, word recognition and repetition, articulation, and swallowing. Although these clinically measurable aspects of daily living have usually been grouped together into three major descriptive categories (aphasia, dysarthria, dysphagia), the development of comprehensive standardized tests of speech and language function and of systematized methods for examining "the peripheral motor mechanism" have led to a better understanding of these disorders, thus allowing a rational, deficit-specific approach to patient care (68–73).

Aphasia: Aphasia treatment is an inter-disciplinary one with close inter-communication between neurologist, neuropsychologist, and speech pathologist. The special province of the neurologist is the physical etiology and the determination of the nature and extent of the lesion and the treatability of the patient's medical conditions (74).

A retraining approach using developmental sequencing, repetition (single letters or sounds progressing to more complex letters or sounds, then to words), or even physical manipulation of the articulators with a spatula and stylet might improve outcome. Therapy that stimulates "word retrieval" may improve the aphasic deficits. Specific programs using gestures, music, and rhythm, such as melodic intonation therapy, or visual stimuli to perform tasks thought to be precursors of symbolic gestures, have been described, and seem to work best with apraxic or globally aphasic patients (75–77).

Descriptions of language recovery after a great variety of lesions show the many brain structures involved in producing and processing language. These lesions include dominant hemispherectomy, basal ganglia, internal capsule, and other cortical sites. This evidence for a multifocal contribution to language underscores the need for better taxonomy, better anatomic–functional correlation, comprehensive aphasia testing, and multiple treatment approaches (74,78–82).

In the 1970s–1980s, treatment studies contributed significantly to resolution of the controversy concerning the efficacy of aphasia rehabilitation. The first contrasted pre- and post-treatment language test scores of 80 treated and 15 untreated aphasics under carefully controlled conditions and was studied by Smith (81). The findings indicate that treated patients improve in language functions beyond the level expected with spontaneous recovery alone. A subsequent study compared 162 treated and 119 untreated aphasics. The findings of both studies suggest that formal language rehabilitation has a positive effect on the course of recovery, especially if it continues for at least six months at the rate of at least three times a week (69). Sarno and Levita (71) showed that even globally aphasic patients improve with speech therapy.

Best forms of speech therapy have not yet been established, but studies are underway to evaluate the impact of intensive specific language stimulation and retraining, with the objective of identifying best practices and achieving best outcomes. Practical experience suggests that some patients can continue to make gains years after their initial stroke. Whether or not this is related to therapy or would have occurred without formal intervention is unknown.

Dysarthria: Dysarthria and dysphasia are frequently confused. Dysarthria from hemispheric lesions frequently improves spontaneously over the first 30–60 days. Dysarthria caused by posterior circulation infarctions may initially improve only to leave significant residual deficits resulting from a combination of muscle weakness and spasticity, vocal cord partial paralysis, dyskinetic motion of the respiratory muscles, difficulty clearing secretions, and palatal myoclonus. ENT consultation may help clarify the contribution of the various components.

Dysarthria is not usually associated with the multi-infarct state caused by lacunae, but it is a prominent feature of pseudobulbar palsy. In the former case, when dysarthria is associated with significant extrapyramidal dysfunction, dopaminergic agents may improve both the motor and coordination deficits and, to a lesser extent, the dysarthria. In the latter case, inappropriate outbursts of laughing and crying may complicate the dysarthria, further frustrating therapeutic efforts. The dysarthric patient may benefit from tongue, mouth, and breathing exercises. The goal is to improve breath control and articulation.

When these measures fail, there are various communication aids (letter boards, computerized voice synthesizers, voice, and amplification devices) that can help the dysarthric patient to communicate more effectively.

Swallowing dysfunction: The first step in this evaluation requires the differentiation of dysphagia from the swallowing apraxias that frequently complicate hemispheric infarctions. Dysphagic patients cannot swallow because of paralysis, spasticity, or dyskinesia of the muscles of the palate, pharynx, or tongue, and because of a depressed or absent gag reflex. Apraxic patients cannot swallow because they have "forgotten" how to swallow, or because they do not have adequate sensory perception to detect food in the mouth. When food is placed in the mouth, it may hang out on the side or remain in the mouth for prolonged periods. It may be partially chewed and then hoarded in the pouch caused by associated facial weakness. Aspiration of this debris is a leading cause of pneumonia in the acute post-stroke patient. All staff providing patient care should be taught to check periodically for retained food.

Apraxic patients improve with a careful, consistent interdisciplinary feeding program. Start with semisolid foods and progress to chopped moist food, cut chunks, and then regular food as tolerated, ensuring no distraction while eating and encouraging the patient not to talk and eat at the same time. Check for retained food after each meal.

Dysphagia occurs when there is a disruption in the sequential motor events required for safe and effective swallowing. Videofluoroscopy may be necessary to ascertain the nature and severity of dysfunction, and to detect silent aspiration. Speech pathologists train the patient and family about appropriate food and drink portions and consistency, and maneuvers which assist in safe and effective mastication and swallowing. These include chin tuck and head positioning. Feeding gastrostomy may be necessary in severe cases for adequate nutrition, but aspiration remains a serious risk.

Orthotist

The orthotist works with the team to provide orthoses for correcting limb position and protecting joints potentially damaged by maladaptive limb movement patterns. Orthoses are external devices for the limbs and spinal column that correct position, protect joint alignment, and enhance functional adaptation. Orthoses can be static or dynamic, mechanical, or power-driven. It is crucial that the principal care provider has fundamental knowledge of the potential benefits, limitations, and complications of orthoses to maximize efficacy and prevent complications. Orthoses are used for supplementation and substitution, protection and correction. Modern braces use a combination of biomechanical principles. They rely on force systems and neurophysiologic principles to assist muscle control and decrease tone. This is accomplished by taking into account the influences of postures and pressure, for example, by increasing the bulk of plastic on one side of a brace to facilitate or inhibit reflexes (83). Sometimes forces must be applied in multiple places on a limb to inhibit a posture. Certain orthoses are meant to facilitate useful reflexes, others to diminish counterproductive ones, always with the goal of promoting functional movement.

Recreational Therapist

Recreational activities are a fundamental component of the human experience and contribute to quality of life. Recreational therapists provide access to activities that the patient may have enjoyed premorbidly (e.g., sporting activities from a wheel chair level or with adaptive equipment) in a nonthreatening environment. Providing guidance and access to community cultural resources, teaching Internet navigation skills, and promoting socialization and exposure to new hobbies are among the many roles of the recreational therapist. Moreover, newly acquired physical skills can be reinforced during recreation therapy sessions.

Vocational Counselor

Vocational rehabilitation programs, though very important, have had limited success in reintegrating the neurologically impaired into the work environment. The goal is to assess, refer, and follow patients who are candidates for vocational training. These programs vary greatly between states. Often a fear of losing healthcare benefits provides a disincentive for the disabled to enter the work force. Unfortunately, a comprehensive, nationally integrated vocational rehabilitation program remains an unrealized goal. Nonetheless, vocational rehabilitation is essential. The post-TBI individual's skills and talents must be identified, and the patient must receive appropriate educational and job placement opportunities if the patient is no longer able to return to premorbid levels of activity. The OT can assist in identifying appropriate adaptive technologies to overcome physical impairments and the social worker can help assure equipment and transportation needs are met. The team can assist in helping the patient return to a former work environment by counseling the employer about changes needed in the physical layout of the workplace, and adjustments that may be necessary to allow successful re-entry to the work force.

Driving: After TBI, people are often eager to regain their independence and get back in the car. For some it is the sole determinant of eventual vocational placement. There are problems that can make it difficult for stroke survivors to drive. The more obvious problems are the easiest to detect and correct. Hand controls can operate throttle and braking functions; a steering wheel hand control now allows one handed steering; cruise controls may prevent fatigue. Lightweight fold-up wheelchairs make it possible for the limited ambulator to get to the car and store the chair in the trunk or back seat. Parking spaces, ramps, and elevators for the handicapped enable them to use the facilities offered in many villages, towns, or cities.

Other deficits make it dangerous to drive. For example, demented patients get lost. Perceptual impairments (visual field losses) may cause drivers to hit objects or pedestrians because of neglect, extinction, or inattention. Apraxic patients cannot coordinate controls. Visual and spatial relationships may become disturbed, making it difficult for some patients to recognize traffic signs and signals. Aphasic patients cannot read signs or signals (although they may recognize shapes or symbols). They may not be able to ask for help if they require assistance. Tremor, dysmetria, and spasticity hamper motor control. Urinary frequency may force frequent stops.

Many states require annual license renewal. At that time, the handicapped driver may be required to notify the Department of Motor Vehicles (DMV) of the handicap. The DMV may then suspend privileges or revoke licenses. Therefore, many stroke survivors are reluctant to notify the DMV of their disabilities. If licenses are suspended, handicapped drivers may again be allowed to drive if they have a letter from their physician stating that they are capable of driving, with or without restrictions (restrictions must be specified). Physicians may be asked to make this determination, even if they are not familiar with the various assessment techniques used to separate safe from unsafe handicapped drivers (e.g., tests of perception, reaction time, coordination). Unless the physican is trained in these assessment techniques, it is wise to consider referral to private driver training programs.

REFERENCES

1. Ayyoub Z, Badawi F, Vasile A, Arzaga D, Cassedy A, Shaw V. Dual diagnosis: spinal cord injury and brain injury. In: ed. Spinal Cord Injury. London: Academic Press, 1980:509–524.
2. Zafonte R, Giap B, Coplin W, Pangilian P. Traumatic brain injury and spinal cord injury: pathophysiology and acute therapeutic strategies. Topics in Spinal Cord Injury Rehabilitation 1999; 5(2):21–22.
3. McIntosh TK, Saatman KE, Raghupathi R, Graham DI, Smith DH, Lee VMY, Trojanowski JQ. The molecular and cellular sequelae of experimental traumatic brain injury: pathogenetic mechanisms. Neuropathology and Applied Neurobiology 1998; 24:251–267.
4. Bramlett HM, Dietrich WD, Green EJ, Busto R. Chronic histooathological conse-quences of fluid-percussion brain injury in rats: effects of post-traumatic hypother-mia. Acta Neuropathol 1997; 93:190–199.
5. Narayan RK, Wilberger JE, Povlishock JT. Neurotrauma. New York: McGraw-Hill, 1996:1078.
6. Sinson G, Voddi M, McIntosh TK. Nerve growth factor administration attenuates cognitive but not neurobehavioral motor dysfunction or hippocampal call loss following fluid-percussion brain injury in rats. J Neurosurg 1995; 65:2209–2216.
7. Sinson G, Voddi M, McIntosh TK. Combined fetal neural transplantation and nerve growth factor infusion: effects on neurological outcome following fluid-percussion brain injury in the rat. J Neurosurg 1996; 84:655–662.
8. Go BK, DeVivo MJ, Richards JS. The epidemiology of spinal cord injury. In: Stover SL, Delisa JA, Whiteneck GG, eds. Spinal Cord Injury Clinical Outcomes from the Model Systems. Aspen Publishers, Gaithersberg, Md, 1995:21–55.
9. Siesjo BK, Bengtsson F. Calcium fluxes, calcium anatagonists, and calscium-related pathology in brain ischemia, hypoglemia, and spreading depression: a unifying hypothesis. J Cereb Blood Flow Metab 1989; 9:127–140.

10. Salzman SK, Chaum JM, Wang L, Puniak MA, Kelley G, Agresta C. S-Emopamil improves functional recovery from experimental spinal trauma. J Neurotrauma 1992; 9:69.
11. Okiyama K, Smith DH, Thomas MJ, McIntosh TK. Evaluation of a novel calcium channel blocker (S)-emopamil on regional cerebral edema and neurobehavioral function after brain injury. J Neurosurg 1992; 77:607–615.
12. De Renzi E, Vignolo LA. The token test: a sensitive test to detect receptive disturbances in aphasics. Brain 1962; 85:665–658.
13. Sun FY, Faden AI. *N*-methyl-d-asparate receptors mediate posttraumatic increases of protein kinase C in rat brain. Brain Res 1994; 661:63–69.
14. Hall ED, Yonkers PA, Andrus PK, Cox JW, Anderson DK. Biochemistry and pharmacology of lipid antioxidants in acute brain and spinal cord injury. J Neurotrauma 1992; 9:S425–S442.
15. Amstad PA, Krupitza G, Cerutti PA. Mechanism of c-fos induction by active oxygen. Cancer Res 1992; 52:3952–3960.
16. Yao Y, Yin D, Jas GS, et al. Oxidative modification of a carboxylterminal vicinal methionine in calmodulin by hydrogen peroxide inhibits calmodulin-dependent activation of the plasma membrane CaATPase. Biochem 1996; 35:2767–2787.
17. Smith SL, Hall ED. Mild pre- and post-traumatic hypothermia attenuates blood–brain barrier damage following controlled cortical impact injury in the rat. J Neurotrauma 1996; 13:1–9.
18. Permutter LS, Gall C, Baudry M, Lynch G. Distribution of calscium-activated protease calpain in the rat brain. J Comp Neurol 1990; 296:269–276.
19. Bartus RT. The calpain hypothesis of neurodegeneration:evidence for a common cytotoxic pathway. The Neuroscientist 1997; 3:314–327.
20. Kampfl A, Postmantur R, Nixon R, et al. U calpian activation and calpain mediated cytoskeletal proteolysis following traumatic brain injury. J Neurochem 1996; 67:1575–1583.
21. Maxwell WL, Polishock JT, Graham DI. A mechanistic analysis of nondisruptive axonal injury: a review. J Neurotrauma 1997; 14:419–440.
22. Conti AC, Raghupathi R, Rink AD, Trojanowski JQ, McIntosh TK. Experimental brain injury induces regionally distinct apoptosis during the acute and delayed post-traumatic period. J Neurosci 1998.
23. Clark RSB, Chen J, Watkins SC, et al. Apoptosis-suppressor gene bcl-2 expression after traumatic brain injury in rats. J Neurosci 1997; 17:9172–91782.
24. Sahs AL, Hartman EC, Aronson SM. Guidelines for Stroke Care. Washington, DC, U.S. Government Printing Office, Department of Health, Education, and Welfare Publication No. (HRA); 76-14017 1976.
25. Feigenson JS. Practical guidelines for stroke rehabilitation. Parts 1 and 2. Neurol Neurosurg Update Series, 2: Lessons 35 and 36, 1981.
26. Granger CV, Greer DS, Liset E, Coulombe J, O'Brien E. Measurement of outcomes of care for stroke patients. Stroke 1975; 6:34–41.
27. Anderson, RS, ed. (1968). Army Medical Specialist Corps. Washington, DC: Government printing office.
28. Rusk H. A World to Care For. The Autobiography of Howard Rusk. New York: Random House. alist corp. Washington DC: Government Printing Office 1977.

29. Kabat H. Studies on neuromuscular dysfunction. XI. New principles of neuromuscular education. Permanente Foundation Medical Bulletin 1947; 5:111–123.
30. Rood MS. Occupational therapy in the treatment of cerebral palsy. Physical Therapy Reviews 1952; 32:76–82.
31. Rood MS. Neurophysiologic reactions as a basis for physical therapy. Physical Therapy Reviews 1954; 34:444–449.
32. Rood MS. The use of sensory receptors to activate, facilitate, and inhibit motor response, autonomic and somatic in developmental sequence. In: Slatterly C, ed. Approaches to the Treatment of Patients with Neuromuscular Deficits. Dubuque, IA: Little Brown, 1964:26–37.
33. Brunnstrom S. Movement Therapy in Hemiplegia: A Neurophysiologic Approach. New York: Harper Row, 1970.
34. Bobath B. The importance of the reduction of muscle tone and the control of mass reflex action in the treatment of spasticity. Occupational Therapy Rehabilitation 1948; 27:371–383.
35. Bobath K. The Motor Deficits in Patients with Cerebral Palsy. London: Heinmann, 1966.
36. Sherrington CS. The Integrative Action of the Nervous System. New Haven, Conn: Yale University Press, 1906:7.
37. Walsche FMP. Contibutions of John Hughlings Jackson to neurology. Archives of Neurology 1961; 5:99–133.
38. Bobath B. Abnormal Postural Reflex Activity Caused by Brain Lesions. Rockville MD: Aspen publishers Inc., 1985.
39. Horak F. Assumptions underlying motor control for neurologic rehabilitation. In: Contemporary management of Motor control problems: Proceedings of the II STEP Confernce (pp. 11–27). Alexandria VA: Foundation for Physical Therapy, 1991.
40. Shepherd RB, Gentile AM. Sit-to-Stand; functional relationship between upper body and lower limb segments. Human Movement Science 1994; 13:817–840.
41. Schmidt RA. Motor learning principles for physical therapists. In: Contemporary management of motor control problems: proceedings of the II STEP Conference. (pp. 49–63). Alexandria VA: Foundation for Physical Therapy, 1991.
42. Bloom FE. CNS plasticity: A survey of opportunities. In: Bignami A, ed. Central Nervous System Plasticity and Repair. New York: Raven Press, 1983.
43. Basso, DM. Neuroplasticity of descending and segmental systems after spinal cord contusion. Neurol Report, 1998; 22(2):48–53.
44. Adams JH, Doyle D, Ford I, Gennarelli TA, Graham DI, McClellan DR. Diffuse axonal injury in head injury: definition, diagnosis, and grading. Histopathology 1989; 15:49–59.
45. Bennett C, Ayers JW, Randolph JF. Electroejaculation of paraplegic males followed by pregnancy. Fertil Steril 1987; 48:1070–1072.
46. Aisen, ML, ed. Orthotics in Neurorehabilitation. New York: Demos Publications, 1992.
47. Aisen ML, Baiges I, Rosen M. Suppression of disabling whole area tremor by application of damping. Proceedings of the European Conference on Parkinson's Disease and Extrapyramidal Disorders, Rome, 1990.

48. Bennett GJ. Applied biomechanics. In: Benzel EC, Tator CH, eds. Contemporary Management of Spinal Cord Injury. American Academy of Neurological Surgeons, Park Ridge, Ill., 1995:46–47.

49. Rossignol S, Barbeau H, Julien C. Locomotion of the adult chronic spinal cat and its modification by monoaminergic agonists and antagonists. In: Goldberger ME, Goirio A, Murrat M, eds. Development and Plasticity of the Mammalian Spinal Cord. Spoleto, Italy: Springer-Verlag, 1986:323–346.

50. Smith JL, Smith LA, Zernicke RF, Hoy M. Locomotion in exercised and non-exercised cats cordotomized at 2 and 12 weeks of age. Exp Neurol 1982; 16:393–413.

51. Finch L, Barbeau H. Influences of partial weightbearing on normal human gait: the development of a gait retraining strategy. Canadian Journal of Neurologic Science, 1985; 12:183.

52. Carr J, Shepherd R. Neurologic Rehabilitation: Optimizing Motor Performance. Chapter 5: Walking. Butterworth-Heineman, oxford.

53. Hesse S, Bertelt C, Jahnke MT. treadmill training with partial body weight support compared with physiotherapy in nonambulatory hemiparetic patients. Stroke 1995; 26:976–981.

54. Kosak MC, Reding MJ. Comparison of partial bodyweight supported gait training versus aggressive braceing assisted walking post stroke. Neurorehabil Neural Repair 2000; 14(1):13–19.

55. Knapp HD, Taub E, Berman AJ. Movements in monkeys with deafferented fore-limbs. Experimental Neurology 1963; (7):305–315.

56. Wolf SL, Lecraw DE, Barton LA, Jann BB. Forced use of hemiplegic upper extremities to reverse the effect of learned nonuse among chronic stroke and head injured patients. Experimental Neurology 1989; 104:125–132.

57. Taub E, Miller NE, Novack TA. Technique to improve chronic motor deficit after stroke. Arch Phys Med Rehabil 1993; 74:347–354.

58. Liepert J, Bauder H, Wolfgang H, Miltner R, Taub E, Weiller C. Treatment Induced cortical reorganization after stroke in humans. Stroke 2000; 31(6):1210.

59. Kozlowski DA, James DC, Schallert T. Use dependent exaggeration of neuronal injury. J Neurosci 1996; 16(15):4776–4786.

60. Peckham PH. Functional electrical stimulation: current status and future prospects of applications to the neuromuscular system in spinal cord injury. Paraplegia 1987; 25:279–288.

61. Marsolais EB, Kobetic R. Functional electrical stimulation for walking in paraplegia. J Bone Joint Surg 1987; 69-A:728–733.

62. Hogan N. Interactive robotic therapist. U.S. Patent Number 5,466,213; MIT, 1995.

63. Aisen ML, Krebs HI, McDowell F, Hogan N, Volpe BT. The effect of robot assisted therapy and rehabilitative training on motor recovery following stroke. Arch Neurol 1997; 54:443–446.

64. Feigenson JS, McDowell FH, Meese P, McCarthy ML, Greenberg SD. Factors influencing outcome and length of stay in a stroke rehabilitation unit. Part I. Analysis of 248 unscreened patients-medical and functional prognostic indicators. Stroke 1977; 8:651–656.

65. Feigenson JS, Scheinberg LC, Catalano M. The cost-effectiveness of multiple scerosis rehabilitation: a model. Neurology 1981; 31:1316–1322.

66. Heilman KM, Valenstein E, ed. Disorders in the Elderly. New York: Stratton, 1975, 103–134.
67. Robinson RG, Price TR. Affective Disorders are Related to Location of Lesion in Acute Stroke Patients. Presented at the Annual Princeton Conference on Stroke, Princeton, 1982.
68. Romano M. Sexuality and the disabled female. Accent on Living, Winter, 1973.
69. Davidoff RA. Antispasticity drugs: a mechanism of action. Neurology 1985; 17:107–116.
70. Goodglass H, Benson FD, Helm N. Aphasia and related disorders: assessment and therapy. In: Siekert RG, ed. Cerebrovascular Survey Report, pp 319–338, Bethesda, National Institute of Neurological and Communicative Disorders and Stroke (NIH), 1980.
71. Roueche JR. Dysphagia.Minneapolis, Sister Kenny Institute, Publication No. 706, 1980.
72. Sarno MT, Levita E. Recovery in treated aphasia in the first year post-stroke. Stroke 1979; 10:663–670.
73. Schuell H. The Minnesota Test for Differential Diagnosis of Aphasia. Minneapolis: University of Minnesota Press, 1965.
74. Spreen O, Benton AL. Neurosensory Center Comprehensive Examination for Aphasia. Victoria, Canada, University of Victoria, 1969.
75. Naeser MA, Alexander MP, Helm-Estrabrooks N, Levine HL, Laughlin SA, Geschwind N. Aphasia with predominantly subcortical lesion sites. Description of three capsular/putaminal aphasia syndromes. Arch Neurol 1982; 39:2–14.
76. Skelly M, Schinsky L, Smith RW, Fust RS. American Indian sign language as a facilitator of verbalization for the oral-verbal apraxic. J Speech Hear Disord 1974; 39:445–456.
77. Sparks R, Helm N, Albert M. Aphasia rehabilitation resulting from melodic intonation therapy. Cortex 1974; 10:303–316.
78. Sparks R, Holland A. Method: melodic intonation therapy for aphasia. J Speech Hear Disord 1976; 41:287–297.
79. Damasio AR, Damasio H, Rizzo M, Varney N, Gersh F. Aphasia with nonhemorrhagic lesions in the basal ganglia and internal capsule. Arch Neurol 1982; 39:15–20.
80. LeDoux JE, Wilson DH, Gazzaniga MS. A divided mind: observations on the conscious properties of the separated hemispheres. Ann Neurol 1977; 2:417–424.
81. Ross ED, Harney JH, deLacoste-Utamsing C, Purdy PD. How the brain integrates affective and propositional language into a unified behavioral function. Arch Neurol 1981; 38:745–748.
82. Smith A, Sugar O. Development of above normal language and intelligence 21 years after left hemispherectomy. Neurology 1975; 25:813–818.
83. Weintraub S, Mesulam M, Kramer L. Disturbance in prosody. A right hemisphere contribution to language. Arch Neurol 1981; 38:742–744.
84. Lima D. Overview of the causes, treatment, and orthotic management of lower limb spasticity. J Prosthe Orthot 1989; 2(1):33–39.
85. Aisen ML, Sevilla D, Fox N, Blau A. Inpatient rehabilitation for multiple sclerosis. J Neurol Rehabil 1996; 10:43–44.
86. Aisen PS, Aisen ML. Shoulder-hand syndrome in cervical spinal cord injury. Paraplegia 1994; 32:588–592.

87. Bennett C, Robinson R, Ohl DA. Electroejaculation: a new therapy for neurogenic infertility. Contemp Urol Nov: 1990; 25–28.

88. Behrman AL, Harkema SL. Locomotor training after human spinal cord injury: a series of case studies. Phys Ther 2000; 80:688–7000.

89. Bernstein N. The Coordination and Regulation of Movements. New York: Pergamonn, 1967.

90. Bracken MB, Freeman DH, Hellenbrandt K. Incidence of acute traumatic hospitalized spinal cord injury in the United States, 1970- 1977. Am J Epidemiol 1981; 133:615–622.

91. Bregman BS, Knkel-Bagden E, Scnell L, Dai D, Shwab ME. Recovery from spinal cord injury mediated by antibodies to neurite growth inhibitors. Nature 1995; 378:498–501.

92. Byrne TN, Waxman SG. Spinal Cord Compression. F. A. Davis Company, Philadelphia, 1990:5–7.

93. Carlos TM, Clark RSB, Franicola-Higgins D, Schiding JK, Kochanek PM. Expression of endothelial adhesion molecules after traumatic brain injury in rats. J Neurotrauma 1995; 12:458.

94. Colello RJ, Scwab ME: The role for oilgodendrocytes in the stabilization of optic axon numbers. J Neurosci 1994; 14:6446–6452.

95. Corcoran PJ, Jebsen RH, Brengelmann GL, Simons BC. Effects of plastic and metal leg braces on speed and energy cost of hemiparetic ambulation. Arch Phys Med Rehabil 1970; 51:69–77.

96. Dhillon HS, Donaldson D, Dempsey RJ, Prasad MR. Activation of phosphatidylinositol bisphosphate signal transduction pathway after experimental brain injury: a lipid study. Brain Res 1995; 698:100–106.

97. Dietrich WD, Alonso O, Halley M. Early microvascular and neuronal consequences of traumatic brain injury: a light and elctron microscopic study in rats. J Neurotrauma 1994; 11:289–301.

98. Dietz V, Quintern J, Boos G, Berger W. Obstruction of the swing phase during gait: Phase-dependent bilateral leg muscle coordination. Brain Res 1986; 384(1):166–169.

99. Dinsdale SM. Decubitus ulcers: role of pressure and friction in causation. Arch Phys Med Rehabil 1974; 55:147.

100. Fishman S, Berger N, Edelstein JE, Springer WP. Lower-limb orthoses. In Atlas of Orthotics. Ed. 2, St. Louis, CV Mosby, 1985:199–237.

101. Freeman JA, Langdon DW, Hobart JC, Thompson AJ. Inpatient rehabilitation in multiple sclerosis: do the benefits carry over to the community? Neurology 1999; 42:236–244.

102. Golberg MP, Choi DW. Combined oxygen and glucose deprivation in cortical cell culture: calcium-dependent and calcium-independent mechanisms of neuronal injury. J Neurosci 1993; 13:3510–3524.

103. Goodglass H, Kaplan EF. The Assessment of Aphasia and Related Disorders. Philadelphia: Lea & Feibiger, 1972.

104. Green D. Prophylaxis of thromboembolism in spinal cord-injured patients. Chest 1994; 102(suppl):649–651.

105. Guttmann L. Spinal Cord Injuries: Comprehensive Management and Research. Oxford: Blackwell Scientific, 1976.

106. Hald T, Bradley WE. The Urinary Bladder: Neurology and Dynamics. Baltimore: William and Willkins, 1982.
107. Heilman KM, Valenstein E, eds. Clinical Neuropsychology. New York: Oxford University Press, 1979.
108. Inman RP. Disability indices, the economic costs of illness, and social insurance: The case of multiple sclerosis. Acta Neurol Scand 1984; 70:(suppl.)46–55.
109. Jankovic J, Brin MF. Theraputic uses of botulinum toxin. N Engl J Med 1991; 324:1186–1194.
110. Johnson RM, Hart DL, Simmons EF, et al. Cervical orthoses. J Bone Joint Surg 1977; 59-A:332–339.
111. Kapfhammer JP, Schwab ME. Inverse patterns of myelination and GAP-43 expression in the adult CNS: neurite growth inhibitors as regulators of neuronal plasticity? J Comp Neurol 1994; 340:194–206.
112. Kaplan LI, Grynbaum BB, Rusk HA, et al. A reappraisal of braces and other mechanical aids in patients with spinal cord dysfunction: results of a follow-up study. Arch Phys Med Rehab 1966; 47:393–405.
113. Kaplan N. Effect of splinting on reflex inhibition and sensorimotor stimulation in treatment of spasticity. Arch Phys Med Rehab 1962; 43:566–568.
114. Knutsson E, Martensson A. Dynamic motor capacity in spastic pareisis and its relation to prime mover dysfunction, spastic reflexes, and antagonist coactivation. Scand J Rehabil Med 1980; 12:93–106.
115. Knutsson E. Topical cryotherapy in spasticity. Scand J Rehabil Med 1970; 2:159–163.
116. Krauss JF, Becker DP, Povlishock JR. Central Nervous System Trauma Status Report. Washington: NIH 1985:313–322.
117. Kreuter M, Sullivan M, Sjosteen A. Sexual adjustment after spinal cord injury (SCI) focusing on partner experiences. Paraplegia 1994; 32:225–235.
118. Lapides J. Neurogenic bladder: principles of treatment. Urologic Clin N Amer 1974; 1:81–97.
119. Lasfargues JE, Custis D, Morrone F, Carswell J, Nguyen T. A model for estimating spinal cord injury prevalence in the United States. Paraplegia 1995; 33:62–68.
120. Lehmann JF. Lower limb orthosis. In: Redford JB, ed. Orthotics Etcetera. Ed. 3, Baltimore: Williams and Wilkins, 1986:278–351.
121. Malick MH, Meyer CMH. Manual on management of the quadriplegic upper extremity. Harmarville Rehabilitation Center, Pittsburgh, PA, 1978; 79–88.
122. Mehrotra RML. An experimental study of the vesical circulation during distension and cystitis. J Pathol Bacteriol 1953; 65:78.
123. Miyai I, Fujimoto Y, Ueda Y, Yamomoto H, Kozaski S, Saito T, Kang J. Treadmill training with body weight support: its effects on Parkinsons disease. Arch Phys Med Rehabil 2000; 81(7):849–852.
124. Narsete TA, Orgel MG, Smith D. Pressure sores. Am Fam Physician 1983; 28:135.
125. Ohl DA, Menge AC, Sonksen J. Penile vibratory stimulation in spinal cord injured men: optimized vibration parameters and prognostic factors. Arch Phys Med Rehabil 1996; 77:903–905.
126. Piepmeier JM, Jenkins NR. Late neurological changes following traumatic spinal cord injury. J Neurosurg 1988; 69:399–402.
127. Pohl JF. The Kenny concept of Infantile paralysis and its treatment. Minneapolis-St. Paul Minn: Bruce, 1943:151–152.

128. Redford JB. Materials for orthotics. In: Redford JB, ed. Orthotics Etcetera. Ed. 3, Baltimore: Williams & Wilkins, 1986:52–79.

129. Rossignol S, Barbeau H. Recovery of locomotion after chronic spinalization in the adult cat. Brain Research 1987; 412:82–95.

130. Rubin BP, Dusart I, Schwab ME. A monoclonal antibody (IN-1) which neutralizes neurite growth inhibitory proteins in the rat CNS recognizes antigens localized in CNS myelin. J Neurocytol 1994; 23:209–217.

131. Sarno MT. The Functional Communication Profile: Manual of Directions, Monograph 42. New York, Institute of Rehabilitation Medicine, New York University Medical Center, 1969.

132. Shea JD. Pressure sores- classification and management. Clin Orthop 1975; 112:89.

133. Sipski M, Alexander CJ. Sexual activities, response and satisfaction in women pre- and post-spinal cord injury. Arch Phys Med Rehabil 1993; 74:1025–1029.

134. Smith CR, Scheinberg LC. Symptomatic treatment and rehabilitation in multiple sclerosis. In: Cook SD, ed. Handbook of Multiple Sclerosis. New York: Marcel Dekker, 1990:327–350.

135. Smith EM, Bodner DR. Sexual dysfunction after spinal cord injury. Urologic Clinics of North America 1993; 20:535–542.

136. Snow BJ, Tsui JKC, Bhatt MH, Varelas M, Hashimoto SA, Calne DB. Treatment of spasticity with botulinum toxin: a double blind study. Ann Neurol 1990; 28:512–515.

137. Solari A, Fillipini G, Gasco P, et al. Physical rehabilitation has a positive effect on disability in multiple sclerosis patients. Neurology 1999; 52:57–62.

138. Spillman AA, Bandtlow CE, Lottspeich F, Schwab M. Identification and characterization of a bovine neurite growth inhibitor. J Biol Chem 1998; 273:19283–19293.

139. Stallman JS, Aisen PS, Aisen ML. Pulmonary embolism presenting as fever in spinal cord injury patients: report of two cases and review of the literature. Journal of the American Paraplegia Society 1993; 16:157–159.

140. Stills M. Thermoformed ankle-foot orthoses. Selected Reading: A Review of Orthotics and Prosthetics. Washington, D.C., The American Orthotic and Prosthetic Association, 1980, pp 305–316.

141. Tator CH, Duncan EG, Edmonds VE, et al. Changes in epidemiology of acute spinal cord injury from 1947 to 1981. Surg Neurol 1993; 40:207–215.

142. Ver Voort S. Infertility in the spinal cord injured male. Urology 1987; 29:157–165.

143. Vinsintin M, Barbeau H. The effects of body weight support on locomotor patterns of spastic paretic patients. Can J Neurol Sci 1989; 16(3):313–325.

144. Voss DE. Proprioceptive neuromuscular facilitation. American Journal of Physical Medicine and Rehabilitation 1967; 46:838–898.

145. Weibel D, Cadelli D, Schwab ME. Regeneration of lesioned rat optic nerve fibers is improved after neutralization of myelin-associated neurite growth inhibitors. Brain Res 1994; 642:259–266.

146. Wernig A, Muller S, Nanassy A, Cagol E. Laufband Therapy based on 'rules of spinal locomotion' in spinal cord injured persons. European Journal of Neuroscience 1995; 7(4):823–829.

147. Yarkony GM, Roth EJ, Heinemann AW, Wu Y, Katz R, Lovell L. Benefits of rehabilitation for traumatic spinal cord injury. Arch Neurol 1987; 44:93–96.

6

Dementia in Multiple Sclerosis

Randolph B. Schiffer

Texas Tech University Health Sciences Center, Lubbock, Texas, U.S.A.

INTRODUCTION

Multiple sclerosis (MS) is a chronic, relapsing, and progressive disease of the central nervous system, which is characterized by heterogeneous patterns of neuropathological damage (1). In some areas of the MS brain, there is perivenular myelin loss with macrophage and T-cell infiltration; in other areas, there is more diffuse demyelination; and still other areas, there is damage and death of oligodendrocytes without remyelination. Later in the disease, glial cell proliferation becomes predominant. Multiple intermediary metabolic impairments are present in and around MS lesions, including diminished *N*-acetyl aspartate and increased glutaminase activity (2,3). MRI abnormalities of brain and spinal cord in MS patients consist of both focal and diffuse changes, reflecting the heterogeneous nature of the underlying molecular alterations in the brain (4).

Approximately 80–100 per 100,000 people have MS in the United States, making it the most frequent cause of disability in early to middle adulthood except for trauma (5). Disease onset typically occurs during young adulthood, with symptoms rarely starting before age 15 or after age 50. Common clinical features include optic neuritis, diplopia, various sensory dysesthesias, spastic patterns of weakness, vertigo and ataxia, alterations of bowel and bladder function, and others. The course of the disease is quite variable, but generally follows a relapsing-remitting pattern early, and converts after a period of years to patterns of accumulating neurologic disability. Life expectancy is not significantly affected, except in the severely debilitated, who are more susceptible to overwhelming infections.

Although the prevalence of MS is roughly 1 per 1000 in the general population, siblings of MS patients have a 2–5% lifetime risk, and parents and children of MS patients have a 1% risk. Linkage studies implicate the major histocompatibility complex and other genes involved in the immune system as some of the determinants of this hereditary risk (6).

NON-COGNITIVE NEUROPSYCHIATRIC SYNDROMES IN MS

A range of non-cognitive neuropsychiatric syndromes occur commonly among people with MS, and these behavioral changes can make it more difficult to recognize and treat the cognitive loss syndromes (7). A list of these non-cognitive syndromes appears in Table 1, followed by a brief discussion of the clinical features of each.

Euphoria

A euphoric alteration in background affective tone occurs in up to 10% of MS patients with more advanced disease (8). The euphoria syndrome almost certainly represents a true neurobehavioral syndrome, related to accumulated lesions in subfrontal and other limbic/diencephalic circuitry (8). This syndrome differs from mania, and variants of other accelerated psychopathology, by the absence of irritating, aggressive, or psychotic emotional features. Euphoria is a clinical marker for the presence of co-occurring cognitive deficits (9).

Pathological Laughing and Weeping

Pathological laughing and weeping is a neurobehavioral syndrome characterized by fluctuating affective expression that is exaggerated, or discordant with the underlying emotional state. Standardized diagnostic criteria have not been established for this syndrome, but the prevalence in MS populations is probably above 10% in patients with advanced disease (10). These symptoms appear to be related to lesions that interrupt the corticobulbar motor pathways bilaterally, releasing reflex mechanisms for facial expression from cortical control (11). Again, the clinical presence of pathological laughing and weeping in MS patients suggests the co-occurrence of one of the cognitive deficit syndromes described subsequently.

Table 1   Non-Cognitive Neuropsychiatric Syndromes in Multiple Sclerosis

Euphoria
Depressive spectrum disorders
Bipolar disorders
Pathological laughing and weeping
Psychosis

Mood Disorders

Bipolar Disorder

As many as 10% of MS patients may fulfill criteria for bipolar disorder, compared to less than 1% of the general population (12,13). Unlike the emotional syndromes described earlier, bipolar disorder may occur throughout the MS disease course, including patients who are mildly affected neurologically. The reasons for the association of this mood cycling disorder with MS are not known.

Depression

The lifetime prevalence of major depression in MS patients is as high as 60% during the disease course (14). Point prevalence rates for major depression syndromes in MS clinic populations are in the range of 14%, but may be even higher in community samples (15). These rates of depressive spectrum disorders are significantly elevated when compared with rates of depression reported in the general U.S. population (16). MS patients have a greater prevalence of depression than patients with comparable disability from other neurological conditions (17,18). The depressive syndromes associated with MS occur with significant frequency across the natural history of the neurological disease, including patients with very mild forms of MS (19). The presence of depressive symptomatology does not correlate well with the severity of neurological disability as measured by instruments such as the Kurtzke scales (20). The suicide rate among MS patients is 7.5 times the rate for the age-matched general population, and is driven substantially by the presence of intercurrent depression (21).

Some of the vulnerability to affective disorders in MS patients may be conferred by the alterations in cognitive function described later. There are reports that MS-associated mood disorders occur more commonly in MS patients with cognitive impairments than in those who are cognitively intact (22). There are several potential interactions between the domains of cognition and mood. For example, visuospatial recognition difficulties could interfere with the interpretation of facial and prosodic emotional states in the faces and behaviors of others. Certain coping strategies that mediate functional achievement could be compromised by poor cognition (23).

Psychosis

The prevalence of psychosis in MS patients is not known, although it occurs much less frequently than affective disorders. A temporal link, with neurological symptoms of MS either preceding or occurring around the time of psychotic manifestation, suggests an etiological association (24). Psychosis also occurs at a later age in MS patients (the mean age is 36 compared with 28 in patients without MS), further supporting the possibility of a causal relationship between MS and psychotic symptoms. Little is known concerning intermediary connections between cognitive impairment in MS and psychotic mental syndromes.

COGNITIVE IMPAIRMENT SYNDROMES

The various syndromes of cognitive impairment associated with MS are receiving increasing attention from the National Multiple Sclerosis Society and other research funding agencies (25). These syndromes are more important detractors from quality of life and employability among MS patients than was thought in the past (26).

Dementia

Impairment of cognitive function on at least one neuropsychological test can be demonstrated in about 50% of MS patients, whether assessed in clinical settings or in community-based studies (27,28). This does not mean that this is the number of MS patients who have dementia. The diagnosis of dementia presently requires the demonstration of significant social or vocational functional impairment attributable to cognitive loss (29). The presence of social or vocational functional loss cannot be discerned from cognitive test results alone, but requires traditional clinical history-taking, preferably with input from a third party, such as a caregiver or employer (30).

The pattern of cognitive deficits seen in MS patients generally affects the cognitive domains listed in Table 2 (31). Basic language skills and verbal intelligence are relatively spared, which contributes to the difficulty of early clinical recognition of these cognitive loss syndromes.

Furthermore, accepted measures of overall impairment in MS, such as the expanded disability status scale (32), do not reflect the presence or extent of cognitive impairment.

Cross-sectional studies of MS patients have found little correlation between the severity of cognitive deficits and disease duration or the degree of physical disability (28). Cognitive impairment may present as an early isolated symptom of MS, or it may be minimal in an otherwise severely affected patient (33,34). Furthermore, clinical activity, as measured by relapse rate or change in disability level, is also a poor predictor of cognitive deficits (35).

The P300, a long-latency component of cortical event-related potentials, is prolonged in MS patients as it is in other neurological disorders that cause cognitive deficits (36). The latency is related to the degree of cognitive impairment, with longer latencies associated with poorer performance, especially on tests sensitive to impairment of learning and memory retrieval (37).

Table 2   Cognitive Domains Affected by Multiple Sclerosis

Information processing
Maintenance of attention
Recent memory
Concept formation and problem-solving

Attention and Information Processing Speed

Simple attention span, measured by rote repetition of brief random number sequences, is generally intact in MS patients (28,38). However, on more complex tests of attention, deficits are consistently observed (39). For example, on the symbol digit modalities test (40), MS patients show deficits in sustained attention and rapid information processing (41). Meta-analysis of neuropsychological test performance in MS patients suggests poorer performance on tasks requiring rapid information processing, regardless of the specific cognitive domain tested (42).

Learning and Memory

MS patients show consistent deficits in recall of verbal and non-verbal information presented minutes to hours previously (38,43). Active recall of previously learned information is usually more impaired than is recognition recall of such information, such as performance on multiple choice or forced choice testing. This discrepancy was initially interpreted as evidence of impaired memory retrieval, with relative preservation of memory encoding and storage (43). More recent studies suggest that the process of memory encoding is also impaired in many MS patients. On learning tasks in which target information is presented repeatedly over a series of trials, MS patients recall less on the initial presentations than do controls, but their overall learning curve is similar to that of the controls (44). That is, the MS patients are slower to learn semantic information under testing conditions, but once acquired, the information can be recalled (45).

These findings suggest that MS patients might be good candidates for types of cognitive rehabilitation, which emphasize repetition, and perhaps time-delayed information acquisition.

Conceptual and Executive Ability

Abstract reasoning and mental flexibility are frequently impaired in MS (38). Rao et al. (28) found significant impairment in 8% to 19% of patients on tests, such as the Wisconsin card sorting test, a measure of conceptual and executive function (16). On this test, MS patients require extra trials to discover the correct sorting principle, and they perseverate, using the same sorting principle when it is no longer effective. Although these behaviors are consistent with dysfunction of the frontal–subcortical axis, conceptual and executive deficits can also result from diffuse brain dysfunction (38).

Visual Information Processing

Observed discrepancies between verbal and performance IQs in MS suggest impairment of visual information processing. On standardized measures of visual information processing, MS patients show impairment compared to healthy controls (28,47). Some of these tests address more than one cognitive, perceptual or motor domain, however, so the nature of the deficits reported remains uncertain.

Language

Classic aphasias have rarely been reported in MS (48,49), but deficits have been noted on confrontation-naming tests and word-list generation tasks (34,47,50). Related abilities, such as reading and writing, have received little empirical attention.

Cognitive Emotional Processing Disorders

The patterns of demyelination in MS heavily affect intrahemispheric and interhemispheric fasciculi and the corpus callosum (51,52). It is not surprising that a variety of higher order processing deficits have been identified in such patients. Interhemispheric transfer deficits are seen in a variety of complex neuropsychological domains involving dichotic listening, and tachistoscopic measures (42,53). Pelletier et al. (54) suggested that specific regions of demyelination in the corpus callosum may lead to specific interhemispheric transfer deficits.

The functional implications of such higher-order neuropsychological deficits are not yet known, but may well affect such interpersonal signaling systems as the interpretation facial and prosodic emotional discrimination system (55). Such deficits in propositional and prosodic emotional communication could confer predispositions to some of the emotional and behavioral difficulties described earlier under Non-Cognitive Neuropsychiatric Syndromes.

Neural Substrates of Cognitive Deficits

There is a modest, positive correlation between the cognitive impairment syndromes of MS and various imaging measures of neurological damage, including total T2 lesion volume, third ventricle enlargement, corpus callosum atrophy, and ventricle-brain ratios (56,57). Bilateral frontal lobe atrophy on imaging may be the best predictor of the presence of cognitive impairments (58).

There are reports of more discrete correlations between the presence of focal lesion patterns by MRI and dysfunction of specific cognitive domains. Studies suggest, for example, that temporal lobe lesions near the hippocampi are associated with anterograde memory deficits (59), and that frontal lobe lesions are associated with conceptual reasoning deficits, as measured by the Wisconsin card sorting test (60). Similarly, corpus callosum size is a strong predictor of impaired information processing speed and tasks requiring interhemispheric transfer, while anterior corpus callosum atrophy is specifically associated with decreased verbal fluency (61,62). Lesion activity, measured using serial MRI scans to determine ongoing pathological changes, is modestly associated with cognitive deterioration over six months (63).

Correlational studies such as these have clinical and scientific limitations imposed by the dynamic and diffuse molecular pathology of the disease. When MR spectroscopy techniques are applied to MS patients with verbal learning deficits, decreased levels of *N*-acetyl aspartate are found in subfrontal areas, apart from lesion counts (64).

Screening and Clinical Assessment

Standard cognitive screening tests, such as the mini-mental state examination, appear quite insensitive to cognitive deficits in MS, even in patients who show cognitive impairment on formal neuropsychological evaluation and in everyday functioning (65).

A number of measures have been devised to assist in screening MS patients for cognitive impairment and in deciding whether to refer for comprehensive neuropsychological evaluation. For example, Beatty et al. (66) devised a screening examination that could be administered in the doctor's office, requiring 5–10 min of professional contact and an additional 20 min of self-administered testing by the patient. The screening examination showed 86% sensitivity and 90% specificity for determining which patients have significant deficits on complete neuropsychological testing. Nevertheless, these screening tests are still fairly cumbersome and are not in widespread use. Furthermore, results from screening tests cannot fully describe the extent and pattern of deficits present, making full neuropsychological testing the established standard for patients with suspected impairment.

A recent consensus conference has recommended a 90-min neuropsychological battery to be used in the assessment of MS patients, called the minimal assessment of cognitive function in MS (MACFIMS) (67).

Treatment of Cognitive Disorders

Pharmacological approaches to the cognitive impairment syndromes of MS initially utilized agents such as 4-aminopyridine, which may improve transmission in demyelinated neuronal systems. Such an approach failed, however (68). It was hoped that the development of the immunomodulator treatments for MS might favorably affect cognition. Accordingly, neuropsychological measures for five cognitive domains were assessed as dependent variables in the pivotal trial of glatiramer acetate in 248 relapsing–remitting MS patients, randomized either to glatiramer or to placebo (69). However, only practice effect improvement in neuropsychological test performance was seen in these patients, and the improvements were equal in treatment and control groups. More favorable results were found in the interferon Beta-1a pivotal trial, where improvement was seen in the treated group on measures of information processing and learning (70).

In general, the same neuropsychological rehabilitation principles established in the care of patients with stroke, brain-injury, and other neurological insults apply to MS. Following thorough evaluation of the deficits present, an individualized plan for restitution of function, compensation with relatively spared cognitive functions, and adaptation using external aids may significantly improve functional ability (71). Physiatrists or neuropsychologists with experience in cognitive therapy are generally best equipped to develop appropriately comprehensive plans. Although preliminary studies suggest that these strategies may be helpful, their overall success and the relative utility of specific interventions in MS patients have not been thoroughly assessed in controlled studies (72).

SUMMARY

MS is associated with a variety of cognitive deficits, including impaired sustained attention, information processing speed, memory retrieval, learning, and executive functions. Depression, bipolar disorder, and other affective disorders are also common. These symptoms appear to be directly related to lesions detected by MRI, suggesting that MS may serve as a model for understanding brain–behavior relationships. Little attention has been paid to specific strategies for the management and rehabilitation of these symptoms, but as new treatments for MS emerge, studies aimed at these issues should be forthcoming.

REFERENCES

1. Ludwin SK. Understanding multiple sclerosis: lessons from pathology. Ann Neurol 2000; 46:691–693.
2. Werner P, Pitt D, Raine CS. Multiple sclerosis: altered glutamate homeostasis in lesions correlates with oligodendrocyte and axonal damage. Ann Neurol 2001; 50:169–180.
3. Bjartmar C, Kidd G, Mork S, et al. Neurological disability correlates with spinal cord axonal loss and reduced N-acetyl aspartate in chronic multiple sclerosis patients. Ann Neurol 2000; 48:893–901.
4. Bergers E, Bot JCJ, van der Valk P, et al. Diffuse signal abnormalities in the spinal cord in multiple sclerosis: direct postmortem in situ magnetic resonance imaging correlated with in vitro high-resolution magnetic resonance imaging and histopathology. Ann Neurol 2002; 51:652–656.
5. Arnason BGW, Wojcik WJ. Multiple sclerosis: an update. Prog Neurol 2000; 2:3–22.
6. Hillert J. Human leukocyte antigen studies in multiple sclerosis. Ann Neurol 1994; 36(suppl):S15–S17.
7. Schiffer RB. Neuropsychiatric problems in patients with multiple sclerosis. In: Lauterbach EC, ed. Psych Ann 2002; 32:128–132.
8. Minden SL, Schiffer RB. Affective disorders in multiple sclerosis. Review and recommendations for clinical research. Arch Neurol 1990; 47:98–104.
9. Surridge D. An investigation into some psychiatric aspects of multiple sclerosis. Br J Psych 1969; 115:749–764.
10. Patterson KM, Weinstein A, Rao SM. Spontaneous emotional expression and subjective emotional experience in MS. Poster presented at National Academy of Neuropsychology meeting. San Francisco, October 1995.

11. Schiffer RB, Herndon RM, Rudick RA. Treatment of pathologic laughing and weeping with amitriptyline. N Eng J Med 1985; 312:1480–1482.

12. Joffe RT, Lippert GP, Gray TA, et al. Mood disorder and multiple sclerosis. Arch Neurol 1987; 44:376–378.

13. Schiffer RB, Wineman NM, Weitkamp LR, et al. Association between bipolar affective disorder and multiple sclerosis. Am J Psych 1986; 143:94–95

14. Feinstein A, Feinstein K. Depression associated with multiple sclerosis. Looking beyond diagnosis to symptom expression. J Affect Disord 2001; 66(2–3):193–198.

15. Chwastiak L, Ehde DM, Gibbons LE, et al. Depressive symptoms and severity of illness in multiple sclerosis: epidemiologic study of a large community sample. Am J Psych 2002; 159:1862–1868.

16. Anthony JC, Folstein M, Romanoski AJ, et al. Comparison of the Lay Diagnostic Interview Schedule and a standardized psychiatric diagnosis. Arch Gen Psych 1995; 42:667–675.

17. Schiffer RB, Babigian HM. Behavioral disorders in multiple sclerosis, temporal lobe epilepsy, and amyotrophic lateral sclerosis. An epidemiologic study. Arch Neurol 1984; 41:1067–1069.

18. Schubert DS, Foliart RH. Increased depression in multiple sclerosis patients. A meta-analysis. Psychosomatics 1993; 34:124–130.

19. Sullivan MJL, Weinshenker B, Mikail S, et al. Depression before and after diagnosis of multiple sclerosis. Multiple Sclerosis 1995; 1:104–108.

20. Moller A, Wiedemann G, Rohde U, et al. Correlates of cognitive impairment and depressive mood disorder in multiple sclerosis. Acta Psychiatr Scand 1994; 89:117–121.

21. Feinstein A. An examination of suicidal intent in patients with multiple sclerosis. Neurology 2002; 59:674–678.

22. Gilchrist AC, Creed FH. Depression, cognitive impairment and social stress in multiple sclerosis. J Psychosom Res 1994; 38:193–201.

23. Arnett PA, Higginson CI, Voss WD, et al. Relationship between coping, depression, and cognitive dysfunction in multiple sclerosis. Clin Neuropsychol. In press.

24. Ron MA, Logsdail SJ. Psychiatric morbidity in multiple sclerosis: a clinical and MRI study. Psychol Med 1989; 19:887–895.

25. LaRocca NG. Solving Cognitive Problems. Monograph, National Multiple Sclerosis Society, 1998.

26. Fischer JS, et al. Recent developments in the assessment of quality of life in multiple sclerosis. Multiple Sclerosis 1999; 5:1–9.

27. McIntosh-Michaelis SA, Roberts MH, Wilkinson SM, et al. The prevalence of cognitive impairment in a community survey of multiple sclerosis. Br J Clin Psychol 1991; 30:333–348.

28. Rao SM, Leo GJ, Ellington L, et al. Cognitive dysfunction in multiple sclerosis: II. Impact on employment and social functioning. Neurology 1991; 41:692–696.

29. American Psychiatric Association. Diagnostic and Statistical Manual of Mental Disorders. 4th ed. Washington, D.C.: American Psychiatric Press, 1994.

30. Morris JC, Storandt M, Miller JP, et al. Mild cognitive impairment represents early-stage Alzheimer disease. Arch Neurol 2001; 58:397–405.

31. Schiffer RB. Cognitive loss. Chapter 9. In: Holland NJ, van den Noort S, eds. Multiple Sclerosis in Clinical Practice. New York: Demos Medical Publishing, 1999:99–105.

32. Kurtzke JF. Rating neurologic impairment in multiple sclerosis: an expanded disability status scale (EDSS). Neurology 1983; 33:1444–1452.
33. Fontaine B, Seilhean D, Tourbah A, et al. Dementia in two histologically confirmed cases of multiple sclerosis: one case with isolated dementia and one case associated with psychiatric symptoms. J Neurol Neurosurg Psych 1994; 57:353–359.
34. Klonoff H, Clark C, Oger J, et al. Neuropsychological performance in patients with mild multiple sclerosis. J Nerv Ment Dis 1991; 179:127–131.
35. Filippi M, Alberoni M, Martinelli V, et al. Influence of clinical variables on neuropsychological performance in multiple sclerosis. Eur Neurol 1994; 34:324–328.
36. van Dijk JG, Jennekens-Schinkel A, Caekebeke JF, et al. Are event-related potentials in multiple sclerosis indicative of cognitive impairment? Evoked and event-related potentials, psychometric testing and response speed: a controlled study. J Neurol Sci 1992; 109:18–24.
37. Giesser BS, Schroeder MM, LaRocca NG, et al. Endogenous event-related potentials as indices of dementia in multiple sclerosis patients. Electroencephalogr Clin Neurophysiol 1992; 82:320–329.
38. Beatty WW. Cognitive and emotional disturbances in multiple sclerosis. Neurol Clin 1993; 11:189–204.
39. Grigsby J, Ayarbe SD, Kravcisin N, et al. Working memory impairment among persons with chronic progressive multiple sclerosis. J Neurol 1994; 241:125–131.
40. Smith A. Symbol Digit Modalities Test. Los Angeles, CA, Western Psychological Services, 1982.
41. Litvan I, Grafman J, Vendrell P, et al. Slowed information processing in multiple sclerosis. Arch Neurol 1988a; 45:281–285.
42. Wishart HA, Strauss E, Hunter M, et al. Interhemispheric transfer in multiple sclerosis. J Clin Exp Neuropsychol 1995; 6:937–940.
43. Beatty WW. Cognitive and emotional disturbances in multiple sclerosis. Neurol Clin 1993; 11:189–204.
44. DeLuca J, Gaudino EA, Diamond BJ, et al. Acquisition and storage deficits in multiple sclerosis. J Clin Exp Neuropsychol 1998; 20:376–390.
45. Demaree HA, Gaudino EA, DeLuca J, et al. Learning impairment is associated with recall ability in multiple sclerosis. J Clin Exp Neuropsychol 2000; 22:865–873.
46. Heaton RK. Wisconsin Card Sorting Test Manual. Odessa, FL, Psychological Assessment, 1981.
47. Caine ED, Bamford KA, Schiffer RB, et al. A controlled neuropsychological comparison of Huntington's disease and multiple sclerosis. Arch Neurol 1986; 43:249–254.
48. Achiron A, Ziv I, Djaldetti R, et al. Aphasia in multiple sclerosis: clinical and radiologic correlations. Neurology 1992; 42:2195–2197.
49. Olmos-Lau N, Ginsberg MD, Geller JB. Aphasia in multiple sclerosis. Neurology 1977; 27:623–626.
50. Beatty WW, Goodkin DE, Monson N, et al. Cognitive disturbances in patients with relapsing remitting multiple sclerosis. Arch Neurol 1989; 46:1113–1119.
51. Huber SJ, Bornstein RA, Rammohan KW, et al. Magnetic resonance imaging correlates of neuropsychological impairment in multiple sclerosis. J Neuropsych Clin Neurosci 1992; 4:152–158.
52. Simon JH, Schiffer RB, Rudick RA, et al. Qualitative Determination of MS-induced corpus callosum atrophy in vivo using magnetic resonance imaging. Am J Neuroradiol 1987; 8:599–604.

53. Lindeboom J, ter Horst R. Interhemispheric disconnection effects in multiple sclerosis. J Neurol Neurosurg Psych 1988; 51:1445–1447.
54. Pelletier J, Habib M, Lyon-Caen O, et al. Functional and magnetic resonance imaging correlates of callosal involvement in multiple sclerosis. Arch Neurol 1993; 50: 1077–1082.
55. Weinstein A, Patterson KM, Rao SM. Hemispheric asymmetrics and processing of affective stimuli: contribution of callosal communication. Brain Cogn 1996; 36:223–225.
56. Swirsky-Sacchetti T, Mitchell DR, Seward J, et al. Neuropsychological and structural brain lesions in multiple sclerosis: a regional analysis. Neurology 1992; 42:1291–1295.
57. Comi G, Filippi M, Martinelli V, et al. Brain MRI correlates of cognitive impairment in primary and secondary progressive multiple sclerosis. J Neurol Sci 1995; 132: 222–227.
58. Benedict HB, Bakshi R, Simon JH, et al. Frontal cortex atrophy predicts cognitive impairment in multiple sclerosis. J Neuropsych Clin Neurosci 2002; 14:44–51.
59. Brainin M, Goldenberg G, Ahlers C, et al. Structural brain correlates of anterograde memory deficits in multiple sclerosis. J Neurol 1988; 235:362–365.
60. Arnett PA, Rao SM, Bernadin L, et al. Relationship between frontal lobe lesions and Wisconsin Card Sorting Test performance in patients with multiple sclerosis. Neurology 1994; 44:420–425.
61. Pozzilli C, Fieschi C, Perani D, et al. Relationship between corpus callosum atrophy and cerebral metabolic asymmetries in multiple sclerosis. J Neurol Sci 1992; 112:51–57.
62. Damian MS, Schilling G, Bachmann G, et al. White matter lesions and cognitive deficits: relevance of lesion pattern? Acta Neurol Scand 1994; 90:430–436.
63. Feinstein A, Ron M, Thompson A. A serial study of psychometric and magnetic resonance imaging changes in multiple sclerosis. Brain 1993; 116:569–602.
64. Foong J, Rosewicz L, Quaghebeur G, et al. Executive function in multiple sclerosis: the role of frontal lobe pathology. Brain 1997; 120:15–26.
65. Beatty WW, Goodkin DE. Screening for cognitive impairment in multiple sclerosis. An evaluation of the Mini-Mental State Examination. Arch Neurol 1990; 47: 297–301.
66. Beatty WW, Paul RH, Wilbanks SL, et al. Identifying multiple sclerosis patients with mild or global cognitive impairment using the Screening Examination for Cognitive Impairment (SEFCI). Neurology 1995; 45:718–723.
67. Benedict HB, Fischer JS, Archibald C I, et al. MAC-FIMS. J Clin Psychol. In press.
68. Smits RC, Emmen HH, Bertelsmann FW, et al. The effects of 4-aminopyridine on cognitive function in patients with multiple sclerosis: a pilot study. Neurology 1994; 44:1701–1705.
69. Weinstein A, Schwid SR, Schiffer RB, McDermott MP, Giang DW, Goodman AD. Neuropsychological status in multiple sclerosis after treatment with Glatiramer. Arch Neurol 1999; 56:319–324.
70. Fischer JS, Priore RL, Jacobs LD, et al. Neuropsychological effects of Interferon Beta 1a I relapsing multiple sclerosis. Ann Neurol 2000; 48:885–892.
71. Prosiegel M, Michael C. Neuropsychology and multiple sclerosis: diagnostic and rehabilitative approaches. J Neurol Sci 1993; 115(suppl):S51–S54.
72. Jonsson A, Korfitzen EM, Heltberg A, et al. Effects of neuropsychological treatment in patients with multiple sclerosis. Acta Neurol Scand 1993; 88:394–400.

7

Dementia in Parkinson's Disease and Dementia with Lewy Bodies

Mark Mapstone and Roger Kurlan

*Department of Neurology, University of Rochester Medical Center,
Rochester, New York, U.S.A.*

INTRODUCTION

The dementia that can occur in Parkinson's disease (PD) and other movement disorders has been characterized as a subcortical dementia (1–3). The subcortical dementias are in contrast to the more well-known cortical dementias, the prototype being Alzheimer's disease (AD). Many have debated the appropriateness of the cortical/subcortical dichotomy in terms of the exclusivity of pathological changes to these regions. Recent research on neuropathology of these dementias reveals less of a dichotomy and more of a continuum from relatively more cortical pathology in the dementias, such as AD, to mixed cortical and subcortical pathology in the case of Dementia with Lewy bodies (DLB), to relatively more subcortical pathology in dementias associated with parkinsonian disorders, such as PD. While the traditional designation of cortical and subcortical may not accurately reflect the underlying pathology of the dementias in question, the concepts are a useful heuristic when applied to the behavioral manifestations of these dementias. Subcortical dementias are characterized behaviorally by slowed mental processing speed (bradyphrenia), attentional and executive deficits, mild retrieval-based memory problems, and neuropsychiatric changes, such as apathy and depression. This contrasts with the deficits in memory and cortical association functions, including aphasias, apraxias, and agnosias, typical of cortical dementias.

A major issue complicating identification of subcortical dementias is the fact that most definitions of dementia are based on conceptual notions derived from the study of cortical dementia phenomenology, which may not be entirely applicable to the subcortical dementias. A commonly used definition for dementia proposed by the *Diagnostic and Statistical Manual of Mental Disorders, Fourth Edition* (DSM-IV) (4) places importance on memory impairment as a defining feature of dementia (Table 1). While these criteria capture the essential elements of the cortical dementias, the emphasis on memory dysfunction is less applicable to other dementing disorders. In the subcortical dementias, memory impairment may not manifest until late in the course of the dementia, it may not be a prominent feature, or it may not be present at all. Application of criteria based on phenomenology of the cortical dementias may only serve to detect late stage dementia in subcortical disease processes. Ultimately, this may result in missed opportunities for therapeutic intervention early in the course of a subcortical dementia.

Another problem with current definitions of dementia is the premium placed on psychometric assessment of cognitive decline. Many of these measures require speeded responses, impose time limits for completion of tests, or require motor responses. For example, verbal fluency is typically defined as the number of verbal responses produced in a 1-min time period. Measures placing a premium of speeded motor responses are problematic in assessing dementia in parkinsonian disorders and may lead to an overestimation of cognitive impairment. A more balanced approach to understanding cognitive and functional decline with less reliance on traditional psychometric assessment is warranted in assessing subcortical dementias.

Table 1   DSM-IV Diagnostic Criteria for Dementia Due to PD

A. The development of multiple cognitive deficits manifested by both:
   (1) memory impairment (impaired ability to learn new information or to recall previously learned information)
   (2) one (or more) of the following cognitive disturbances:
      (a) aphasia (language disturbance)
      (b) apraxia (impaired ability to carry out motor activities despite intact motor function)
      (c) agnosia (failure to recognize or identify objects despite intact sensory function)
      (d) disturbance in executive functioning (i.e., planning, organizing, sequencing, abstracting)
B. The cognitive deficits in criteria A1 and A2 each cause significant impairment in social or occupational functioning and represent a significant decline from a previous level of functioning
C. There is evidence from the history, physical examination, or laboratory findings that the disturbance is the direct physiological consequence of PD
D. The deficits do not occur exclusively during the course of a delirium

---

Source: From Ref. 4.

Disease-Related Cognitive Deficits

In general, the cortical dementias are characterized by prominent retentive memory impairments, with associated deficits in language, visuospatial function, and praxis. However, it is clear that even with substantial overlap in phenomenology, there are different behavioral profiles within the cortical dementias (5). For example, primary progressive aphasia is a cortical dementia characterized by an isolated impairment of language in which memory is intact for the first period of the illness (6). There is even some evidence that mild cognitive impairment (MCI), thought by many to be an early manifestation of AD, may be characterized by different subtypes, with some involving primarily non-mnemonic abilities (7). It is possible that subcortical dementia syndromes might present with isolated cognitive deficits as well.

For the purposes of this chapter, we will define dementia as "a chronic and usually progressive decline of intellect and/or comportment, which causes a gradual restriction of customary daily living activities unrelated to changes of alertness, mobility, or sensorium" (8). The change of mental state should not be secondary to sensory deficits, physical limitations, or preoccupation with psychiatric symptomatology, such as stress, anxiety, depression, or paranoia. The existence of actual (not just perceived) intellectual and personality deficits should be determined either by history or examination. In this chapter, we will review the dementias associated with PD and DLB in an attempt to highlight the continuum of neuropathological and clinical changes in these disorders.

DEMENTIA IN PD

PD is an extrapyramidal movement disorder with a well-known clinical tetrad of tremor, rigidity, bradykinesia, and postural instability. Cognitive symptoms are prominent in many non-demented PD patients and may consist of mental slowing (bradyphrenia), executive deficits (9,10), working memory deficits (11,12), visuospatial deficits (13,14), and a memory deficit typically characterized as retrieval-based (15). The evolution of dementia in PD is often quite difficult to distinguish from these relatively circumscribed cognitive deficits.

Incidence and Prevalence of Dementia in PD

The prevalence of dementia in PD has been reported to be as low as 8% (16) and as high as 93% (17). An early literature review encompassing more than 2500 patients among 17 studies suggested a prevalence rate of 15% (18). More recent studies, however, report higher rates of 20–40% (19–23). The wide range of prevalence estimates is attributed to a variety of methodological issues, including retrospective analysis of patient charts, ascertainment from case records rather than direct assessments, absence of uniform criteria for diagnosis, variable inclusion of lesser forms of cognitive impairment, and failure to adjust for age. In some reports, standardized cognitive testing batteries were not employed. Incidence, not prevalence, may be a much better measure of dementia in PD, because dementia reduces survival in PD and thus detection of dementia is less likely in prevalence surveys (24).

Relatively few studies have measured the incidence of dementia in PD patients. One study found the cumulative probability of dementia over a 5-year period to be 21% for incident cases of PD, compared to a rate of 5.7% for matched controls without PD (25). In another study (26), the authors followed a cohort of 203 PD patients and found that 31% met the criteria for dementia after 12 years. In a third study, Mayeaux et al. (27) re-evaluated a cohort of clinic-based PD patients 5 years after the prevalence date and found an incidence of dementia of 69 per 1000 person years of observation, six times higher than expected in an age-matched cohort without PD. Another study identified an incidence rate of 47.6 per 1000 person years of observation (20). Another study reports an incidence rate of 95.3 per 1000 person years (28). In addition, these authors report the risk for development of dementia in patients with PD relative to the control subjects after adjusting for age, sex, and education as 5.9.

Neuropathology Associated with Dementia in PD

There does not appear to be a common neuropathological mechanism for dementia in PD. In a recent study of 100 cases at autopsy, dementia was related to AD-like pathology in approximately 30% of the cases, cortical and subcortical Lewy bodies in 10% of cases, and "typical" PD pathology in approximately half of the cases (29). Functionally, disruption of multiple parallel feedback-dependent circuits connecting basal ganglia structures with cortex (30) is thought to be a primary mechanism for cognitive deficits observed in PD (31–33). Disruption of dorsolateral prefrontal cortex, for example, is thought to be the underlying mechanism of working memory and set-shifting deficits seen in idiopathic PD (11,12). However, it is unclear at what point in the neuropathological process these isolated deficits evolve that represent a dementia.

The primary neuropathological marker of PD is the Lewy body, which is found in various brainstem regions of PD patients. The presence of this inclusion body in surviving neurons of the substantia nigra distinguishes PD from other parkinsonian disorders. Lewy bodies can also be found in the cortex and up until recently were not thought to be present in large numbers in PD. However, new staining techniques have provided the means to identify these Lewy bodies, which appear to be widely distributed in cortex of demented PD patients (34,35). A recent study (36) found α-synuclein positive cortical Lewy bodies to be a more sensitive and more specific marker for dementia in PD than ubiquitin positive Lewy bodies. Furthermore, they found that these Lewy bodies were a better predictor of dementia than Alzheimer-like changes, including neurofibrillary tangles, amyloid plaques, and dystrophic neurites. Several other pathological characteristics, such as degeneration of the medial substantia nigra (37), neurites in the CA2 region and entorhinal cortex (38), and neuropil threads in entorhinal cortex (39) have also been linked to dementia in PD. Overall, the underlying basis for progression of cognitive dysfunction in patients with PD appears to be heterogeneous (40), with variable contributions from cholinergic deficits (41), and extension of the α-synuclein positive Lewy bodies to limbic and neocortical regions (36).

Risk Factors for Developing Dementia in PD

Certain risk factors for the development of dementia in patients with PD have been reported. With the exception of older age at onset of PD (20,22,23,42–44), the results have been somewhat inconsistent. In many studies, duration of illness appears to be related to the development of dementia in PD with increased incidence of dementia as duration increases. For example, longitudinal studies have shown that dementia accrues at the rate of 40–70 cases per 1000 years of observation, representing a relative risk of almost four times that of age-matched peers without PD (20,45,46).

The relationship between duration of illness and increased risk for developing dementia raises the question of the relationship between severity of motor symptoms and the development of dementia in PD. Many studies have suggested that the severity of motor features, particularly akinetic features, such as brady-kinesia and rigidity, is related to the development of dementia (20,43,45,47). One study found that prevalence of dementia in PD was related to the Hoehn and Yahr stage with 0% prevalence at Stage I, 6% at Stage II, 16% at Stage III, 35% at Stage IV, and 57% at Stage V (48). Other studies have shown that dementia is associated with the presence of axial as opposed to appendicular symptoms (49–51). Another study found that initial presentation of masked facies may be a risk factor (52). However, the relationship between motor symptoms and the presence of dementia is not necessarily a negative one. For example, one study found that the presence of significant tremor may protect against dementia (53).

Several studies have suggested that non-motor features are related to the development of dementia in PD. For example, some studies have shown a relationship between the presence of dementia and low education or low socio-economic status (43) and male gender (54,55). The presence of depression, particularly poorly controlled depression, has been identified as a risk factor for development of dementia in PD (21,23,47,51,56,57). However, the exact nature of the relationship between depression and dementia in PD is not at all clear. These states may share overlapping neuroanatomical mechanisms or they may represent processes independently affected by separable subcortical–cortical networks.

Finally, there appears to be a moderate role of genetic factors in the development of dementia in PD. One study demonstrated that siblings of demented PD patients were three times more likely to develop AD than siblings of normal individuals (58). Moreover, when examining the risk to siblings over the age of 65, the authors revealed a fivefold increased risk of AD. A single family has been identified with autosomal dominant inheritance of parkinsonism with prominent dementia and early age of onset (59). Evidence for linkage was found on the short arm of chromosome 4. The apolipoprotein gene ε4 allele is thought to be a moderate risk factor in developing AD, but the relationship between alleles of this gene and PD dementia is less clear. There is some evidence, however, that the apolipoprotein ε2 allele increases risk of dementia in PD patients (60), while the apolipoprotein ε4 allele has little influence (60,61).

Clinical Characteristics of Dementia in PD

Dementia in PD must be differentiated from the specific cognitive impairments that are known to exist in idiopathic PD. It has been reported that a majority of PD patients have some objective cognitive impairment (62). In one study, Huber et al. (63) found that 35% of their sample of PD patients met the criteria for dementia. However, an additional 50% had measurable cognitive impairment, which did not fully meet the criteria. Thus, in this sample, nearly 85% of the patients had some form of cognitive impairment. Early in the course of the illness, PD patients demonstrate a characteristic pattern of neuropsychological impairment, which is very similar to deficits seen in patients with focal lesions of the frontal lobe. The most consistently reported cognitive deficits in non-demented PD patients are in executive function (i.e., initiating, planning, sequencing, monitoring, and shifting cognitive sets). This executive deficit can manifest as impaired memory organization during encoding and retrieval processes (31,64,65), working memory deficits (11,12,66), and problems with temporal ordering of new information (67). In non-demented PD patients, retentive memory is relatively intact. Memory dysfunction in PD appears to be primarily a retrieval deficit, compared to the deficits in consolidation and storage evident in patients with AD (52,68). Careful neuropsychological evaluation of memory function is important in distinguishing the more common retrieval-based deficits seen in PD from the retentive-based deficits characteristic of a cortical dementia. Other authors have reported deficits in other cognitive abilities including visuospatial and visuomotor skills (69) and verbal fluency (70–72).

In PD patients who go on to develop dementia, these isolated cognitive deficits worsen and additional cognitive domains are affected (73). Some authors have attributed expanding deficits in domains, such as memory, visuospatial function, and language in demented PD patients to a primary worsening of executive abilities. For example, in a recent study of demented PD patients the authors demonstrated that prominent deficits seen in recall of information could be significantly improved when cues used to help encoding were provided to facilitate retrieval (74). These authors also found that memory scores were related to performance on several tests of executive function. However, not all cognitive deficits in demented PD patients are easily explained by increasing disruption of executive abilities. For example, neuropsychiatric symptoms, such as hallucinations and delusions are common in PD patients with dementia (75). Many of these symptoms are more severe than those of patients with cortical dementias, such as AD (75). Many authors suggest that the evolution of dementia from circumscribed cognitive deficits reflects an evolution of neuropathological change beyond the substantia nigra and affecting neurotransmitter systems other than dopamine.

Treatment/Management Issues

Dementia is the aspect of PD most often precipitating nursing home placement and caregiver stress (23,76). The emergence of dementia greatly complicates therapy due to the need to reduce or eliminate anti-parkinsonian medications (e.g., anticholinergics) because of adverse mental effects of the drugs. The effect of levodopa therapy on cognitive function in non-demented PD patients is thought to be negligible, possibly due to separable subcortical–cortical mechanisms (77). However, some studies have shown task-specific improvements following levodopa therapy, especially on tasks of frontal lobe function (78). Anticholinesterase inhibitors, such as tacrine, donepezil, and rivastigmine, have shown some promise in treating dementia associated with PD (79–82). The efficacy of these medications in PD dementia may speak to the role of neurotransmitter systems other than dopamine in the evolution of dementia. The role of estrogen in prevention of dementia is not clear. However, one recent study demonstrated that it can be protective for the development of dementia within the setting of PD and may even be of some benefit for patients who are already demented (83).

DEMENTIA WITH LEWY BODIES

DLB is a diagnostic entity that has only recently come into the vernacular. This term subsumes a variety of clinical diagnoses used previously, including diffuse Lewy body disease (84), Lewy body variant of AD (85), and Lewy body dementia (86). With regard to pathology, DLB is said to be the second most common etiology of dementia following AD (87).

Consensus criteria for clinical diagnosis of dementia with Lewy bodies were proposed by McKeith et al. (88) and are shown in Table 2. While these consensus criteria have undoubtedly brought some coherence to our understanding of the clinical manifestation of the illness, DLB nonetheless is a complicated disease process and appears to represent a continuum of clinical presentations, varying based on the brain regions affected by deposition of Lewy bodies and associated cell loss (89). The sensitivity and specificity of these relatively new consensus criteria have not been adequately examined. However, in a single prospective sample of 50 dementia cases presenting to autopsy, application of these criteria resulted in 83% sensitivity and 95% specificity (90). McKeith et al. concluded that the consensus criteria might be useful for confirmation of diagnosis, but of lesser value in screening for DLB. In another study, Serby and Samuels (91) challenged the validity of these consensus criteria by analyzing 242

Table 2   Consensus Criteria for the Clinical Diagnosis of Probable and Possible DLB

---

(1) Progressive cognitive decline of sufficient magnitude to interfere with normal social or occupational function. Prominent or persistent memory impairment may not necessarily occur in the early stages, but is usually evident with progression of the disease. Deficits on tests of attention, fronto-subcortical skills, and visuospatial ability may be prominent.

(2) Two of the following core features are necessary for a diagnosis of probable DLB and one is necessary for a diagnosis of possible DLB:
  - Fluctuating cognition with pronounced variation in attention and alertness
  - Recurrent visual hallucinations that are typically well formed and detailed
  - Spontaneous motor features of parkinsonism

(3) Features supportive of the diagnosis are:
  - Repeated falls
  - Syncope
  - Transient loss of consciousness
  - Neuroleptic sensitivity
  - Systematized delusions
  - Hallucinations in other modalities

(4) A diagnosis of DLB is less likely in the presence of:
  - Strokes (e.g., positive neurologic signs or vascular lesions on brain imaging)
  - Evidence on physical examination or laboratory investigation of any physical illness or other brain disorder that sufficiently accounts for the clinical picture

---

Source: From Ref. 90.

published cases with clinico-pathological correlation of DLB. The authors found that 64% of the subjects had parkinsonism, 66% had parkinsonism with co-morbid dementia, 39% had visual hallucinations, and 30% had cognitive fluctuations. They concluded that the presence of both parkinsonism and dementia most consistently correlated with the pathological diagnosis of DLB. In a clinico-pathological correlation study, Richard et al. (92) provided evidence that the timing of clinical features best distinguishes PD from DLB, with early dementia and variably present PD motor features characterizing DLB and late dementia with early PD motor features characterizing PD or PD with dementia.

Prevalence

Several studies have suggested that DLB is the second most common form of dementia in the elderly following AD (87,90). Up to 20% of all the cases referred to specialty clinics for neuropathological assessment meet criteria for DLB (87). Rosenberg et al. (93) reported that DLB pathological changes were found in 31% of the 277 patients in a retrospective neuropathological analysis. One study reported that 26% of referrals to a dementia clinic met criteria for DLB (94), and another found 24% met criteria in an adult day hospital setting (95). Age at onset of clinical symptoms varies widely with a range of 50–83 according to one study (96). Several studies have reported that the illness results in a much faster decline than AD (97,98). However, other studies have failed to replicate a reduced survival rate (99,100). Nonetheless, there appears to be great variation in the rate of decline with some individuals showing a particularly rapid course (101).

Risk Factors

There appears to be a genetic risk for DLB with several authors reporting familial cases (e.g., 102,103). In a recent study, Tsuang et al. (103) found DLB-affected individuals in each of two pedigrees carried at least 1 apolipoprotein ε4 allele. The authors found no nucleotide alterations in α-, β-, or γ-synuclein, or parkin genes in affected individuals. There may also be an association between a specific chromosome 21 amyloid precursor protein mutation and Lewy body formation, possibly mediated by environmental or genetic factors (104). Like in AD, apolipoprotein ε4 is overrepresented in DLB (104,105). However, this overrepresentation of the ε4 allele is also linked to the presence of amyloid deposition in cortex in both AD and DLB (106) and the issue of whether the overrepresentation of ε4 is merely indicative of the emergence of co-morbid AD patholology or is linked to DLB-specific neuropathology is unclear. While there does appear to be evidence for a genetic component to DLB, no specific genetic markers have been identified. Many investigators have reported a greater preponderance of male patients with DLB (93,107–110). Kosaka et al. (109) reported nearly a 3:1 ratio of males over females.

Clinical Characteristics of Dementia in DLB

The core feature of DLB is a dementia, which has mixed subcortical and cortical characteristics. In over half of the cases, cognitive impairment is the presenting symptom (111,112). As the disease progresses, most patients will develop a severe dementia. The dementia has a fluctuating course with alterations in cognitive function occurring over periods of hours, days, or weeks. In addition to dementia, DLB is usually associated with mild parkinsonism including bradykinesia, rigidity, or masked facies. Resting tremor is usually not present. The time of onset of these mild extrapyramidal features is debated, but recent studies have suggested that they tend to occur early in the course (92). This clinical picture is in contrast to that of PD or PD with dementia in which motor symptoms precede cognitive changes. Finally, DLB is often accompanied by prominent psychiatric disturbance, including visual hallucinations, delusions, and mood alteration, most commonly depression. Recent studies suggest that of all psychiatric symptoms, visual hallucinations may be the best symptom for discriminating between DLB and AD (113).

The overall clinical picture of DLB is often very difficult to discriminate from early AD with extrapyramidal features. This difficulty is likely the result of the mixed subcortical and cortical pathology evident in these patients on autopsy.

Nonetheless, there are some unique cognitive characteristics that may aid in the clinical distinction of these other disorders. For example, in a recent study, Ballard et al. (114) found that two symptoms, delusional misidentification and hallucinations, in the early stages of dementia best identified patients with DLB from a sample of 270 DLB and AD patients. The authors report that the presence of psychiatric symptoms at presentation was a better discriminator between DLB and AD than the emergence of these symptoms over the course of the disease.

Most studies comparing DLB patients to AD patients on neuropsychological measures have reported disproportionate deficits in visuoconstruction/visuospatial abilities and frontally mediated abilities, such as basic attention and executive function in DLB patients even when matched for overall dementia severity (85,115–117). In one study by Hansen et al. (85), nine autopsy-confirmed DLB patients were compared to AD subjects matched in age, education, overall dementia severity, and interval from test to death. The authors report similar levels of poor performance on tests of episodic memory, naming, semantic fluency, and arithmetic between the groups, but the DLB subjects performed much worse on tests of attention and visuoconstruction. Furthermore, the DLB patients were significantly worse on a phonemic fluency test suggesting a specific deficit in sustained verbal output. These general findings were replicated in a larger study of 50 autopsy-confirmed DLB patients and 95 autopsy-confirmed AD patients (117). The authors report that the DLB and AD subjects were equally impaired on measures of episodic knowledge, confrontation naming, and semantic knowledge. However, the DLB subjects were significantly more impaired on tests of psychomotor processing speed, visuoconstruction, verbal fluency, and abstract reasoning. Using a logistic regression model, the authors were able to correctly classify 60% of DLB patients and 88% of AD patients based on performance on tests of phonemic fluency, WAIS-R block design, clock drawing, trail-making test (part A), and semantic knowledge.

In a recent study, Doubleday et al. (118) characterized cognitive performance in a group of 41 clinically diagnosed DLB patients and compared this to 26 AD patients matched for age and duration and severity of cognitive deficits. The authors report that inattention, visual distractibility, difficulties shifting cognitive set, perseveration, confabulations, and intrusions on tests of memory were significantly higher in the DLB group. While rare in the AD group, over 75% of the DLB patients produced intrusions on tests of memory. The authors were able to correctly classify the patients based largely on deficits in subcortical/frontally mediated skills. The presence of mental inflexibility, perseveration, and intrusions together correctly classified 79% of the patients.

Neuropathology

The neuropathological hallmark of DLB is the cortical Lewy body. Cortical Lewy bodies can be found in wide areas of neocortex, limbic, and paralimbic regions. They lack the core and halo appearance, which is typical of brainstem

Lewy bodies and were previously difficult to identify in cortex. The development of anti-ubiquitin immunostains in the 1980s led to easier identification of cortical Lewy bodies. Antibodies to ubiquitin are more specific to cortical Lewy bodies as they do not also stain neurofibrillary tangles. Staining for cortical Lewy bodies with α-synuclein is now considered the state of the art. Small numbers of cortical Lewy bodies can be found in non-demented PD patients, so the presence of Lewy bodies in the cortex does not appear to be the defining neuropathological feature of DLB. Rather, the disease-specific distribution of cortical Lewy bodies appears to be critical. For example, a recent study demonstrated that the severity and duration of dementia in a sample of DLB subjects was related to increasing para-hippocampal Lewy body densities and not neocortical densities (119). Still, the relationship between specific clinical symptoms and regional cortical, limbic, and paralimbic distribution of Lewy bodies is far from clear. One study found that the density of cortical Lewy bodies in mid-frontal cortex negatively corre-lates with MMSE score (120).

In addition to cortical Lewy bodies, DLB may also be associated with other pathological features, including βA4 amyloid plaques similar to that of AD (121), neurofibrillary tangles often found in entorhinal cortex, and Lewy neurites found in the CA2/3 region of the hippocampus (122). The most common type of cortical plaque found in DLB patients is the "diffuse plaque," which is in contrast to the neuritic plaque characteristic of AD. Mild-to-moderate aggregation of cortical plaques occurs in about two-thirds of DLB cases (110). In the remaining one-third of DLB cases, there are very few senile plaques present.

Cortical atrophy typically occurs in DLB. A recent study using voxel-based MRI morphometry showed that patients with DLB had greater regional gray matter volume loss bilaterally in the temporal and frontal lobes and insular cortex compared to control subjects (123). While some authors have speculated that the prominent hallucinations of DLB are due to primary occipital lobe path-ology, recent imaging work suggests that the occipital lobe is relatively free of gross pathology in DLB (124).

A recent study provides interesting results about the progression of Lewy body pathology in the cerebral cortex. Marui et al. (125) studied Lewy bodies and Lewy body neurites in the cerebrum of 27 DLB patients using α-synuclein staining. Their results demonstrate that Lewy body pathology begins in the amyg-dala, progresses to limbic cortex, and eventually to the neocortex. They further demonstrate that Lewy pathology begins in cortical layers V and VI, progressing to layer II and eventually to layer I. Finally, they report that the more advanced pathology was associated with concurrent AD pathological changes, suggesting that AD pathology exacerbates Lewy body pathology.

Treatment/Management Issues

Levodopa has moderate efficacy in treating the motor disturbance of DLB with approximately 40–50% of patients demonstrating significant improvement (126).

With regard to the cognitive changes in DLB, several studies have pointed to cholinesterase inhibitors as a potential avenue for treatment. In general, cholinesterase inhibitors are well-tolerated and provide a modicum of efficacy for fluctuating confusion, cognition, and psychiatric symptoms. In a placebo-controlled trial of rivastigmine in 120 DLB patients (127), the authors found significant improvement in psychiatric features, including a reduction in hallucinations, delusions, apathy, and anxiety. While these authors did not report significant worsening of parkinsonian features in this study, several other studies have reported that anticholinesterase inhibitors can lead to a worsening of parkinsonism (128).

DLB patients may display an unusual sensitivity to typical antipsychotic medications. Treatment with typical neuroleptics may be poorly tolerated and can result in irreversible worsening of parkinsonian motor symptoms. Severe neuroleptic sensitivity can result in exacerbation of hallucinations, clouding of consciousness, and autonomic dysfunction. These reactions have been reported to occur in 40–50% of neuroleptic-treated DLB patients and can significantly increase mortality (129).

There is conflicting evidence about the efficacy of the new atypical antipsychotics, such as risperidone and olanzapine. In several early studies, these medications resulted in roughly the same side-effect profile as classical neuroleptics (130,131). However, in a recent study, Cummings et al. (132) found no increase in parkinsonian symptoms in DLB patients treated with 5, 10, or 15 mg of olanzapine in a double-blind randomized controlled trial. The results demonstrated a dose-dependent response, with 5 mg of olanzapine significantly reducing hallucinations and delusions, 10 mg significantly reducing delusions, and 15 mg not differing from placebo.

ACKNOWLEDGMENT

We thank Maria Fagnano for her assistance in preparing this manuscript.

REFERENCES

1. Albert ML, Feldman RG, Willis AL. The 'subcortical dementia' of progressive supranuclear palsy. J Neurol Neurosurg Psych 1974; 37:121–130.
2. McHugh PR, Folstein MF. Psychiatric syndromes of Huntington's chorea: a clinical and phenomenologic study. In: Benson DF, Blumer D, eds. Psychiatric Aspects of Neurologic Diseases. New York: Grune and Stratton, 1975:267–286.
3. Cummings JL, Benson DF. Subcortical dementia: review of an emerging concept. Arch Neurol 1984; 41:874–879.
4. American Psychiatric Association. Diagnostic and Statistical Manual of Mental Disorders, 4th ed. Washington, DC: American Psychiatric Publishing, 1994.
5. Weintraub S, Mesulam MM. Four neuropsychological profiles in dementia. In: Boller F, Grafman J, eds. Handbook of Neuropsychology, Vol. 8. Amsterdam: Elsevier, 1993:253–281.

6. Mesulam MM. Slowly progressive aphasia without generalized dementia. Ann Neurol 1982; 11:592–598.
7. Mapstone M, Steffenella T, Duffy CJ. A visuospatial variant of mild cognitive impairment: getting lost between aging to AD. Neurology 2003; 60:802–808.
8. Mesulam MM. Aging, Alzheimer's disease and dementia: clinical and neurobiological perspectives. In: Mesulam MM, ed. Principles of Behavioral and Cognitive Neurology. New York: Oxford University Press, 2000:439–506.
9. Cronin-Golomb A, Corkin S, Growdon JH. Impaired problem solving in Parkinson's disease: impact of a set-shifting deficit. Neuropsychologia 1994; 32:579–593.
10. Jacobs DM, Marder K, Cote LJ, Sano M, Stern Y, Mayeux R. Neuropsychological characteristics of preclinical dementia in Parkinson's disease. Neurology 1995; 45:1691–1696.
11. Postle BR, Jonides J, Smith EE, Corkin S, Growdon JH. Spatial, but not object, delayed response is impaired in early Parkinson's disease. Neuropsychology 1997; 11:171–179.
12. Owen AM, Iddon JL, Hodges JR, Summers BA, Robbins TW. Spatial and non-spatial working memory at different stages of Parkinson's disease. Neuropsychologia 1997; 35:519–532.
13. Finton MJ, Lucas JA, Graff-Radford NR, Uitti RJ. Analysis of visuospatial errors in patients with Alzheimer's disease or Parkinson's disease. J Clin Exp Neuropsychol 1998; 20:186–193.
14. Levin BE, Llabre MM, Reisman S, Weiner WJ, Sanchez-Ramos J, Singer C, Brown MC. Visuospatial impairment in Parkinson's disease. Neurology 1991; 41:365–369.
15. Breen EK. Recall and recognition memory in Parkinson's disease. Cortex 1993; 29:91–102.
16. Taylor A, Saint-Cyr JA, Lang AE. Dementia prevalence in Parkinson's disease. Lancet 1985; 1:1037.
17. Pirozzolo F, Hansch C, Mortimer. Dementia in Parkinson's disease: Neuropsychological analysis. Brain Cogn 1982; 1:71–83.
18. Brown RG, Marsden CD. How common is dementia in Parkinson's disease? Lancet 1984; ii:1262–1265.
19. Mayeux R, Denaro J, Hemenegildo N, Marder K, Tang MX, Cote LJ, Stern Y. A population-based investigation of Parkinson's disease with and without dementia. Relationship to age and gender. Arch Neurol 1992; 49:492–497.
20. Biggins CA, Boyd JL, Harrop FM, Madeley P, Mindham RH, Randall JI, Spokes EG. A controlled, longitudinal study of dementia in Parkinson's disease. J Neurol Neurosurg Psych 1992; 55:566–571.
21. Friedman A, Barcikowska M. Dementia in Parkinson's disease. Dementia 1994; 5:12–16.
22. Tison F, Dartigues JF, Auriacombe S, Letenneur L, Boller F, Alperovitch A. Dementia in Parkinson's disease: a population-based study in ambulatory and institutionalized individuals. Neurology 1995; 45:705–708.
23. Aarsland D, Tandberg E, Larsen JP, Cummings JL. Frequency of dementia in Parkinson disease. Arch Neurol 1996; 53:538–542.
24. Marder K, Leung D, Tang M, Bell K, Dooneief G, Cote L, Stern Y, Mayeux R. Are demented patients with Parkinson's disease accurately reflected in prevalence surveys? A survival analysis. Neurology 1991; 41:1240–1243.

25. Rajput AH, Offord KP, Beard CM, Kurland LT. A case-control study of smoking habits, dementia, and other illnesses in idiopathic Parkinson's disease. Neurology 1987; 37:226–232.
26. Elizan TS, Sroka H, Maker H, Smith H, Yahr MD. Dementia in idiopathic Parkinson's disease. Variables associated with its occurrence in 203 patients. J Neural Transm 1986; 65:285–302.
27. Mayeux R, Chen J, Mirabello E, Marder K, Bell K, Dooneieff G, Cote L, Stern Y. An estimate of the incidence of dementia in idiopathic Parkinson's disease. Neurology 1990; 40:1513–1417.
28. Aarsland D, Andersen K, Larsen JP, Lolk A, Nielsen H, Kragh-Sorensen P. Risk of dementia in Parkinson's disease: a community-based, prospective study. Neurology 2001; 56:730–736.
29. Hughes AJ, Daniel SE, Kilford D, Lees AJ. Accuracy of clinical diagnoses of idiopathic Parkinson's disease: a clinico-pathological study of 100 cases. J Neurol Neurosurg Psych 1992; 55:181–184.
30. Alexander GE, DeLong MR, Strick PL. Parallel organization of functionally segregated circuits linking basal ganglia and cortex. Annu Rev Neurosci 1986; 9:357–381.
31. Taylor AE, Saint-Cyr JA, Lang AE. Frontal lobe dysfunction in Parkinson's disease. The cortical focus of neostriatal outflow. Brain 1986; 109:845–883.
32. Mohr E, Fabbrini G, Williams J, Schlegel J, Cox C, Fedio P, Chase TN. Dopamine and memory function in Parkinson's disease. Movement Disord 1989; 4:113–120.
33. Malapani C, Pillon B, Dubois B, Agid Y. Impaired simultaneous cognitive task performance in Parkinson's disease: a dopamine-related dysfunction. Neurology 1994; 44:319–326.
34. Lennox G, Lowe J, Morrell K, Landon M, Mayer RJ. Anti-ubiquitin immunocytochemistry is more sensitive than conventional techniques in the detection of diffuse Lewy body disease. J Neurol Neurosurg Psych 1989; 52:67–71.
35. Hansen L, Salmon D, Galasko D, Masliah E, Katzman R, DeTeresa R, Thal L, Pay MM, Hofstetter R, Klauber M, et al. The Lewy body variant of Alzheimer's disease: a clinical and pathologic entity. Neurology 1990; 40:1–8.
36. Hurtig HI, Trojanowski JQ, Galvin J, Ewbank D, Schmidt ML, Lee VM-Y, Clark CM, Glosser G, Stern MB, Gollomp SM, Arnold SE. Alpha-synuclein cortical Lewy bodies correlate with dementia in Parkinson's disease. Neurology 2000; 54:1916–1921.
37. Rinne JO, Rummukainen J, Paljarvi L, Rinne UK. Dementia in Parkinson's disease is related to neuronal loss in the medial substantia nigra. Ann Neurol 1989; 26: 47–50.
38. Churchyard A, Lees AJ. The relationship between dementia and direct involvement of the hippocampus and amygdala in Parkinson's disease. Neurology 1997; 49:1570–1576.
39. Kim H, Gearing M, et al. Ubiquitin-positive CA2/3 neurites in hippocampus coexist with cortical Lewy bodies. Neurology 1995; 45:1768–1770.
40. Jellinger KA, Bancher C. Proposals for re-evaluation of current autopsy criteria for the diagnosis of Alzheimer's disease. Neurobiol Aging 1997; 18:S55–S65.
41. Braak H, Braak E. Neuropathological stageing of Alzheimer-related changes. Acta Neuropathologica (Berl) 1991; 82:239–259.

42. Mayeux R, Stern Y, Rosentein R, Marder K, Hauser WA, Cote L, Fahn S. An estimate of the prevelance of dementia in idiopathic Parkinson's disease. Arch Neurol 1988; 45:260–263.
43. Glatt SL, Hubble JP, Lyons K, Paolo A, Troster AI, Hassanein RE, Koller WC. Risk factors for dementia in Parkinson's disease: effect of education. Neuroepidemiology 1996; 15:20–25.
44. Reid WG. The evolution of dementia in idiopathic Parkinson's disease: neuropsychological and clinical evidence in support of subtypes. Int Psychogeriatr 1992; 4(suppl 2):147–160.
45. Ebmeier KP, Calder SA, Crawford JR, Stewart L, Besson JA, Mutch WJ. Clinical features predicting dementia in idiopathic Parkinson's disease: a follow-up study. Neurology 1990; 40:1222–1224.
46. Mindham RH, Ahmed SW, Clough CG. A controlled study of dementia in Parkinson's disease. J Neurol Neurosurg Psych 1982; 45:969–974.
47. Marder K, Tang MX, Cote L, Stern Y, Mayeux R. The frequency and associated risk factors for dementia in patients with Parkinson's disease. Arch Neurol 1995; 52:695–701.
48. Growdon JH, Corkin S, Rosen TJ. Distinctive aspects of cognitive dysfunction in Parkinson's disease. Adv Neurol 1990; 53:365–376.
49. Taylor AE, Saint-Cyr JA, Lang AE. Parkinson's disease. Cognitive changes in relation to treatment response. Brain 1987; 110:35–51.
50. Pillon B, Dubois B, Cusimano G, Bonnet AM, Lhermitte F, Agid Y. Does cognitive impairment in Parkinson's disease result from non-dopaminergic lesions? J Neurol Neurosurg Psych 1989; 52:201–206.
51. Hobson P, Meara J. The detection of dementia and cognitive impairment in a community population of elderly people with Parkinson's disease by use of the CAMCOG neuropsychological test. Age Aging 1999; 28:39–43.
52. Stern Y, Marder K, Tang MX, Mayeux R. Antecedent clinical features associated with dementia in Parkinson's disease. Neurology 1993; 43:1690–1692.
53. Mortimer JA, Pirozzolo FJ, Hansch EC, Webster DD. Relationship of motor symptoms to intellectual deficits in Parkinson disease. Neurology 1982; 32:133–137.
54. Bower JH, Maraganore DM, McDonnell SK, Rocca WA. Influence of strict, intermediate, and broad diagnostic criteria on the age- and sex-specific incidence of Parkinson's disease. Mov Disord 2000; 15:819–825.
55. Hughes TA, Ross HF, Musa S, Bhattacherjee S, Nathan RN, Mindham RH, Spokes EG. A 10-year study of the incidence of and factors predicting dementia in Parkinson's disease. Neurology 2000; 54:1596–1602.
56. Starkstein SE, Mayberg HS, Leiguarda R, Preziosi TJ, Robinson RG. A prospective longitudinal study of depression, cognitive decline, and physical impairments in patients with Parkinson's disease. J Neurol Neurosurg Psych 1992; 55:377–382.
57. Starkstein SE, Sabe L, Petracca G, Chemerinski E, Kuzis G, Merello M, Leiguarda R. Neuropsychological and psychiatric differences between Alzheimer's disease and Parkinson's disease with dementia. J Neurol Neurosurg Psych 1996; 61:381–387.
58. Marder K, Tang MX, Alfaro B, Mejia H, Cote L, Louis E, Stern Y, Mayeux R. Risk of Alzheimer's disease in relatives of Parkinson's disease patients with and without dementia. Neurology 1999; 52:719–724.

59. Muenter MD, Forno LS, Hornykiewicz O, Kish SJ, Maraganore DM, Caselli RJ, Okazaki H, Howard FM Jr, Snow BJ, Calne DB. Hereditary form of parkinsonism-dementia. Ann Neurol 1998; 43:768–781.

60. Harhangi BS, De Rijk MC, Van Duijn CM, Van Broeckhoven C, Hofman A, Breteler MM. APOE and the risk of PD with or without dementia in a population-based study. Neurology 2000; 54:1272–1276.

61. Koller WC, Glatt SL, Hubble JP, Paolo A, Troster AI, Handler MS, Horvat RT, Martin C, Schmidt K, Karst A, et al. Apolipoprotein E genotypes in Parkinson's disease with and without dementia. Ann Neurol 1995; 37:242–245.

62. Mohr E, Juncos J, Cox C, Litvan I, Fedio P, Chase TN. Selective deficits in cognition and memory in high-functioning parkinsonian patients. J Neurol Neurosurg Psych 1990; 53:603–606.

63. Huber SJ, Freidenberg DL, Shuttleworth EC, Paulson GW, Christy JA. Neuro-psychological impairments associated with severity of Parkinson's disease. J Neuropsychiatry Clin Neurosci 1989; 1:154–158.

64. Flowers KA, Pearce I, Pearce JM. Recognition memory in Parkinson's disease. J Neurol Neurosurg Psych 1984; 47:1174–1181.

65. Whittington CJ, Podd J, Kan MM. Recognition memory impairment in Parkinson's disease: power and meta-analyses. Neuropsychology 2000; 14:233–246.

66. Petrides M, Milner B. Deficits on subject-ordered tasks after frontal- and temporal-lobe lesions in man. Neuropsychologia 1982; 20:249–262.

67. Cooper JA, Sagar HJ, Sullivan EV. Short-term memory and temporal ordering in early Parkinson's disease: effects of disease chronicity and medication. Neuro-psychologia 1993; 31:933–949.

68. Troster AI, Butters N, Salmon DP, Cullum CM, Jacobs D, Brandt J, White RF. The diagnostic utility of savings scores: differentiating Alzheimer's and Huntington's diseases with the logical memory and visual reproduction tests. J Clin Exp Neuro-psychol 1993; 15:773–788.

69. Cronin-Golomb A, Braun AE. Visuospatial dysfunction and problem solving in Parkinson's disease. Neuropsychology 1997; 11:44–52.

70. Raskin SA, Borod JC, Tweedy J. Neuropsychological aspects of Parkinson's disease. Neuropsychol Rev 1990; 1:185–221.

71. Cooper JA, Sagar HJ, Jordan N, Harvey NS, Sullivan EV. Cognitive impairment in early, untreated Parkinson's disease and its relationship to motor disability. Brain 1991; 114:2095–2122.

72. Dubois B, Boller F, Pillon B, Agid Y. Cognitive deficits in Parkinson's disease. In: Boller F, Grafman J, eds. Handbook of Neuropsychology. Vol. 5. Amsterdam: Elsevier, 1991:195–240.

73. Stern Y, Tang MX, Jacobs DM, Sano M, Marder K, Bell K, Dooneief G, Schofield P, Cote L. Prospective comparative study of the evolution of probable Alzheimer's disease and Parkinson's disease dementia. J Int Neuropsychol Soc 1998; 4:279–284.

74. Pillon B, Deweer B, Agid Y, Dubois B. Explicit memory in Alzheimer's, Huntington's, and Parkinson's diseases. Arch Neurol 1993; 50:374–379.

75. Aarsland D, Cummings JL, Larsen JP. Neuropsychiatric differences between Parkinson's disease with dementia and Alzheimer's disease. Int J Geriatr Psych 2001; 16:184–191.

76. Goetz CG, Stebbins GT. Risk factors for nursing home placement in advanced Parkinson's disease. Neurology 1993; 43:2227–2279.
77. Growdon JH, Kieburtz K, McDermott MP, Panisset M, Friedman JH. Levodopa improves motor function without impairing cognition in mild non-demented Parkinson's disease patients. Parkinson Study Group. Neurology 1998; 50:1327–1331.
78. Owen AM, James M, Leigh PN, Summers BA, Marsden CD, Quinn NP, Lange KW, Robbins TW. Fronto-striatal cognitive deficits at different stages of Parkinson's disease. Brain 1992; 115:1727–1751.
79. Mori S. Responses to donepezil in Alzheimer's disease and Parkinson's disease. Ann NY Acad Sci 2002; 977:493–500.
80. Werber EA, Rabey JM. The beneficial effect of cholinesterase inhibitors on patients suffering from Parkinson's disease and dementia. J Neural Transm 2001; 108: 1319–1325.
81. Reading PJ, Luce AK, McKeith IG. Rivastigmine in the treatment of parkinsonian psychosis and cognitive impairment: preliminary findings from an open trial. Movement Disorders 2001; 16:1171–1174.
82. Aarsland D, Laake K, Larsen JP, Janvin C. Donepezil for cognitive impairment in Parkinson's disease: a randomized controlled study. J Neurol Neurosurg Psych 2002; 72:708–712.
83. Marder K, Tang MX, Alfaro B, Mejia H, Cote L, Jacobs D, Stern Y, Sano M, Mayeux R. Postmenopausal estrogen use and Parkinson's disease with and without dementia. Neurology 1998; 50:1141–1143.
84. Kosaka K, Yoshimura M, Ikeda K, Budka H. Diffuse type of Lewy body disease: progressive dementia with abundant cortical Lewy bodies and senile changes of varying degree-a new disease? Clin Neuropathol 1984; 3:185–192.
85. Hansen I, Salmon D, Galasko D et al. The Lewy body variant of Alzheimer's disease: a clinical and pathologic entity. Neurology 1990; 40:1–8.
86. Gibb WRG, Esiri MM, Lees AJ. Clinical and pathological features of diffuse cortical Lewy body disease (Lewy body dementia). Brain 1987; 110:1131–1153.
87. Jellinger KA Structural basis of dementia in neurodegenerative disorders. J Neural Transm 1996; 47:1–29.
88. McKeith IG, Galasko D, Kosaka K, et al. Consensus guidelines for the clinical and pathologic diagnosis of dementia with Lewy bodies (DLB): report of the consortium on DLB international workshop. Neurology 1996; 47:1113–1124.
89. Lowe JS, Mayer RJ, Landon M Pathological significance of Lewy bodies in dementia. In: Perry R, McKeith I, Perry E, eds. Dementia with Lewy Bodies. New York: Cambridge University Press, 1996:195–203.
90. McKeith IG, Ballard CG, Perry RH, et al. Prospective validation of consensus criteria for the diagnosis of dementia with Lewy bodies. Neurology 2000; 54: 1050–1058.
91. Serby M, Samuels SC. Diagnostic criteria for dementia with lewy bodies reconsidered. Am J Geriatr Psych 2001; 9:212–216.
92. Richard IH, Papka M, Rubio A, Kurlan R. Parkinson's disease and Dementia with Lewy bodies: One disease or two? Movement Disorders 2002; 17:1161–1165.
93. Rosenberg CK, Cummings TJ, Saunders AM, Widico C, McIntyre LM, Hulette CM. Dementia with Lewy bodies and Alzheimer's disease. Acta Neuropathologica 2001; 102:621–626.

94. Shergill S, Mullan E, D'ath P, Katona C. What is the clinical prevalence of Lewy body dementia? Int J Geriatr Psych 1994; 9:907–912.
95. Ballard CG, Mohan RNC, Patel A, Bannister C. Idiopathic clouding of consciousness— do the patients have cortical Lewy body disease? Int J Geriatr Psych 1993; 8:571–576.
96. Papka M, Rubio A, Schiffer RB. A review of Lewy body disease, an emerging concept of cortical dementia. J Neuropsych Clin Neurosci 1998; 10:267–279.
97. McKeith IG, Perry RH, Fairbairn AF, Jabeen S. Perry EK. Operational criteria for senile dementia of Lewy body type (SDLT). Psychological Medicine 1992; 22:911–922.
98. Lippa CF, Smith TW, and Swearer JM. Alzheimer's disease and Lewy body disease: a comparative clinico-pathological study. Ann Neurol 1994; 35:81–88.
99. Weiner MF, Risser RC, Cullum CM, et al. Alzheimer's disease and its Lewy body variant: a clinical analysis of postmortem verified cases. Am J Psych 1996; 153:1269–1273.
100. Ala TA, Yang K-H, Sung JH, Frey WHI. Hallucinations and signs of Parkinsonism help distinguish patients with dementia and cortical Lewy bodies from patients with Alzheimer's disease. J Neurol Neurosurg Psych 1997; 62:16–21.
101. Armstrong TP, Hansen LA, Salmon DP, et al. Rapidly progressive dementia in a patient with the Lewy body variant of Alzheimer's disease. Neurology 1991; 41:1178–1180.
102. Mark MH, Dickson DW, Sage JI, et al. The clinicopathological spectrum of Lewy body disease. Adv Neurol 1996; 69:315–318.
103. Tsuang DW, Dalan AM, Eugenio CJ, Poorkaj P, Limprasert P, La Spada AR, Steinbart EJ, Bird TD, Leverenz JB. Familial dementia with lewy bodies: a clinical and neuropathological study of 2 families. Arch Neurol 2002; 59:1622–1630.
104. Rosenberg CK, Pericak-Vance MA, Saunders AM, Gilbert JR, Gaskell PC, Hulette CM. Lewy body and Alzheimer pathology in a family with the amyloid β precursor protein APP717 gene mutation. Acta Neuropathologica 2000; 100:145–152.
105. Benjamin R, Leake A, Edwardson JA et al. Apolipoprotein E genes in Lewy body and Parkinson's disease. Lancet 1994; 343:1565.
106. Olichney J, Hansen L, Galasko D, Saitoh T, Hofstetter C, Katzman R, Thal L. The apolipoprotein E epsilon4 allele is associated with increased neuritic plaques and cerebral amyloid aniopathy in Alzheimer's disease and Lewy body variant. Neurology 1996; 47:190–196.
107. Okazaki H, Lipton LS, Aronson SM. Diffuse intracytoplasmic ganglionic inclusions (Lewy type) associated with progressive dementia and quadrapesis in flexion. J Neurol Neurosurg Psych 1961; 20:237–244.
108. Kosaka K. Lewy bodies in the cerebral cortex. Report of three cases. Acta Neuropathologica (Berlin) 1978; 42:127–134.
109. Kosaka K, Yoshimura M, Ikeda K, Budka H. Diffuse type of Lewy body disease: progressive dementia with abundant cortical Lewy bodies and senile changes of varying degree- a new disease? Clin Neuropathol 1984; 3:185–192.
110. Dickson D, Crystal H, Mattiace L, et al. Diffuse Lewy body disease: light and electron microscopic immunocytochemistry of senile plaques. Act Neuropathologica 1989; 78:572–584.
111. Gibb WRG, Luthert PJ, Janota I, Lantos PL. Cortical Lewy body dementia: clinical features and classification. J Neurol Neurosurg Psych 1989; 52:185–192.

112. Kosaka K. Diffuse Lewy body disease in Japan. J Neurol 1990; 237:197–204.
113. Ballard CG, O'Brien JT, Swann AG, Thompson P, Neill D, McKeith IG. The natural history of psychosis and depression in dementia with Lewy bodies and Alzheimer's disease: persistence and new cases over 1 year of follow-up. J Clin Psych 2001; 62:46–49.
114. Ballard C, Holmes C, McKeith I, Neill D, O'Brien J, Cairns N, Lantos P, Perry E, Ince P, Perry R. Psychiatric morbidity in dementia with Lewy bodies: a prospective clinical and neuropathological comparative study with Alzheimer's disease. Am J Psych 1999; 156:1039–1045.
115. Rice V, Salmon D, Galasko D, Connor D, Thal L, Butters N. Neuropsychological deficits in patients with clinically diagnosed Lewy body variant of Alzheimer's disease [abstr]. J Int Neuropsychol Soc 1996; 2:31.
116. Walker Z, Allen R, Shergill S, Katona C. Neuropsychological performance in Lewy body dementia and Alzheimer's disease. Br J Psych 1997; 170:156–158.
117. Galasko D, Salmon DP, Lineweaver T. Hansen L, Thal LJ. Neuropsychological measures distinguish patients with Lewy body variant from those with Alzheimer's disease. Neurology 1998; 50:A181.
118. Doubleday EK, Snowden JS, Varma AR, Neary D. Qualitative performance characteristics differentiate dementia with Lewy bodies and Alzheimer's disease. J Neurol Neurosurg Psych 2002; 72:602–607.
119. Harding AJ, Halliday GM. Cortical Lewy body pathology in the diagnosis of dementia. Acta Neuropathologica 2001; 102:355–363.
120. Samuel W, Galasko D, Masliah E, Hansen LA. Neocortical Lewy body counts correlate with dementia in the Lewy body variant of Alzheimer's disease. J Neuropathol Exp Neurol 1996; 55:44–52.
121. Hansen LA, Masliah E, Galasko D, Terry RD. Plaque only Alzheimer's disease is usually the Lewy body variant and vice versa. J Neuropathol Exp Neurol 1993; 52:648–654.
122. Dickson DW, Schmitt ML, Lee VM, Zhao ML, Yen SH, Trojanowski JC. Immunoreactivity profile of hippocampal CA2/3 neurites in diffuse Lewy body disease. Acta Neuropathologica 1994; 87:269–276.
123. Burton EJ, Karas G, Paling SM, Barber R, Williams ED, Ballard CG, McKeith IG, Scheltens P, Barkhof F, O'Brien JT. Patterns of cerebral atrophy in dementia with Lewy bodies using voxel-based morphometry. Neuroimage 2002; 17:618–630.
124. Middelkoop H, van der Flier WM, Burton EJ, Lloyd AJ, Paling S, Barber R, Ballard C, McKeith IG, O'Brien JT. Dementia with Lewy bodies and AD are not associated with occipital lobe atrophy on MRI. Neurology 2001; 57:2117–2120.
125. Marui W, Iseki E, Nakai T, Miura S, Kato M, Ueda K, Kosaka K. Progression and staging of Lewy pathology in brains from patients with dementia with Lewy bodies. J Neurol Sci 2002; 195:153–159.
126. Louis E, Klatka L, Lui Y et al. Comparison of extrapyramidal features in 31 pathologically confirmed cases of diffuse Lewy body disease and 34 pathologically confirmed cases of Parkinson's disease. Neurology 1997; 48:376–380.
127. McKeith IG, Del Ser T, and Spano P. Efficacy of rivastigmine in dementia with Lewy bodies: a randomized, double-blind, placebo-controlled international study. Lancet 2002; 356:2031–2036.

128. Shea C, MacKnight C, Rockwood K. Donepezil for treatment of dementia with Lewy bodies: a case series of nine patients. Int Psychogeriatr 1998; 10:229–238.
129. McKeith IG, Fairbairn A, Perry RH, Thompson P, Perry EK. Neuroleptic sensitivity in patients with senile dementia of Lewy body type. Br Med J 1992; 305:673–678.
130. McKeith IG, Ballard CG, Harrison RW. Neuroleptic sensitivity to risperidone in Lewy body dementia. Lancet 1995; 346:699.
131. Walker Z, Grace J, Overshot R, Satarasinghe S, Swan A, Katona CL, McKeith IG. Olanzapine in dementia with Lewy bodies: a clinical study. Int J Geriatr Psych 1999; 14:459–466.
132. Cummings JL, Street J, Masterman D, Clark WS. Efficacy of olanzapine in the treatment of psychosis in dementia with lewy bodies. Dementia & Geriatric Cognitive Disorders 2002; 13:67–73.

8

Huntington's Disease (HD)

Peter G. Como

Department of Neurology, University of Rochester Medical Center, Rochester, New York, U.S.A.

Huntington's disease (HD) is an autosomal, dominant, neurodegenerative disorder that results from an unstable expansion of the trinucleotide repeat CAG in the gene *IT-15* on chromosome 4 (1–8). HD has a prevalence of 5–10 per 100,000 population. In the United States, there are approximately 30,000 individuals with clinical features of HD and approximately 200,000 individuals felt to be at an immediate risk for HD. The clinical features of HD usually emerge in adulthood (mean age of 37 years) characterized by the primary motor features of chorea, abnormal eye movements, dystonia, and in later-stage disease bradykinesia. It is well established that 100% of the patients experience progressive intellectual dysfunction culminating in global dementia. Psychiatric and behavioral symptoms also occur in a majority of patients. Symptoms of HD lead to progressive functional disability and death over a period of 10–30 years. The stage of HD is classified by the total functional capacity (TFC) scale based upon the patient's capacity to engage in employment, attend to finances, maintain domestic and personal daily activities, and ability to remain cared for in the primary residence (9). The TFC has been reliably shown to decline on average between 0.75 and 1.0 points per year and correlates with radiographic abnormalities, severity of the movement disorder, and cognitive dysfunction (10,11).

By tradition, the clinical diagnosis of HD has relied upon the emergence of abnormal motor signs in a person at risk (by virtue of a known family history of HD). The motor signs of emerging HD typically include dyskinesias (chorea, athetosis, dystonia), oculomotor abnormalities (especially slowed volitional saccadic eye movements), and alterations in tone (rigidity), spontaneous movement and alternating movements, and alterations in gait (associated arm swing) and reflexes (hyperreflexia). No single sign is pathognomonic of HD, but the constellation of these extrapyramidal abnormalities, especially their persistence or progression, provides a reliable basis for benchmarking the clinical onset of illness. In the absence of other causes of extrapyramidal dysfunction, such as exposure to neuroleptic medications, motor abnormalities remain the sine qua non for the diagnosis of HD.

Although chorea is the most conspicuous symptom of HD, cognitive deterioration and psychiatric impairment are largely responsible for the functional decline in HD, which typically includes loss of job, inability to maintain finances, inability to complete domestic and personal daily activities, and incapacity to remain in the home (12). While it is commonly accepted that severe cognitive deterioration and global dementia is characteristic of advanced HD, patients with early onset of symptoms tend to demonstrate the so-called "subcortical" dementing pattern (13) with predominant involvement of basal ganglia and anterior cortical areas. The so-called fronto-striatal-mediated cognitive dysfunction is characteristic of several neurological movement disorders, notably Parkinson's disease. The relationship between the cognitive disorder and the movement disorder of HD, particularly chorea, remains somewhat unclear. Brandt et al. (14) showed that the severity of the memory disorder is predicted more accurately by the severity of voluntary motor impairment and, to a lesser extent, by the severity of chorea than by duration of illness. Other investigators (15–17) have reported that the cognitive performance of HD patients is correlated with voluntary motor skills (e.g., reaction time, praxis) but not by ratings of chorea, dystonia, or bradykinesia. Thus, although the motor signs of HD are by far the most observable distinguishing features of HD, it is likely these motor features are secondary to brain mechanisms quite separate from those responsible for the cognitive syndrome (18).

There have been relatively few longitudinal studies of cognitive decline in HD patients. Most published studies have attempted to define a slope of cognitive decline. In a cohort of mild HD patients (TFC Stages I and II), performance in episodic and semantic memory remained stable over a period of 1 year whereas tests of verbal fluency and short-term memory/new learning declined (19). Using four grouping tests (psychomotor speed, short-term memory, visuospatial function, and semantic knowledge), Bamford et al. (20) conducted a 42-month prospective testing of early stage HD patients. Decline was observed primarily in psychomotor tasks in this cohort. More recently, Bachoud-Levi et al. (21) assessed 32 early stage HD patients as part of their intracerebral transplantation program. Patients were followed with serial neuropsychological examinations at yearly intervals from two to four years. A significant decline in overall cognitive function was noted, primarily with attention and executive function but also with language comprehension and immediate visual memory.

The largest HD database maintained by the Huntington Study Group using the unified Huntington's disease rating scale (UHDRS) includes assessment of motor, cognitive, psychiatric, and functional capacity (22). To date this database contains information on over 7000 HD patients followed for several years. Cross-sectional cognitive performance in subjects grouped by UHDRS motor ratings revealed a consistent linear decline in psychomotor speed, verbal fluency, and executive function (23–25). Moreover, in a subset of nearly 3000 HD patients, Nehl and Paulsen (23) reported that cognitive and psychiatric symptoms accounted for a unique and statistically significant portion of the variance on decline in functional capacity beyond that of motor and demographic variables.

NEUROPSYCHOLOGICAL IMPAIRMENT IN HD

Attention and Concentration

Attention and concentration are among the first to deteriorate in HD. It has consistently been demonstrated that HD patients perform most poorly on subtests of the WAIS and WAIS-R that comprise the concentration or "freedom from distraction" factor (arithmetic, digit span, and digit symbol) (26–31). It also appears that complex attentional tasks, such as the Stroop color word test and the brief test of attention, are among the most sensitive tasks in early HD and show the most decline over time (23,32).

Memory

Memory disturbances are a very prominent and early-appearing cognitive feature of HD (33–36). Deficits are noted in the learning and retention of new information (33,37,38), as well as in the retrieval of previously acquired information (39–42). In addition to these problems with explicit memory, there is now considerable evidence that specific forms of implicit memory are also impaired in HD (43,44).

Early studies of short-term memory/new learning in HD patients found poor recall of verbal material after short delays (33,45). HD patients have poor encoding strategies during learning trials resulting in poor storage and subsequent recall of new information (37). However, these deficits do not seem to be as severe as those found in Alzheimer's disease (AD) patients. Moreover, HD patients benefit from being supplied verbal mediation strategies for enhancing memory (46,47).

There are consistent findings that suggest relatively preserved recognition of recently presented material, despite marked deficits in recall. Investigators using various paradigms (e.g., free recall of word lists, selective reminding tasks, paired-associate learning) have reported that on-demand recall of new material is often in HD (33,34,48,49). However, HD patients demonstrate significantly better memory for the same information, often approaching that of healthy controls, when recognition paradigms are used (48,50–52). This consistent finding of relatively preserved recognition memory in HD has led to the hypothesis that inefficient retrieval is the major source of poor memory performance in HD (34,44,53).

Studies using the California verbal learning test (CVLT) (54), a standardized verbal list-learning task, have reported similar dissociations between recall and recognition performance in HD (55–57). Although HD patients perform as poorly as do AD and amnesic patients on the five recall trials of the 16-word list, their scores on the 44-item recognition test (16 targets and 28 distractors) are superior to those of the AD and amnesic patients (57). It is not certain, however, whether this difference between recognition and recall performance in HD is evident throughout the disease's progression. Kramer et al. (55) reported that this superiority of recognition memory may be limited to early stage HD patients. However, Brandt et al. (58) raised the possibility that this phenomenon may be test-specific as matched groups of AD and HD patients did not differ in recognition accuracy on the Hopkins verbal learning test (HVLT).

Few studies have examined visuospatial memory in HD. Moss et al. (48) assessed visual recognition of spatial positions, colors, patterns, faces, and words in normal controls and in HD, AD, and Korsakoff's syndrome patients. The HD patients performed significantly worse than normal subjects for all types of memoranda except words, again reinforcing the relative preservation of verbal recognition in HD. Jacobs et al. (59,60) found immediate visual memory to be only mildly affected in early HD patients. On the visual reproductions subtest of the Wechsler memory scale-revised, HD patients recalled and reproduced as many line drawings as control subjects, and significantly more than AD patients matched for level of dementia.

Two other features of HD patients' short-term memory deficits are of some clinical importance. In comparison with AD and amnesic patients, HD patients make few intrusion errors on recall tasks and manifest relatively intact retention over a 30-min delay period. On a test of memory for short passages (34), on the CVLT (57), and on the visual reproduction subtest (59,60), AD patients produce more intrusion errors than do HD patients. Similarly, studies assessing patients' retention of verbal and figural materials over a 25- to 30-min delay have found that HD patients forget significantly less information than AD and amnesic patients (57,61). Massman et al. (62) reported that when parameters of intrusion errors and forgetting rate are combined with differences between recall and recognition performance in a discriminant function analysis, HD and AD patients can be differentiated with better than 80% accuracy.

Memory for past events in HD is qualitatively different from that in several other memory-disordered populations. For example, Korsakoff's patients display a marked temporal gradient of retrograde amnesia, with events from the recent past more severely affected than events from the distant past (63,64). In contrast, patients with HD, even early in the course of the disease, appear to be equally impaired in remembering public events from all periods of time (65,66).

Language

Despite the progressive nature of the dementia of HD, clinically significant aphasia is rarely seen. This stands in marked contrast to the dementia of AD, and may serve as a distinguishing feature of the cortical and subcortical dementias more generally (67,68). Nevertheless, motor speech impairment is commonly observed in HD patients. Dysarthria and dysprosodia are most common, affecting approximately 50% of the early-stage patients. These speech disorders become more pronounced as the disease progresses, often precluding intelligible communication late in the disease (69–73). HD patients are also impaired in the comprehension of both affective and propositional prosody (74).

Although HD patients do not typically demonstrate aphasic syndromes, they can develop specific abnormalities in the use of the language. Caine et al. (75) compared patients with HD to those with multiple sclerosis (MS) and reported that the HD group was more impaired than the MS group in confrontation naming, repetition, and narrative language. Like patients with frontal lobe lesions (76), HD patients do not initiate verbal communication and sparsely participate in ongoing conversations, which may also reflect other cognitive dysfunction, such as attention and memory. They tend to demonstrate long response latencies and pronounced intervals between phrases, resulting in conversation that is interspersed with long gaps of silence. Syntactic complexity of both spoken and written language is reduced, and phrase length is progressively restricted (71). In advanced HD, spoken language consists of single words or short phrases that often do not constitute complete sentences. Difficulties with speech production can also be compromised by involuntary choreiform movements of the diaphragm.

Early in the course of HD, there is a reduction in verbal fluency as demonstrated on tasks such as the controlled oral word association test (COWA) (77) and category fluency tasks (e.g., naming of animals, fruits, and vegetables) (34,52,78). When HD and AD patients matched for severity of dementia are compared on word list generation tasks, significant differences emerge (78,79). Patients with HD are impaired equally on letter and category fluency tasks, whereas AD patients are more impaired on category than on letter fluency (80) Indices of sensitivity and specificity have shown that letter and category fluency differentiate HD patients from normal individuals. Since HD patients have marked deficits in retrieval and little, if any, breakdown in semantic knowledge, they have as much difficulty retrieving and generating exemplars of animals as they do have in generating words beginning with a specific.

Contrary to early reports, confrontation naming is clearly affected in HD (75,81). Performance on the Boston naming test (BNT) and other similar tests becomes poorer as the disease progresses, but patients' errors are rarely paraphasic in nature until the advanced stages. More often, patients misperceive the stimulus drawings or give responses based on only a portion of the stimuli (34,71,82,83), which may reflect either the known visuospatial impairment in

HD and/or an executive dysfunction phenomenon known as being stimulus-bound (tendency to be drawn to a salient aspect of a scene rather than integrate all visual percepts). Hodges et al. (83) compared the performance of 16 HD patients, 52 AD patients, and 52 healthy control subjects on the BNT. In addition to recording the number of errors made by each individual, errors on this task were classified as visual, semantic-superordinate, semantic associative, or phonemic. A double dissociation was found between the patient groups and error type. AD patients made more semantic-superordinate errors (e.g., calling a *harmonica* a "musical instrument") and semantic-associative errors (e.g., responding with "ice" when shown a picture of an igloo), whereas HD patients made more visual errors (e.g., calling a *stethoscope* a "tie"). Previously, Podoll et al. (71) found that 65% of all visual confrontation errors made by HD patients suggested impaired visual recognition, rather than impaired lexical selection. That is, the errors made by HD patients were primarily due to perceptual rather than linguistic impairments.

Visuospatial Function

Deficits in visuomotor performance are evident in even mild HD patients, although true constructional apraxia is rarely noted. The ability to copy even simple geometric designs is impaired in early-stage HD. Patients early in the disease also take significantly longer than age- and education-matched controls to copy the Rey-Osterrieth complex figure and typically produce less than adequate renditions (84). Deficits are also noted on the block design and object assembly subtests of the WAIS-R, which assess spatial analysis and visuoconstructional abilities.

Visuospatial difficulties in HD do not appear to be fully attributable to chorea, as they often appear prior to clinically significant movement disorders (85). Deficits are also observed on visuospatial tests that do not require speed or motor responses. Using an untimed, motor-free visuospatial task, Fedio et al. (86) found HD patients to be less efficient than normal controls in identifying differences between checkerboard-like grids. In addition, as mentioned earlier, many of the visual confrontation errors of HD patients may reflect perceptual misidentifications secondary to executive dysfunction.

Mohr et al. (87) administered a battery of six spatial tasks, plus the WAIS-R performance subtests, to 20 mildly demented HD patients and healthy control subjects. The spatial test battery was reduced by principal components analysis to three factors, together accounting for 70% of the variance. The HD and normal control groups differed significantly on Factor 1 (general visuospatial processing) and Factor 3 (mental rotation and manipulation). They did not differ on Factor 2 (consistency of spatial judgment). Factor 1 was significantly correlated with performance on the dementia rating scale, attesting to its status as a general factor. Only Factor 3, requiring the imagined movement of objects, was correlated with duration of illness.

A major visuospatial defect in HD involves the mental manipulation of personal, or egocentric, space (84). This was demonstrated vividly in an early experiment by Potegal (88). Patients with HD and healthy control subjects viewed a visual target on a table; they were then blindfolded and instructed to point to the target. The patients were as accurate as the control subjects in localizing the target when standing in front of it. Unlike the normal subjects, however, the HD patients were significantly less accurate after moving one step to the left or right.

Patients with HD are also impaired on tasks where adjustments must be made for imagined alterations in their body position in space. For example, HD patients perform more poorly on the standardized road map test of directional sense (89) than either the normal control subjects or AD patients matched for education and IQ (84,86). It is of interest that HD patients display their greatest deficits on the "toward" portion of the road map test, where greater mental rotation is required (84).

Bylsma et al. (90) replicated the finding of impaired road map test performance in HD; although patients made no more errors than control subjects, they required significantly more time to complete the task. Bylsma et al. also found early- to mid-stage HD patients to be impaired on a route-walking task. Patients and control subjects were handed maps depicting routes to be walked on a nine-location grid (3 × 3) marked on the floor. The routes varied in the number of moves required (from 6 to 11). On half the trials, subjects were required to always orient their bodies forward while traversing the route (no-turn condition); on the other half, they were required to turn their bodies in the direction they were traveling (turn condition). The HD patients were especially impaired on the turn condition. Because the turn condition requires the subject to mentally rotate the map to its original position to select the next move, these results support the interpretation of a defect in egocentric or personal orientation in HD.

Executive Function

The pattern of executive dysfunction in HD is similar in many ways to that seen in individuals with prefrontal cortical lesions and other movement disorders (e.g., Parkinson's disease or PD). These parallels are not entirely unexpected, given the reciprocal connections between the frontal cortex and the basal ganglia. At least five functionally specific, anatomically discrete pathways connecting the frontal lobes to the striatum have been described; three of them involve the caudate nucleus (91).

Many early-stage HD patients describe difficulties with planning, organizing, and scheduling day-to-day activities. Spouses and family members report that patients become less adaptable and behaviorally rigid; they tend to get "stuck" on an idea or task. In early HD, impairment of daily functioning is more likely to result from these cognitive deficits than from motor impairment (92,93). Similarities between HD and patients with frontal lobe injury are reflected on neuropsychological tests of executive function. Both types of patients display impaired attention, decreased verbal fluency, poor motor programming, difficulty in compensating for postural adjustments, inability to switch cognitive sets, and difficulties with abstraction (34,76,85,86,88).

Cognitive Function in At-Risk HD Individuals

More than 30 neuropsychological studies of individuals at risk for HD have been published since the 1970s. Despite mixed findings (94,95), the evidence is clear that cognitive and behavioral changes can be detected prior to diagnosis in individuals at risk for HD (96–102). This is consistent with patient and family reports of subjective changes in cognitive function antedating the onset of motor symptoms of HD and contributing to a decline in occupational performance and domestic daily activities (e.g., handling finances, bill paying, etc.). The available studies have varied significantly in terms of the samples and specific cognitive measures utilized, limiting comparison across studies. Thus, the magnitude and time-course of early changes in HD are unclear. Cognitive impairment in presymptomatic individuals is most robust when the sample is genetically characterized with CAG repeat length and the cognitive tests are well standardized and carefully targeted on specific, known functions of the basal ganglia and/or its connections.

Paulsen et al. (103) studied longitudinal cognitive decline in at-risk individuals from the UHDRS database. This study included 260 subjects considered at-risk for HD and not gene-tested who initially showed no motor symptoms of HD and have had at least one subsequent evaluation on an average of two years later. Based upon their motor examination, 70 of these subjects converted to definite HD subsequent to the initial visit. Baseline cognitive performance was consistently worse for the at-risk group that showed phenoconversion to manifest HD compared with those who did not. Average cognitive performance scores on the symbol digit modalities test and the Stroop interference test were consistently worse in the group nearer to disease conversion. By comparison, longitudinal change scores revealed that the at-risk group which did not phenoconvert during the follow-up study period showed improvement in all cognitive tests (likely due to practice effects), whereas performances in the at-risk group which converted to manifest disease showed decline in all cognitive domains. Moreover, the average scores for these cognitive measures were below normative expectations, ranging between 1.5 and 2.0 standard deviation below age-expected level. These results suggested that there is evidence of cognitive impairment in persons at risk for HD and the difference is most pronounced with close proximity to motor onset.

The potential underlying mechanisms of cognitive decline in HD are still poorly understood; however, findings of impaired neuropsychological function in asymptomatic, gene-positive individuals, notably those in close proximity to motor onset, may parallel striatal neuronal loss similar to that noted in neuroimaging studies of at-risk individuals (104,105). Lawrence et al. (106) found a significant relationship between striatal dopamine receptor binding on PET and cognitive performance in 17 presymptomatic individuals known to carry the HD mutation.

The fact that specific impairment in neuropsychological function may serve as a potential neurobiological marker in HD has potentially great promise in identifying disease onset, particularly if evidence of cognitive impairment antedates motor symptoms by several years. As therapeutic candidates continue to be studied, which may delay onset or slow down progression, the earliest identification of disease markers is crucial. The NIH/NINDS sponsored study, Neurobiological Predictors of Huntington's Disease (PREDICT-HD), will examine over 600 individuals with the known genetic mutation, who are asymptomatic at study entry with detailed neuroimaging, neuropsychological testing, neurological, and psychiatric assessment to more reliably identify the earliest (and most reliable) markers of disease onset. This study is a five-year observational investigation which began enrollment in the middle of 2002.

PSYCHIATRIC SYNDROMES IN HD

Psychosis

Patients with HD experience psychotic symptoms more frequently than the general population. The clinical picture includes a broad spectrum of disorders including paranoia, isolated delusional states, and psychotic states. The challenge to the clinician is to be able to recognize and treat psychotic symptoms in HD patients who have been diagnosed with this disorder, and also to consider these symptoms as the earliest manifestation of HD in patients who are at risk, as it is becoming increasingly apparent that psychiatric disturbance can antedate the onset of motor symptoms of HD.

Some patients with HD present with psychotic symptoms resembling various types of schizophrenia (107). A retrospective study of 110 patients with HD in 30 families found a lifetime prevalence of schizophrenia in 9% of the HD patients (1). In another study of 30 patients with HD, schizophrenia and atypical psychosis were seen in five patients (108). In a review of 11 studies, Mendez noted that the prevalence of psychotic symptoms in HD ranged from 3.4% to 12% (109). Other studies revealed that psychotic symptoms may be found in up to 30% of the HD patients (110). The prevalence of schizophrenia-like symptoms in HD patients is much higher than the expected 1% prevalence of schizophrenia in the general population. There is a familial aggregation of schizophrenia-like syndromes in HD families (111). There has been no clear association between the presence of psychotic symptoms and the severity of motor manifestations or CAG repeat length (112). Psychosis is more common among early onset cases than among those whose disease begins in midlife or old age, suggesting that an early age of onset may be associated with an increased risk for psychosis (113–115).

The underlying neuropathology leading to psychosis in HD is not well understood, but there are several hypotheses. The psychosis may be due to dysfunction in the basal ganglia itself with the known pathological changes that occur in the caudate nucleus or to the altered pathways linking the basal ganglia to the limbic-associated cortex. It is possible that the psychosis may be due directly to cortical disease. Psychosis in HD has been correlated with medial caudate pathology and reduced anterior hemispheric metabolism (116,117). Neurotransmitter alterations in these brain regions may also contribute to the occurrence of psychosis in HD. Dopamine has been implicated in the pathogenesis of psychosis. Dopamine, however, is relatively preserved in HD while other neurochemical systems are affected. It has been postulated that the disproportionate preservation of dopamine may facilitate the occurrence of psychosis in HD (113).

It may be difficult to diagnose schizophrenia versus a psychotic disorder due to HD in patients who have HD or are at risk for HD. It is possible that there may be an overrepresentation of schizophrenia in HD patients (118). Psychosis can be the first manifestation in some cases and is part of the clinical spectrum (119). It is also possible that there are other genetic factors that might predispose HD patients to psychosis (112,115).

In patients with HD, the most common psychotic presentation is poorly systematized paranoia that is commonly seen with aggression, irritability, and poor impulse control. Patients tend to underreport paranoia and need to be asked specifically about increased suspiciousness and distrustfulness during their clinical evaluation. Family members may not be aware of the paranoia or minimize it. Overvalued ideas, such as preoccupation with marital infidelity, are seen and may border on psychotic states. Isolated, well-defined delusional states and schizophrenia-like psychotic states are less common. For individuals who are at risk for HD and present with psychosis, it is difficult to make a diagnosis in the absence of other symptoms of HD, such as chorea. Symptoms such as apathy and flat affect are present in HD as well as in schizophrenia and are not helpful in the differential diagnosis. In patients with HD, typical psychotic symptoms are more commonly persecutory delusions, which typically do not interfere with the daily activities. Patients with HD-psychosis typically do not report hallucinations as part of their psychosis, suggesting that the presence of auditory and visual hallucinations might indicate a diagnosis of schizophrenia rather than a psychotic disorder due to HD.

Psychotic symptoms in HD patients have a more benign course, and respond well to neuroleptic treatment, compared to patients with schizophrenia. Another differentiating feature may be the age of presentation of the psychosis. HD patients may present much later in life with psychosis after having had many years of successfully employment, becoming ill in their 40s or 50s. This would be an unusual presentation of schizophrenia.

The differential diagnosis of psychotic disorder due to HD includes psychotic depression, severe obsessive–compulsive disorder (OCD), drug-induced psychotic states (cocaine-induced paranoia), mania with psychotic features, and delirium. Acute onset of confusion, agitation, and waxing and waning of the mental status are features of delirium. As in any other neurodegenerative disorder, patients with HD are susceptible to toxic or metabolic encephalopathy. In these cases, a medical cause, such as an infection, should be considered. Aspiration pneumonia can be seen in HD patients with swallowing difficulties and urinary tract infections in patients with incontinence are common causes of acute delirium in patients with HD. Other medical problems that should be considered include electrolyte imbalance and drug-induced encephalopathy secondary to medications and/or illicit drugs. In patients with gait problems and frequent falls, the possibility of a subdural hematoma should be considered.

Treatment of Psychosis in HD

Treatment for psychotic disorders in HD patients typically involves the use of antipsychotic medications. The so-called typical neuroleptic agents are often used in HD to treat the psychotic symptoms as well as chorea. Side effects of the typical neuroleptics are very common, including lethargy, extrapyramidal side effects (EPS), and tardive dyskinesia (TD) (120). Exacerbation of swallowing problems may worsen with the initiation of the typical neuroleptics. Hypokinesia with typical antipsychotic agents may be a significant side effect, especially as the HD advances in severity. Van Vugt et al. (121) reported that patients with HD who were on typical antipsychotic agents had more hypokinesia and lower scores of functional status compared with patients who were not on antipsychotics. Typical antipsychotics have also been reported to induce and worsen dystonia in patients with HD (122). This emphasizes the potential problem with the use of neuroleptic agents in HD. It is recommended to use these agents only when clinically necessary and to use the smallest dose possible. Typically HD patients respond to much smaller doses, compared to other patients with schizophrenia or other psychiatric disorders.

Atypical antipsychotics cause less extrapyramidal side effects, such as dystonia, TD, and parkinsonian symptoms (123). Clozapine has a superior extrapyramidal side effect profile as compared with other neuroleptics, but has the major disadvantage of blood monitoring for bone marrow suppression. Clozapine may be useful in treatment-resistant cases (124) and has been shown to decrease choreiform movements (125,126). The need to check blood counts due to the possibility of agranulocytosis makes it difficult to use in patients with chorea and severe behavioral disturbances. Quetiapine also has a lower incidence of producing EPS symptoms and does not have the bone marrow suppression problems associated with clozapine. It is also useful for irritability, agitation, and insomnia in HD, although there are no reported studies indicating its efficacy in psychosis in HD. Olanzapine is another atypical neuroleptic with a benign EPS profile which has been used in HD to help with psychosis, irritability, insomnia, and obsessional thinking (127). Currently, either quetiapine or olanzapine are considered the first-line choices for the treatment of psychosis in HD patients.

When treating HD patients with neuropleptic agents, potential serious adverse events, such as neuroleptic malignant syndrome (NMS), can occur. The symptoms of NMS include acute mental status changes, lead-pipe rigidity, autonomic dysfunction, and increased creatinephosphokinase (CPK). Patients may also experience neuroleptic-induced catatonia with mutism, waxy flexibility, psychomotor retardation or agitation, and autonomic instability. Patients treated with neuroleptics may also develop TD; however, the exact incidence in the HD population is unknown and may be difficult to diagnose in the setting of existing choreiform movements.

In summary, psychosis is more common in HD than in the general population. The type of psychotic symptoms, their frequency, and relationship to other variables have not been well studied. It is possible that there are genetic factors that might predispose to psychosis. Psychosis may be the first manifestation of HD in some patients. There are numerous methodological problems with the current literature in this area. This includes small sample sizes, variability of diagnostic criteria, definition of psychosis, referral bias and lack of prospective, controlled clinical trials of antipsychotic agents in HD populations.

Mood and Anxiety Disorders

HD is associated with many neuropsychiatric sequella, among which mood disorders feature prominently. As with psychosis, there remains debate whether or not psychiatric changes represent the onset of disease manifestations in advance of the characteristic motor changes. In HD, there is a dearth of methodologically robust treatment trials to guide clinicians in their choice of the appropriate antidepressant or mood stabilizer. Most studies of mood disorders in HD have been small, open-label trials.

Anxiety symptoms and more defined anxiety syndromes are also commonly seen in HD. As with depression, anxiety has been reported as a relatively frequent prodrome to the motor symptoms of HD (128). Untreated anxiety has significant implications: it can worsen the expression of the motor symptoms of HD; it can increase the risk of alcohol and other substance abuse; and it can have an adverse effect on the quality of life. Hence, the recognition and management of anxiety in HD is crucial.

Depression

Folstein et al. (114) noted that 42% of all HD patients in their state-wide sample ($n = 88$) had either a major depression or dysthymic disorder. This figure overlaps with that of Shiwach (129), who reported that the lifetime prevalence of major depression in 110 HD patients was 39%. The relatively small sample sizes, for epidemiological purposes, are offset by the confluence of findings, suggesting that a significant minority of HD patients, almost one in two, will suffer a clinically significant depressive illness during the course of their lifetime. These figures are similar to that for other disabling, degenerative neurological disorders, such as PD (130), MS (131), and AD (132). The suicide rate in HD disease is 4 to 6 times higher than in the general population and accounts for over 2% of deaths in a large sample of HD patients (133).

Bipolar Affective Disorder

The prevalence of bipolar affective disorder has not been well researched in HD. However, Folstein et al. (114) noted hypomanic or manic episodes in 10% of 88 patients, while Mendez examined seven studies of HD patients and, using a variable definition of mania, estimated the rate as 4.8% (109).

Anxiety

Detailed epidemiological studies of the prevalence and incidence of anxiety in HD are lacking. However, clinical experience suggests that anxiety syndromes, such as social phobia and generalized anxiety disorders, are particularly prevalent. Panic attacks and more generalized "anxiety attacks" also occur. In addition, the frequent losses of all kinds experienced by those afflicted with HD often lead to adjustment disorders with anxiety. Obsessions and compulsions in HD have been reported in the literature (134) and are commonly seen clinically. Most patients with HD report worry over financial loss, guilt about passing the HD gene to their offspring, and uncertainty regarding the course and prognosis of their disease as common sources of anxiety.

Obsessive–Compulsive Behavior

Common to many involuntary movements disorders is the presence of OCD. A review of 960 patients who were followed at 43 HD centers found that 22.3% had evidence of obsessive-compulsive behavior at their first visit to a Huntington's Center (135,136) when simply asked during general evaluation whether or not they had obsessive–compulsive behavior. The lifetime prevalence for primary OCD is 2% to 3% (137). Thus, obsessive compulsive behavior may have a higher than normal prevalence in HD. In support of this, Anderson et al. (135,138) found that up to 50% of a group of 27 HD patients reported obsessive–compulsive behavior when administered the Yale-Brown obsessive compulsive scale (Y-BOCS), suggesting that these symptoms may be among the most common behavioral features of HD. In this study, presence of obsessive–compulsive behavior did not correlate with motor symptoms, duration of disease, or impairment in function, but more executive dysfunction was evident in the OCD group on neuropsychological tests. It is important to recognize that not all HD patients with obsessive–compulsive behavior meet full criteria for OCD. However, these unrecognized symptoms may still cause major disability in HD and impose additional burdens on caregivers. Improper characterization of obsessive–compulsive behavior as psychosis or other behaviors may lead to inappropriate treatment.

Several case reports describe the features of obsessive–compulsive behavior in HD. Cummings and Cunningham (139) described two patients with HD who had OCD. Both were belligerent when prevented from acting on their compulsions. Onset of symptoms began in mid-life, in contrast to primary OCD, which generally begins in the early 20s. Scicutella (140) also reports on a patient with onset of OCD and mild choreiform movements at age 70, who was subsequently diagnosed with HD. Dewhurst et al. (138) listed "obsessional features" among a list of prodromal personality changes seen in HD patients. A case reported by Tonkonogy and Barreira (141) involved a clinical history and neuroimaging compatible with HD in a patient who had washing compulsion. De Marchi et al. (142) reported a family with HD and a 34% lifetime prevalence of OCD. In their discussion of why obsessive–compulsive behavior is rarely reported in HD, they suggest that it may be an embarrassing symptom for patients, who do not volunteer information about it (143). Cummings and Cunningham (139) suggest several reasons why obsessive–compulsive behavior is seldom reported in HD. These include lack of specific questioning, assignment of the symptoms to other categories of behavior (e.g., perseveration, psychosis), or the possibility that only a small number of HD patients develop obsessive–compulsive behavior.

Examples of the types of obsessive–compulsive behavior seen in HD include sexual images, aggressive obsessions (usually directed at others), compulsive consumption of cigarettes, or beverages, frequently caffeinated, and "just so" or symmetry obsessions (which often produced compulsions to rearrange things to suit the obsessive feelings). At times, the obsessive–compulsive behavior may border on delusional beliefs, as may occur when a physical complaint is the focus of the obsession. There does not appear to be any stage of HD at which these symptoms are more likely to appear, but obsessive–compulsive behavior, like other psychiatric manifestations of HD may, in some cases, predate the emergence of an obvious movement disorder.

Neuropathological Basis for Mood Disorder in HD

A number of key frontal-subcortical neural circuits are known to regulate mood and behavior (144). The pathophysiology of HD disrupts the integrity of these pathways, leading to neuropsychiatric sequellae. Functional neuroimaging (PET) has shown that HD patients with depression have lower metabolic activity in the orbitofrontal and inferior prefrontal cortex compared with euthymic HD controls (145). The importance of frontal system pathology in the pathogenesis of depression has also been noted in other neuropsychiatric disorders, such as PD (146). Furthermore, these PET findings concur with data from patients with primary depression (147). Interruption in the neural circuits probably translates into mood disturbance via a dysregulation in pivotal neurotransmitter, such as serotonin, dopamine and glutamate, among others.

There is evidence to suggest that depression in HD may be linked to early neuronal loss in the medial caudate, an area richly connected to limbic structures subserving mood and affect. Indeed, the part of the neostriatum damaged earliest in HD, the dorsal medial caudate, may provide a clue as to why mood disorder may be the first symptom of HD.

These early neuroanatomical changes without prominent motor features may also correlate with the onset of mood disorders in HD. Shiwach et al. reported that a third of their depressed sample of HD patients presented with mood change on average 4.3 years (range 1–8 years) before the onset of motor symptoms (129). Mindham et al. (148) compared psychopathology prior to onset of confirmed disease in HD and Alzheimer patients and noted that the former were twice as likely to have a mood disorder, suggesting a more integral association between HD and depression as opposed to mood change as a non-specific prodrome.

Treatment of Mood Disorders in HD

Treatment of mood disorders in HD may be divided into two synergistic modalities, the pharmacologic and the psychosocial. In general, there is a paucity of literature pertaining to both and, as such, evidence obtained from primary psychiatric disorders or other neuropsychiatric conditions may help guide the treatment of mood disorders in HD. Several caveats warrant consideration regarding the treatment of HD patients:

1. HD patients may have an increased sensitivity to the side effects of medication, namely dehydration and/or delirium with lithium carbonate, and agitation with the selective serotonin re-uptake inhibitors (SSRIs). In addition, central nervous system toxicity may be aggravated when the neurologic patient is depressed or already sedated by other drugs used, for example, to treat chorea (149).
2. Metabolism of drugs may be altered in HD for a number of reasons, such as low serum albumin, impaired renal clearance, and general physical debilitation
3. Psychotropic medication may further compromise an already impaired neurological status, that is, the anticholinergic effects of tricyclic antidepressant (TCA) medication may aggravate cognitive impairment, while orthostatic hypotension, another side effect of TCA, may further impair gait and balance.
4. Dosage regimes should be conservative, that is, start low and go slow.
5. Patients should have a physical examination and work-up prior to treatment as some medical problems may affect the mental state and mislead the clinician. Examples are hypothyroidism mistaken for depression, and hyperactive delirium caused by a pneumonia or urinary tract infection which can be misdiagnosed as mania.

6.   Adequate attention should be directed at symptoms of HD that may be aggravating mood difficulties, that is, insomnia leading to fatigue and demoralization; movement difficulties promoting irritability and frustration; anorexia and weight loss exacerbating low self-esteem and fatigue.

Pharmacologic Treatment

There are no randomized, controlled trials of treatment for either depression or mania in HD. Two published sets of guidelines (150,151) are based on anecdotal evidence and clinical expertise.

Depression

SSRIs are the first choice when it comes to treating depression (major depression and dysthymia). While there are no treatment trials with these drugs reported in the HD literature, there are data from other neuropsychiatric disorders, such as AD (152) and MS (153), which suggest that sertraline is effective. Anecdotal reports suggest that other SSRI drugs, such as fluoxetine (154), are just as effective in patients with secondary depression. The SSRIs are generally well tolerated. Problems may, however, occasionally occur with gastrointestinal side effects, in particular nausea and diarrhea, and vigilance is called for in HD patients with anorexia and weight loss. Treatment may increase agitation in some patients because of akathisia-like effects, but in others the SSRIs may have a calming effect by ameliorating irritability (155). Rarely, the SSRI drugs may induce apathy (156).

Theoretically, all the SSRIs may improve motor symptoms probably by inhibiting dopamine release in the basal ganglia secondary to 5HT2 stimulation (157).

Other classes of antidepressants, including serotonin and noradrenaline re-uptake inhibitors, serotonin antagonism and re-uptake inhibitors, noradrenaline and dopamine re-uptake inhibitors and TCAs, are typically used as second-line agents in patients who fail SSRIs. There are no controlled trials of these agents, with the exception of TCAs, in HD.

The longevity of the TCAs, as much as their utility, explains their prominence in the HD literature published to date. While these drugs are no less effective than the SSRIs in treating depression, their more troublesome side effects, particularly within the anticholinergic spectrum, have demoted them from their first choice slot, occupied until the late 1980s. A series of early case reports and one open trial in HD patients demonstrated their effectiveness in treating depression (102,108,159,160), but sample sizes were small, and dosages plus length of treatment were not always stipulated. In HD patients, desipramine and nortriptyline are drugs of choice, given their lesser propensity for anticholinergic side effects.

There are a number of other antidepressant drugs available, but data on their effectiveness in HD are again lacking. Mirtazepine has the advantage of increasing appetite and may thus prove useful in depression associated with anorexia and weight loss. It is also sedating, suggesting a possible use in the agitated, depressed patient.

A last resort for treating refractory depression is electroconvulsive therapy (ECT). There are limited data from three published studies suggesting that ECT is effective in treating depression in HD. Folstein and Folstein (161) in a single case study and Folstein (158) in a retrospective series of two patients found treatment to be effective and without side effects. Ranen (162) noted that five of six patients improved with ECT; however, delirium and deterioration in movements were reported in two patients. Evans (163) reported a single case of psychotic depression refractory to medication, but responsive to ECT. There was no associated cognitive worsening and choreiform movements were only slightly exacerbated. On the basis of this limited data, ECT can be tried in HD, but only after failed treatment with an antidepressant medication.

Mania

The treatment for mania typically involves the use of mood stabilizing agents. Concern has been expressed about the use of lithium carbonate because of poor response and possible toxicity that may arise should the patient become dehydrated, a not infrequent situation in HD patients (151). However, there is, as yet, not enough evidence suggesting that the hazards of lithium outweigh the benefits. Alternatives to lithium carbonate include carbamazepine and valproic acid, although treatment trials in HD have not been carried out; valproic acid may help with irritability, however, attention to increased gait impairment and falls is required.

Anxiety Disorders

There are no controlled clinical trials of anxiety disorders in HD patients. Clinical consensus of HD experts recommend that in episodic anxiety, such as that triggered by short-term environmental changes, the use of short-acting benzodiazepines as needed can be effective. These include lorazepam, oxazepam, and temazepam. Benzodiazepines should be used with caution as they may worsen gait and cognition, and may even lead to delirium.

For chronic anxiety, consensus opinion suggests the use of SSRIs as first-line agents. Within the SSRI class, activating agents, such as fluoxetine, should be avoided as they may worsen anxiety. Since these agents do not provide immediate relief of anxiety symptoms, short-term benzodiazepines can be used as adjunctive agents. Other antidepressants, which may be beneficial for chronic anxiety, include venlafaxine, nefazodone, and mirtazepine.

HD patients with significant OCD typically respond to SSRIs similar to that reported in primary OCD populations, however, no controlled clinical trials documenting the efficacy of any SSRI in HD patients with OCD are available.

Psychosocial Treatment

Similar to pharmacological treatment, there are no controlled studies that have investigated the efficacy of psychosocial treatment in HD. Nevertheless, a host of treatment modalities may prove useful, either as adjunct to medication, or else as stand-alone approaches. Supportive psychotherapy, grief counselling, and support groups for patients have potential utility, but may be limited by the presence of cognitive dysfunction and other markers of disease severity. Thus, traditional insight-oriented psychotherapy may be less useful in a cognitively compromised individual. In addition, varying degrees of motor disability might inadvertently increase mood disturbance among patients attending group counselling sessions who might infer their future course by observing the severity of HD among their fellow patients.

PSYCHIATRIC CONSEQUENCES OF PRESYMPTOMATIC DNA TESTING

The availability of a direct gene test in presymptomatic at-risk individuals has been available since 1993. Despite the relative ease by which gene testing can now be completed, there has not been a dramatic increase in the number of at-risk individuals seeking presymptomatic gene testing. Nonetheless, as the agents that may delay the onset or slow disease progression become available in the coming years, the number of individuals who pursue gene testing will undoubtedly increase. The treatment of mood dysfunction associated with presymptomatic gene testing will likely become an additional activity for the HD clinician.

A fairly substantial literature exists regarding the psychological consequences of gene testing in HD. There is consensus among published studies that psychological dysfunction is the potential consequence of both gene-positive and gene-negative results. More striking is the finding by Decruyenaere (164) that 15% of participants in their predictive DNA program had at least mild depression or elevated scores for general anxiety during the pre-test period. These authors concluded that individuals who are close to the perceived age of onset of HD and who have pessimistic risk perception (along with clinical features of depression and/or anxiety) are at increased risk for post-test psychological distress. Long term follow-up of individuals with a positive gene test demonstrate that they appear to have greater psychological distress (165). Codori (166) found that individuals with greater mood disturbance and poor adjustment had tested positive, were married, had no children, and were closer to their estimated age of disease onset.

Among the individuals who receive a gene positive result, depression and anxiety are the most commonly reported psychiatric symptoms typically occurring two to three months following the test result (167–169), but are reported to occur within 10 days following the test result (170). These individuals are considered to be at a high risk for psychological dysfunction. However, there is no reported increased rate of catastrophic events, such as psychiatric hospitalization, increased suicide rate, or increased suicide attempts. Still, evidence of anxiety and depression observed during the pre-testing phase have been reported to persist up to a year following testing (171).

Among individuals with a gene-negative result, psychological problems are reported to occur anywhere from 2 to 12 months following the result being made known. Approximately 10% of individuals with gene-negative results require on-going psychological treatment (168). Common reasons for psychological dysfunction in the gene-negative group include survivor guilt, results contradicting expected outcome and regret over past decisions (e.g., sterilization). However, psychological test scores on depression and anxiety inventories competed during the pre-testing phase are reported to normalize after 1-year post-test results (171).

Despite compelling evidence of increased mood and anxiety symptoms among individuals who pursue predictive testing, regardless of the test result, there are no reported treatment studies of this population. Several factors must be considered regarding the treatment of mood disorders in this population. These include, but are not limited to evidence of pre-test mood disorder, level of psychosocial support and proximity to disease onset. Without published studies of treatment in this population, treatment efforts should focus on "target" symptoms. Individuals with clinical evidence of an adjustment disorder (either with depressed mood, with anxiety, or with mixed anxiety and depressed mood) should receive short-term psychiatric intervention (e.g., 6 to 12 months) following the test result, which may include both psychopharmacological and psychotherapeutic intervention. The choice of pharmacological agent is similar to that described earlier for patients with manifest HD. In general, serotonergic agents tend to be well tolerated with good efficacy. Re-evaluation of the need for pharmacological intervention in these individuals should be done on a regular basis given the results of long-term follow-up studies, which suggest a general resolution of psychiatric dysfunction over time, regardless of the result.

In summary, psychiatric disorders are common in patients with HD, contributing significantly to the morbidity and mortality associated with the disease. Despite the lack of empirical data on the treatment of psychiatric syndromes in HD, these features of the disorder can be successfully ameliorated if properly diagnosed. Further research is clearly needed to elucidate best clinical practice, however, there is in place a body of evidence, drawn from anecdotal evidence, clinical trials, and other neuropsychiatric disorders that can provide working therapeutic guidelines.

REFERENCES

1. The Huntington's Disease Collaborative Research Group. A novel gene containing a trinucleotide repeat that is expanded and unstable on Huntington's disease chromosomes. Cell 1992; 72:971–983.
2. MacDonald ME, Gusella JF. Huntington's disease: translating a CAG repeat into a pathogenic mechanism. Curr Opin Neurobiol 1996; 6:638–643.
3. Nance MA. Huntington disease—another chapter rewritten [invited editorial]. Am J Hum Genet 1996; 59:1–6.
4. Ross CA et al. Huntington disease and the related disorder, dentatorubral-pallidoluysian atrophy (DRPLA). Medicine 1997; 76:305–308.

5. Ross CA. Intranuclear neuronal inclusions: a common pathogenic mechanism for glutamine-repeat neurodegenerative disease? [minireview]. Neuron 1997; 19:1147–1150.

6. Ross CA. When more is less: pathogenesis of glutamine repeat neurodegenerative diseases. Neuron 1995; 15:493–496.

7. Price DL, Sisodia SS, Borchelt DR. Genetic neurodegenerative diseases: the human illness and transgenic models. Science 1998; 282:1079–1083.

8. Hardy J, Gwinn-Hardy K. Genetic classification of primary neurodegenerative disease. Science 1998; 282:1075–1079.

9. Shoulson I, Fahn S. Huntington's disease: clinical care and evaluation. Neurology 1979; 29:1–3.

10. Shoulson I, Kurlan R, Rubin AJ, Goldblatt D, Behr J, Miller C, Kennedy J, Bamford KA, Caine ED, Kido DK, Plumb S, Odoroff C. Assessment of functional capacity in neurodegenerative movement disorders: Huntington's disease as a prototype. In: TL Munsat, ed. Quantification of Neurologic Deficit. Boston: Butterworths, 1989, pp. 285–309.

11. Shoulson I. Huntington's disease: Cognitive and psychiatric features. Neuropsychiatry, Neuropsychol Behav Neurol 1990; 3:15–22.

12. Storey E, Beal MF. Neuropsychological aspects of Huntington's disease. In: Thal LJ, Moos WH, Gamzu ER, eds. Cognitive Disorders: Pathophysiology and Treatment. New York: Marcek Dekker, 1992, pp. 93–132.

13. Huber SJ, Shuttleworth EC, Paulson GW. Dementia in Parkinson's disease. Arch Neurol 1986; 43:987–990.

14. Brandt J. Access to knowledge in the dementia of Huntington's disease. Dev Neuropsychol 1985; 1:335–348.

15. Girotti F, Marano R, Soliveri P, Geminiani G, Scigliano G. Relationship between motor and cognitive disorders in Huntington's disease. J Neurol 1998; 235: 454–457.

16. Heindel WC, Butters N, Salmon DP. Impaired learning of a motor skill in patients with Huntington's disease. Behav Neurosci 1998; 102:141–147.

17. Heindel WC, Salmon DP, Shults CW, Walicke PA, Butters N. Neuropsychological evidence for multiple implicit memory systems: A comparison of Alzheimer's, Huntington's, and Parkinson's disease patients. J Neurosci 1989; 9:582–587.

18. Brandt J, Butters N. The neuropsychology of Huntington's disease. Trends Neurosci 1986; 9:118–120.

19. Hodges JR, Salmon DP, Butters N. Differential impairment of semantic and episodic memory in Alzheimer's and Huntington's diseases: a controlled prospective study. J Neurol Neurosurg Psych 1990; 53:1089–1095.

20. Bamford KA, Caine ED, Kido DK et al. A prospective evaluation of cognitive decline in early Huntington's disease: functional and radiological correlates. Neurology 1995; 45:1867–1873.

21. Bauchoud-Levi AC, Maison P, Bartolomeo P, Boisse MF, Barba GD, Ergis AM, Baudic S, Degos JS, Cesaro P, Peschanski M. Retest effects and cognitive decline in longitudinal follow-up of patients with early HD. Neurology 2001; 56:1052–1058.

22. Huntington Study Group. Unified Huntington's disease rating scale: reliability and consistency. Mov Disord 1996; 11:136–142.

23. Nehl C, Paulsen JS, Huntington Study Group. Cognitive and psychiatric aspects of Huntington's disease contribute to functional capacity. J Nerv Ment Dis 2004; 192:72–74.

24. Marder K, Zhao H, Myers RH, Cudkowicz M, Kayson E, Kieburtz K, Orme C, Paulsen J, Penney JB, Siemers E, Shoulson I. Rate of functional decline in Huntington's disease. Neurology 2000; 54:452–458.

25. Feigin A, Kieburtz K, Bordwell K, Como P, Steinberg K, Sotack J, Zimmerman C, Hickey C, Orme C, Shoulson I. Functional decline in Huntington's disease. Mov Disord 1995; 10:211–214.

26. Boll TJ, Heaton R, Reitan R. Neuropsychological. and emotional correlates of Huntington's chorea. J Ment Nerv Disord 1974; 158:61–69.

27. Brandt J. Cognitive investigations in Huntington's disease. In: Cermak L. ed. Neuropsychological Explorations of Memory and Cognition: Essays in Honor of Nelson Butters. New York: Plenum Press, 1990, pp. 135–146.

28. Brandt J. Cognitive impairments in Huntington's disease: Insights into the neuropsychology of the striatum. In: Boller F, Grafman J, eds. Handbook of Neuropsychology, Vol. 5. Amsterdam: Elsevier Scientific Publisher, 1991, pp. 241–264.

29. Strauss ME, Brandt J. Attempt at preclinical identification of Huntington's disease using the WAIS. J Clin Exp Neuropsychol 1986; 8:210–218.

30. Schretlen D, Bobholz J. Standardization and initial validation of a brief test of executive attentional ability. J Clin Exp Neuropsychol 1992; 14:65.

31. Brandt J, Butters N. The neuropsychology of Huntington's disease. Trends Neurosci 1986; 9:118–120.

32. Brandt J, Strauss ME, Larus J, Jensen B, Folstein SE, Folstein MF. Clinical correlates of dementia and disability in Huntington's disease. J Clin Neuropsychol 1984; 6:401–412.

33. Caine ED, Ebert MH, Weingartner H. An outline for the analysis of dementia. The memory disorder of Huntington's disease. Neurology 1977; 27:1087–1092.

34. Butters N, Sax DS, Montgomery K, Tarlow S. Comparison of the neuropsychological deficits associated with early and advanced Huntington's disease. Arch Neurol 1978; 35:585–589.

35. Wilson RS, Como PG, Garron DC, Klawans HL, Barr A, Klawans D. Memory failure in Huntington's disease. J Clin Exp Neurol 1987; 9:147–154.

36. Moses JA, Jr., Golden CJ, Berger PA, Wisniewski AM. Neuropsychological deficits in early, middle, and late stages of Huntington's disease as measured by the Luria Nebraska Neuropsychological Battery. Int J Neurosci 1981; 14:95–100.

37. Weingartner H, Caine ED, Ebert MH. Encoding processes, learning, and recall in Huntington's disease. In: Chase TN, Wexler NS, Barbeau A, eds. Advances in Neurology. Vol. 23. Huntington's Disease. New York: Raven Press, 1979, pp. 215–226.

38. Randolph C. Implicit, explicit, and semantic memory functions in Alzheimer's disease and Huntington's disease. J Clin Exp Neuropsychol 1991; 13:479–494.

39. Beatty WW, Salmon DP, Butters N, Heindel WC, Granholm EL. Retrograde amnesia in patients with Alzheimer's disease or Huntington's disease. Neurobiol Aging 1988; 9:181–186.

40. Bylsma FW, Brandt J, Strauss ME. Aspects of procedural memory are differentially impaired in Huntington's disease. Arch Clin Neuropsychol 1990; 5:287–297.

41. Bylsma FW, Rebok G, Brandt J. Long-term retention of implicit learning in Huntington's disease. Neuropsychologia 1991; 29:1213–1221.
42. Cohen NJ, Squire LR. Preserved learning and retention of pattern-analyzing skill in amnesia: Dissociation of knowing how and knowing that. Science 1980; 210: 207–210.
43. Butters N, Heindel WC, Salmon DP. Dissociation of implicit memory in dementia: Neurological implications. Bull Psychonom Soc 1990; 28:359–366.
44. Butters N, Salmon DP, Heindel WC. Processes underlying the memory impairments of demented patients. In: Goldberg E, ed. Contemporary Neuropsychology and the Legacy of Luria. Hillsdale, NJ: Lawrence Erlbaum, 1990, pp. 99–126.
45. Granholm E, Butters N. Associative encoding and retrieval in Alzheimer's and Huntington's disease. Brain Cognit 1988; 7:335–347.
46. Butters N, Albert MS, Sax DS, Miliotis P, Nagode J, Sterste A. The effect of verbal mediators on pictorial memory in brain-damaged patients. Neuropsychologia 1983; 21:307–323.
47. Heindel WC, Butters N, Salmon DP. Impaired learning of a motor skill in patients with Huntington's disease. Behav Neurosci 1988; 102:141–147.
48. Moss MB, Albert MS, Butters N, Payne M. Differential patterns of memory loss among patients with Alzheimer's disease, Huntington's disease, and alcoholic Korsakoff s syndrome. Arch Neurol 1986; 43:239–246.
49. Heindel WC, Salmon DP, Shults CW, Walicke PA, Butters N. Neuropsychological evidence for multiple implicit memory systems: A comparison of Alzheimer's, Huntington's, and Parkinson's disease patients. J Neurosci 1989; 9:582–587.
50. Caine ED, Hunt RD, Weingartner H, Ebert MH. Huntington's dementia. Clinical and neuropsychological features. Arch Gen Psychiatry 1978; 35:378–384.
51. Butters N, Wolfe J, Granholm E, Martone M. An assessment of verbal recall, recognition and fluency abilities in patients with Huntington's disease. Cortex 1986; 22:11–32.
52. Butters N, Wolfe J, Martone M, Granholm E, Cermak LS. Memory disorders associated with Huntington's disease: Verbal recall, verbal recognition, and procedural memory. Neuropsychologia 1985; 23:729–743.
53. Butters N. The clinical aspects of memory disorders: Contributions from experimental studies of amnesia and dementia. J Clin Neuropsychol 1984; 6:17–36.
54. Delis DC, Kramer JH, Kaplan E, Ober BA. The California Verbal Learning Test. San Antonio, TX: The Psychological Corporation, 1987.
55. Kramer JH, Delis DC, Blusewicz MJ, Brandt, J, Ober BA, Strauss M. Verbal memory errors in Alzheimer's and Huntington's dementias. Dev Neuropsychol 1988; 4:1–15.
56. Kramer JH, Levin B, Brandt J, Delis DC. Differentiation of Alzheimer's, Huntington's, and Parkinson's diseases on the basis of verbal learning characteristics. Neuropsychol 1989; 3:111–120.
57. Delis DC, Massman PJ, Butters N, Salmon DP, Cermak LS, Kramer JH. Profiles of demented and amnesic patients on the California Verbal Learning Test: Implications for the assessment of memory disorders. Psychol Assess: J Consult Clin Psychol 1991; 3:19–26.
58. Brandt J, Corwin J, Krafft L. Is verbal recognition memory really different in Huntington's and Alzheimer's disease? J Clin Exp Neuropsychol 1992; 14:773–784.

59. Jacobs D, Salmon DP, Tröster AI, Butters N. Intrusion errors in the figural memory of patients with Alzheimer's and Huntington's disease. Arch Clin Neuropsychol 1990; 5:49–57.

60. Jacobs D, Tröster AI, Butters N, Salmon DP, Cermak LS. Intrusion errors on the visual reproduction test of the Wechsler Memory Scale and the Wechsler Memory Scale-Revised: An analysis of demented and amnesic patients. Clin Neuropsychol 1990; 4:177–191.

61. Butters N, Salmon DP, Cullum CM, Cairns P, Tröster A, Jacobs D, Moss M, Cermak L. Differentiation of amnesic and demented patients with the Wechsler Memory Scale-Revised. Clin Neuropsychol 1988; 2:133–148.

62. Massman PJ, Delis DC, Butters N, Levin BE, Salmon DP. Are all subcortical dementias alike?: Verbal learning and memory in Parkinson's and Huntington's disease patients. J Clin Exp Neuropsychol 1990; 12:729–744.

63. Albert MS, Butters N, Levin J. Temporal gradients in the retrograde amnesia of patients with alcoholic Korsakoff s disease. Arch Neurol 1979; 36:211–216.

64. Kopelman MD. Remote and autobiographical memory, temporal context memory and frontal atrophy in Korsakoff and Alzheimer patients. Neuropsychologia 1989; 27:437–460.

65. Albert MS, Butters N, Brandt J. Patterns of remote memory in amnesic and demented patients. Arch Neurol 1981; 38:495–500.

66. Albert MS, Butters N, Brandt J. Development of remote memory loss in patients with Huntington's disease. J Clin Neuropsychol 1981; 3:1–12.

67. Cummings JL. Subcortical Dementia. New York: Oxford University Press, 1990.

68. Folstein SE, Brandt J, Folstein, MF. Huntington's disease. In: Cummings JL, ed. Subcortical Dementia. New York: Oxford University Press, 1990:87–107.

69. Gordon WP, Illes J. Neurolinguistic characteristics of language production in Huntington's disease: A preliminary report. Brain Lang 1987; 31:1–10.

70. Ludlow CL, Connor NP, Bassich CJ. Speech timing in Parkinson's and Huntington's disease. Brain Lang 1987; 32:195–214.

71. Podoll K, Caspary P, Lange HW, Noth J. Language functions in Huntington's disease. Brain 1988; 111:1475–1503.

72. Wallesch CW, Fehrenbach RA. On the neurolinguistic nature of language abnormalities in Huntington's disease. J Neurol Neurosurg Psychiatry 1988; 51:367–373.

73. Illes J. Neurolinguistic features of spontaneous language production dissociate three forms of neurodegenerative disease: Alzheimer's, Huntington's, and Parkinson's. Brain Lang 1989; 37:628–642.

74. Speedie LJ, Brake N, Folstein SE, Bowers D, Heilman KM. Comprehension of prosody in Huntington's disease. J Neurol Neurosurg Psychiatry 1990; 53:607–610.

75. Caine ED, Bamford KA, Schiffer RB, Shoulson I, Levy S. A controlled neuropsychological comparison of Huntington's disease and multiple sclerosis. Arch Neurol 1986; 43:249–254.

76. Alexander MP, Benson DF, Stuss DT. Frontal lobes and language. Brain Lang 1989; 37:656–691.

77. Borkowski JG, Benton AL, Spreen O. Word fluency and brain damage. Neuropsychologia 1967; 5:135–140.

78. Butters N, Granholm E, Salmon DP, Grant I, Wolfe J. Episodic, and semantic memory: A comparison of amnesic and demented patients. J Clin Exp Neuropsychol 1987; 9:479–497.
79. Monsch AU, Bondi MW, Butters N, Paulsen JS, Salmon DP, Brugger P, Swenson MR. A comparison of category and letter fluency in Alzheimer's and Huntington's Disease. Neuropsychol 1994; 8:25–30.
80. Barr AE, Brandt J. Verbal fluency deficits in dementia. J. Clin Exp Neuropsychol 1993; 15:27.
81. Smith S, Butters N, White R, Lyon L, Granholm E. Priming semantic relations in patients with Huntington's disease. Brain Lang 1988; 33:27–40.
82. Bayles KA, Tomoeda CK. Confrontation naming impairment in dementia. Brain Lang 1983; 19:98–114.
83. Hodges JR, Salmon DP, Butters N. Differential impairment of semantic and episodic memory in Alzheimer's and Huntington's diseases: A controlled prospective study. J Neurol Neurosurg Psychiatry 1991; 53:1089–1095.
84. Brouwers P, Cox C, Martin A, Chase T, Fedio P. Differential perceptualspatial impairment in Huntington's and Alzheimer's dementias. Arch Neurol 1984; 41:1073–1076.
85. Josiassen RC, Curry LM, Mancall EL. Development of neuropsychological deficits in Huntington's disease. Arch Neurol 1983; 40:791–796.
86. Fedio P, Cox CS, Neophytides A, CanalFrederick G, Chase TN. Neuropsychological profile of Huntington's disease. In: Chase TN, Wexler NS, Barbeau A, eds. Advances in Neurology. Vol. 23. Huntington's Disease. New York: Raven Press, 1979: 239–255.
87. Mohr E, Brouwers P, Claus JJ, Mann UM, Fedio P, Chase TN. Visuospatial cognition in Huntington's disease. Mov Disord 1991; 6:127–132.
88. Potegal M. A note on spatial-motor deficits in patients with Huntington's disease: A test of a hypothesis. Neuropsychologia 1971; 9:233–235.
89. Money J. A Standardized Road Map Test of Directional Sense. San Rafael, CA: Academic Therapy Publications, 1976.
90. Bylsma FW, Brandt J, Strauss ME. Personal and extrapersonal orientation in Huntington's disease patients and those at risk. Cortex 1992; 28:113–122.
91. Alexander GE, DeLong MR, Strick PL. Parallel organization of functionally segregated circuits linking basal ganglia and cortex. Annu Rev Neurosci 1986; 9:357–381.
92. Bamford KA, Caine ED, Kido DK, Plassche WM, Shoulson I. Clinical-pathologic correlation in Huntington's disease: A neuropsychological and computed tomography study. Neurology 1989; 39:796–801.
93. Rothlind JC, Bylsma FW, Peyser C, Folstein SE, Brandt J. Cognitive and motor correlates of everyday functioning in early Huntington's disease. J Nerv Ment Dis 1993; 181:194–199.
94. Strauss ME, Brandt J. Are there neuropsychologic manifestations of the gene for Huntington's disease in asymptomatic, at-risk individuals? Arch Neurol 1990; 47:905–908.
95. Giordani B et al. Longitudinal neuropsychological and genetic linkage analysis of persons at risk for Huntington's disease. Arch Neurol 1995; 52:59–64.
96. Campodonico JR, Codori AM, Brandt J. Neuropsychological stability over two years in asymptomatic carriers of the Huntington's disease mutation. J Neurol Neurosurg Psychiatry 1996; 61:621–624.
97. Diamond R et al. Evidence of presymptomatic cognitive decline in Huntington's disease. J Clin Exp Neuropsychol 1992; 14:961–975.

98. Foroud T et al. Cognitive scores in carriers of Huntington's disease gene compared to noncarriers. Ann Neurol 1995; 37:657–664.
99. Jason GW et al. Presymptomatic neuropsychological impairment in Huntington's disease. Arch Neurol 1988; 45:769–73.
100. Lyle OE, Gottesman II. Premorbid psychometric indicators of the gene for Huntington's disease. J Consult Clin Psychol 1977; 45:1011–1022.
101. Siemers E et al. Motor changes in presymptomatic Huntington disease gene carriers. Arch Neurol 1996; 53:487–492.
102. Kirkwood SC et al. Longitudinal cognitive and motor changes among presymptomatic Huntington disease gene carriers. Arch Neurol 1999; 56:563–568.
103. Paulsen JS, Zhao H, Stout JC, Brinkman RR, Guttman M, Ross CA, Como P, Manning C, Hayden MR, Shoulson I. Clinical markers of early disease in persons near onset of Huntington's disease. Neurology 2001; 57:658–662.
104. Alyward EH, Codori A, Barta P et al. Basal ganglia volume and proximity to onset in presymptomatic Huntington's disease. Arch Neurol 1996; 53:1293–1296.
105. Antonini A, Lenders KL, Speigel R et al. Striatal glucose metabolism and dopamine D2 receptor binding in asymptomatic gene carriers of Huntington's disease. Brain 1996; 119:2085–2095.
106. Lawrence AD, Hodges JR, Rosser AE et al. Evidence for specific cognitive deficits in preclinical Huntington's disease. Brain 1998; 121:1329–1341.
107. Shiwach RS, Norbury CG. A controlled psychiatric study of individual at risk for HD. Br J Psychiatry 1994; 165:500–505.
108. Caine ED, Shoulson I. Psychiatric symptoms in HD. Am J Psychiatry 1994; 140:728–733.
109. Mendez MF. HD: update and review of neuropsychiatric aspects. Int J Psychiatry Med 1994; 24:189–208.
110. Bolt, JMW. Huntington's chorea in the west of Scotland. Br J Psychiatry 1970; 116:259–270.
111. Tsuang D, Almqvist EW, Lipe H, Strgar F, DiGiacomo L, Hoff D, Eugenio C, Hayden MR. Bird Familial aggregation of psychotic symptoms in Huntington's disease. Am J Psychiatry 2000; 157(12):1955–1959.
112. Weigell-Weber M, Schmid W, Spiegel R. Psychiatric symptoms and CAG expansion in Huntington's disease. Am J Med Genet 1996; 67(1):53–57.
113. Cummings JL. Behavioral and psychiatric symptoms associated with Huntington's disease. Neurology 1995; 65:179–186.
114. Folstein SE, Chase GA, Wahl WE et al. HD in Maryland: clinical aspect of racial variation. Am J Hum Genet 1987; 41:168–179.
115. Lovestone S, Hodgson S, Sham P, Differ AM, Levy R. Familial psychiatric presentation of Huntington's disease. J Med Genet 1996; 33(2):128–131.
116. Vonsattel JP, Myers RH, Stevens TJ et al. Neuropathological classification of HD. J Neuropath Exp Neurol 1985; 44:559–577.
117. Kuwert T, Lange HW, Langen KJ et al. Cerebral glucose consumption measured by PET in patient with and without psychiatric symptoms of HD. Psychiatry Res 1989; 29:361–362.
118. De Marchi N, Mennella R. Huntington's disease and its association with psychopathology. Harv Rev Psychiatry 2000; 7(5):278–289.
119. Folstein S. Huntington disease: a disorder of families. The John Hopkins University Press, 1989.

120. Shoulson I. HD: functional capacities in patients treated with neuroleptic and antidepressant drugs. Neurology 1981; 31:1333–1335.
121. van Vugt JP, van Hilten BJ, Roos RA. Hypokinesia in Huntington's disease. Mov Disord 1996; 11:384–388.
122. Schott K, Ried S, Dichgans J. Antipsychotically induced dystonia in Huntington's disease: A case report. Eur Neurol 1989; 29:39–40.
123. Kapur S, Seeman P. Does fast dissociation from the dopamine d(2) receptor explain the action of atypical antipsychotics?: A new hypothesis. Am J Psychiatry 2001; 158:360–369.
124. Sajatovic M, Verbanac P, Ramirez LF et al. Clozapine treatment of psychiatric symptoms resistant to antipsychotic treatment in patients with Huntington's chorea. Neurology 1991; 41:156.
125. Van Vugt JP, Siesling S, Vergeer M, van der Velde EA, Roos RA. Clozapine versus placebo in Huntington's disease: a double blind randomised comparative study. J Neurol Neurosurg Psychiatry 1997; 63:35–39.
126. Bonuccelli U, Ceravolo R, Maremmani C, Nuti A, Rossi G, Muratorio A. Clozapine in Huntington's chorea Neurology 1994; 44(5):821–823.
127. Squitieri F, Cannella M, Porcellini A et al. Short-term effects of olanzapine in Huntington's Disease. Neuropsychiatry Neuropsychol Behav Neurol 2001; 14:69–72.
128. Dewhurst K, Oliver JE, McKnight AL. Socio-psychiatric consequences of Huntington's disease. Br J Psych 1970; 116:255–258.
129. Shiwach R. Psychopathology in Huntington's disease in patients. Acta Psychiatr Scand 1994; 90:241–246.
130. Starkstein SE, Robinson RG. Depression and Parkinson's disease, in Aging and Clinical Practice: Depression and co-existing disease. In: Robinson RG, Rabins PV, eds. Igaku-Shoi, New York, pp. 213–248.
131. Sadovnik AD, Remick RA, Allen J et al. Depression and multiple sclerosis. Neurol 1996; 46:628–632.
132. Loreck DJ, Folstein MF. Depression in Alzheimer's disease, in Depression and neurologic disease. In: Starkstein SE, Robinson G, eds. Baltimore: John Hopkins Press, pp. 50–62.
133. Schoenfield M, Meyers RH, Cupples RA, Barkman B et al. Increased rate of suicide among patients with Huntington's disease. J Neurol Neurosurg Psychiatry 1984; 47:1283–1287.
134. Cummings JL, Cunningham K. Obsessive-compulsive disorder in Huntington's Disease. Biol Psychiatry 1992; 31:263–270.
135. Anderson K, Louis E, Stern Y, Marder K. Cognitive Correlates of Obsessive and Compulsive Symptoms in Huntington's Disease. Am J Psychiatry 2001; 158: 799–801.
136. Marder K, Zhao H, Myers RH et al. Rate of functional decline in Huntington's disease. Neurology 2000; 54(2):452–458.
137. Karno M, Goldin JM, Sorenson SB, Burnom A. The epidemiology of obsessive compulsive disorder in five U.S. communities. Arch Gene Psychiatry 1988; 45:1094–1099.
138. Dewhurst K, Oliver J, Trick K et al. Neuro-psychiatric aspects of Huntington's disease. Confin Neurol 1969; 31:258–268.

139. Cummings JL, Cunningham K. Obsessive-Compulsive disorder in Huntington's Disease. Biol Psychiatry 1992; 31:263–270.
140. Scicutella A. Late life obsessive compulsive disorder and Huntington's disease. J Neuropsychiatry Clin Neurosci 2000; 12(2):288–289.
141. Tonkonogy J, Barreira P. Obsessive-compulsive disorder and caudate frontal lesion. Neuropsychiatry Neuropsychol Behav Neurol 1989; 2:203–209.
142. De Marchi N, Morris M, Mennella R, La Pia S, Nestadt G. Association of obsessive-compulsive disorder and pathological gambling with Huntington's disease in an Italian pedigree: possible association with Huntington's disease mutation. Acta Psychiatria Scandia 1998; 97:62–65.
143. De Marchi N, Mennella R. Huntington's disease and its association with psychopathology. Harvard Rev Psychiatry 2000; 7:278–289.
144. Alexander GE, Crutcher MD. Functional architecture of basal ganglia circuits: neural substrates of parallel processing. Trends Neurosc 1990; 13:266–271.
145. Mayberg HS, Starkstein SE, Peyser CE, Brandt J et al. Paralimbic frontal lobe hypometabolism in depression associated with Huntington's disease. Neurology 1992; 42:1791–1797.
146. Mayberg HS, Starkstein SE, Sadzot B et al. Selective hypometabolism in the inferior frontal lobe in depressed patients with Parkinson's disease. Ann Neurol 1990; 28:57–64.
147. Baxter LR, Schwartz JM, Phelps ME et al. Reduction of prefrontal cortex metabolism common to three types of depression. Arch Gen Psychiatry 1989; 46: 243–250.
148. Mindham RHS, Steele C, Folstein MF, Lucas J. A comparison of the frequency of major affective disorder in Huntington's disease and Alzheimer's disease. J Neurol Neurosurg Psychiatry 1985; 48:1172–1174.
149. Fogel BS. Drug therapy in neuropsychiatry. In: Fogel BS, Schiffer RB, Rao SM, eds. Neuropsychiatry. Williams & Waverly, 1996.
150. Peyser CE, Folstein SE. Depression in Huntington's disease, In: Starkstein SE, Robinson RG, eds. Depression in Neurologic Disease. Baltimore: John Hopkins University Press, 1993:117–139 .
151. Ranen NG, Peyser CE, Folstein SE. A Physician's Guide to the Management of Huntington's Disease: Pharmacologic and Non-pharmacologic Interventions. Huntington's Disease Society of America, 1993.
152. Lyketsos CG, Sheppard JM, Steele CD et al. Randomized, placebo controlled, double blind clinical trial of sertraline in the treatment of depression complicating Alzheimer's disease: initial results from the depression in Alzheimer's Disease study. Am J Psych 2000; 157:1686–1689.
153. Scott TF, Nussbaum P, McConnell H et al. Measurement of treatment response to sertraline in depressed multiple sclerosis patients using the Carrol scale. Neurol Res 1995; 1:421–422.
154. Flax JW, Gray J, Herbert J. Effects of fluoxetine on patients with multiple sclerosis. Am J Psych 1991; 14:1603.
155. Ranen NG, Lipsey JR, Treisman G et al. Sertraline in the treatment of severe aggressiveness in Huntington's disease. J Neuropsychiatry Clin Neurosci 1996; 8:338–340.
156. Hoehn-Saric R, Lipsey JR, McLeod DR. Apathy and indifference in patients in patients on fluoxetine and fluvoxamine. J Clin Psychopharmacol 1990; 10: 343–345.

157. Kapur S, Remington G. Serotonin-dopamine interaction and its relevance to schizophrenia. Am J Psych 1996; 153:466–476.
158. Folstein SE, Folstein MF, McHugh PR. Psychiatric syndromes in Huntington's disease. In: Chase TN et al. eds. Adv Neurol. Raven Press, NY, 23:281–289.
159. Folstein SE, Abbott MH, Chase GA, Jensen BA, Folstein MF. The association of affective disorder with Huntington's disease in a case series and in families. Psychol Med 1983; 13:537–542.
160. Moldawsky RJ. Effect of amoxapine on speech in a patient with Huntington's disease. Am J Psych 1984; 141:150.
161. Folstein S, Folstein M. Diagnosis and treatment of Huntington's disease. Compr Ther 1981; 7:60–66.
162. Ranen NG, Peyser CE, Folstein SE. ECT as a treatment for depression in Huntington's disease. J Neuropsych 1994; 6:154–158.
163. Evans DL, Pedersen C, Tancer ME. ECT in the treatment of organic psychosis in Huntington's disease. Convulsive Ther 1987; 3:145–150.
164. Decruyenaere M, Evers-Kiebooms G, Boogaerts A, Cassiman JJ, Cloostermans T, Demyttenaere K, Dom R, Fryns JP. Psychological functioning before testing for Huntington's disease: the role of the parental disease, risk, perception, and subjective proximity of the disease. J Med Genet 1999; 36:897–905.
165. Taylor CA, Myers RH. Long-term impact of Huntington's disease linkage testing. Amer J Med Genet 1997; 70:365–370.
166. Codori AM, Slavney PR, Young C, Miglioretti DL, Brand J. Predictors of psychological adjustment to genetic testing for Huntington's disease. Health Psychol 1997; 16:36–50.
167. Almquist EW, Bloch M, Brinkman R, Craufurd D, Hayden MR. A worldwide assessment of the frequency of suicide, suicide attempts, or psychiatric hospitalization after predictive testing for Huntington's disease. Am J Hum Genet 1999; 64:1293–1304.
168. Hayden MR, Bloch M, Wiggins S. Psychological effects of predictive testing for Huntington's disease. In: Weiner WJ, Lang AE. eds. Advances in Neurology, Vol. 65. Behavior Neurology of Movement Disorders. New York: Raven Press, 1995:201–210.
169. Mandich P, Jacopini G, DiMaria E, Sabbadini, G, Chimirri F, Bellone E, Novelleto A, Ajmar F, Frontali M. Predictive testing in Huntington's disease: ten years experience in two Italian centers. Italian J Neurol Sci 1998; 19:68–74.
170. Lawson K, Wiggins S, Green T, Adam S, Bloch M, Hayden MR. Adverse psychological events occurring in the first year after predictive testing for Huntington's disease: The Canadian collaborative predictive testing. J Med Genet 1996; 33:862–862.
171. Decruyenaere M, Evers-Kiebooms G, Boogaerts A, Cassiman JJ, Cloostermans T, Demyttenaere K, Dom R, Fryns JP, Van den Berghe H. Prediction of psychological functioning one year after the predictive test for Huntington's disease and impact of the test result on reproductive decision making. J Med Genet 1996; 33:737–743.

9

Dementia in Neuromuscular Disorders

Valeria Sansone and Giovanni Meola

University of Milan, San Donato Hospital, Milan, Italy

INTRODUCTION

Patients with neuromuscular disorders very often have disabling conditions that may interfere with everyday activities. The disabilities caused by a neuromuscular disorder may affect mood: depression and anxiety may develop. These symptoms are often a reactive response to the underlying medical condition and are usually not considered part of the neuromuscular disorder. There are, however, a number of neuromuscular disorders in which behavioral and cognitive studies have demonstrated a selective impairment of brain function. This may be the result of the absence or deficiency of a membrane structural protein (like dystrophin) present in brain and muscle or of a ubiquitous protein kinase (like that involved in myotonic dystrophy type 1 or Steinert's disease). Alternatively, tissues like brain, in which oxidative metabolism is very active, may be affected just like muscle in the mitochondrial encephalomyopathies. Channelopathies may involve muscle and nerve, but also brain function if the ion channels responsible for the neuromuscular symptoms are present in brain neurons. There is growing evidence that clinical manifestations of amyotrophic lateral sclerosis (ALS) can include a frontotemporal dementia, which may correlate with the extent of ubiquitin-immunoreactive intraneural inclusions in cortical regions (Table 1).

Traditionally considered muscle-selective disorders, behavioral and cognitive studies have demonstrated that some neuromuscular diseases are also brain diseases. This may have important implications for the clinical management of patients with these neuromuscular disorders.

Table 1   Classification of Neuromuscular Disorders Associated with a Dementia Syndrome

---

Hereditary
Dystrophinopathies (Duchenne and Becker muscular dystrophy)
Myotonic dystrophies (myotonic dystrophy type 1, DM1, and myotonic dystrophy type 2, DM2/PROMM)
Congenital muscular dystrophies
Familial amyotrophic lateral sclerosis (fALS)
Mitochondrial encephalomyopathy
Acquired
Sporadic amyotrophic lateral sclerosis
Neuromyotonia

SPECIFIC DISORDERS

Brain Function in the Dystrophinopathies

The dystrophinopathies are the most common form of muscle disease. Clinically, they present with progressive proximal muscle weakness associated with high levels of creatinephosphokinase (CPK). The dystrophin gene is the largest gene identified to date (2.5 million base pairs) and is susceptible to a very high spontaneous mutation rate. The gene resides on the X chromosome, so that the disease affects males only. Complete absence of dystrophin causes Duchenne muscular dystrophy (DMD). Patients present symptoms in early childhood and are usually wheelchair-bound by age 11. Death occurs in teenage years from cardiac or respiratory failure unless the patient is ventilated. Patients with milder symptoms, presenting later in childhood and still ambulatory in young adulthood, usually display deletion mutations of the dystrophin gene that are still compatible with translation of a semifunctional protein [Becker muscular dystrophy (BMD)]. The protein is dystrophin, a 427-kDa component of the membrane cytoskeleton of muscle fibers, smooth muscle, and neurons. The primary function of the dystrophin molecule in muscle is to reinforce the muscle membrane against contraction-induced injury and its action is supported by a number of dystrophin-associated glycoproteins (actin, dystroglycan, sarcoglycans). Insights into dystrophin physiology and pathophysiology have been gained through the study of dystrophin-deficient animals, particularly the mdx mouse.

An important aspect of DMD that deserves attention is the role played by the absence or deficiency of dystrophin on CNS function (1). Seven promoters scattered throughout the huge DMD/BMD gene locus normally code for distinct isoforms of dystrophin that exhibit nervous system developmental, regional, and cell-type specificity. Regulation of dystrophin and associated glycoproteins in brain seems to be different than in muscle. For instance, there is evidence that dystrophin and utrophin are separately regulated in brain and that dystrophin deficiency does not result in utrophin upregulation, suggesting that they may have distinct roles in CNS neurons (2). In muscle, dystrophin anchors several glyco-proteins, including alpha- and beta-dystroglycans, syntrophins, and dystrobre-vins. In contrast to muscle, little is known about the localization and the molecular interactions of dystrophin and dystrophin-associated glycoproteins in brain. In the brain, these molecules may have a role in the organization of CNS synapses (3). It has been well established that full-length dystrophin and specific smaller isoforms appear in the synapses of some neurons and, in particu-lar, in the synapes of the rods and bipolar cells of the retina (4–6). These isoforms are Dp260 and Dp71, expressed in rod spherules and in other brain regions. Dysfunction of these isoforms in the retina is responsible for the abnormalities observed on the retinogram (reduction in B/A wave amplitude ratio) (4–8).

Less clear is the role of dystrophin or its isoforms in brain function. This issue is complicated by the number of different dystrophin isoforms expressed by different neuronal cell types (9,10). In brain, Dp71 is the major protein product of the dystrophin gene, but there is evidence that Dp71 isoforms may have different functions in the same cell or organelle (11). Different neuronal subtypes and glial cells may express dystroglycan in complexes where full-length or truncated dystrophin is variably associated with the other glycoproteins, such as full-length or truncated utrophin. By bridging the extracellular matrix and the cytoskeleton, dystroglycan may play an important role in synapses and at the blood–brain barrier, areas where the membrane structural and functional organ-ization need to be strictly maintained (12).

There is growing clinical evidence linking the absence of dystrophin with cognitive dysfunction. Duchenne in his initial descriptions (13) noted that some boys displayed cognitive impairment and there is now overwhelming evidence supporting these original observations. The average IQ of a boy with DMD is 85, and 30% of boys with the disease have an IQ <70 (14–28). Regardless of IQ, a specific cognitive profile, namely poor performance in digit span, story recall, and comprehension, was observed in a sample of 80 boys with DMD (29). Genotype–phenotype correlations between deletion mutation and degree of cognitive impairment have not been conclusive. Distal dystrophin deletions involving Dp140 are associated with intellectual impairment, suggesting that this brain distal isoform plays a role in normal cognitive development (30). Del-etions towards the 3' end have been shown to have a higher incidence of cognitive impairment (31,32). Others found that deletions in exon 52 are associated with cognitive impairment in 70% of the patients (33), while still other authors (9) have correlated cognitive impairment with the presence of a mutation in the Dp71 isoform. The variable degree of cognitive impairment may be related to the different dystrophin gene mutations present in the boys tested in the different studies. In any case, mental retardation in DMD does not seem to be progressive. For this reason, transient ischemia during development or at birth resulting from a direct effect of dystrophin deficiency in vascular smooth muscle in arteries and arterioles has been proposed as a possible alternative explanation for the cognitive impairment. Consistent with a vascular etiology of mental retardation in DMD is the finding of dystrophin isoforms on the pericapillary endfeet of astrocytes at the blood–brain barrier in hippocampus and cerebral cortex (34–34c). The alterations occurring in the brain vessel wall of the mdx mouse, affect both endothelial and astroglial cells and are associated with opened tight junctions associated proteins and specific water channels (aquaporin-4) suggesting that part of the pathomechanisms associated with brain changes may be related to changes in brain osmotic equilibrium (34d–36).

Functional studies of brain in mdx mouse and in patients with DMD are contradictory. Initial studies suggested that Mdx mice seemed to act normally for both spatial learning and hippocampal long-term potentiation (37). More recent studies however, suggest that dystrophin deficiency in mdx mice impairs long-term memory and spatial learning, at least in part due to altered synaptic plasticity mechanisms, and suggest that the severity of the deficits may depend on the nature of the training process (37a).

Clear evidence correlating clinical evidence of brain dysfunction and brain structural changes is lacking. Histological abnormalities have been observed in 14% (39) to 65% of the cases (40–44) and consist of neuronal loss, heterotopias, gliosis, neurofibrillary tangles, Purkinje cell loss, abnormal dendritic length, branching and intersection abnormalities, disordered architecture, astrocytosis, and perinuclear vacuolation. No correlation has been found between neuropsychological deficits and brain MRI in some studies (28,43), while others have found a relationship to measured cortical thickness and ventricular size (45).

Biochemical disturbances underlying the mental deficit associated with the lack of dystrophin are yet to be determined. A PET study (28) and a 31P-magnetic resonance spectroscopy (46) study showed the cerebellum to be the focus of biochemical abnormalities. This finding is particularly interesting because there is a high expression of dystrophin in neurons in this region and because the cognitive deficits in patients with DMD, specifically deficits in verbal working memory (29), are known to have a cerebellar component (47).

Cognitive and Behavioral Findings in the Myotonic Dystrophies

The myotonic dystrophies are the most common muscular dystrophies of adult life and are distinguished from other muscular dystrophies by the presence of myotonia and by a wide range of abnormalities in other organs. They can be classified into myotonic dystrophy type 1 known as DM1 or Steinert's disease and myotonic dystrophy type 2 (or DM2/PROMM, where PROMM is an eponym describing proximal myotonic myopathy) (48–50). They are genetically distinct disorders that share common clinical features and pathophysiology (51–55).

DM1 is caused by an abnormal triplet expansion (CTG repeat) on the myotonic dystrophy protein kinase (DMPK) gene on chromosome 19q13 (56–60). The larger the expansion, the more severe is the phenotype. No correlation has been found, however, between degree of leukocyte (CTG)n expansion and cardiac or CNS involvement. DM2 is caused by a tetraplet expansion CCTG on chromosome 3q21 (61–62c).

Both DM1 and DM2 are characterized by autosomal dominant inheritance, clinical and EMG myotonia, posterior iridescent cataracts, and muscle weakness. In DM1, weakness is predominantly distal, whereas in DM2, it may be predominantly proximal. Both are multisystem disorders, characterized by the involvement of the neuromuscular, cardiovascular, and the endocrine systems, as well as by cognitive and personality abnormalities (51–55,58,63).

Myotonic Dystrophy Type 1: DM1 (Fig. 1)

Congenital form: This is clinically distinctive from the classical adult form of myotonic dystrophy and is associated with very large (CTG)n expansions (usually >1000). This form of the disease is generally maternally transmitted, although paternal transmission has also been reported (64). It is recognized as one of the major neuromuscular causes of respiratory insufficiency. Clinically, the disorder presents in utero with hydramnios and decreased fetal movements. At birth, many skeletal and neuromuscular manifestations distinguish these children from their affected parents. Facial diplegia is prominent and jaw weakness is also. This is in striking contrast to skeletal muscle strength, which may be diminished but only to a minor degree. No myotonia is present; rather, these patients

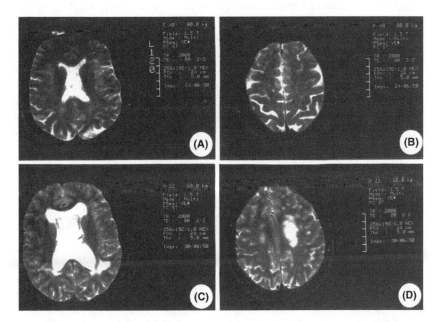

Figure 1 Brain MRI scans of a 53-year-old female patient with adult onset myotonic dystrophy type 1 (**A, B**) with the typical cognitive and behavioral abnormalities described in the text. Brain MRI of the 15-year-old son of the patient in **A** and **B**, with congenital myotonic dystrophy (**C, D**).

display hypotonia. In the neonatal period, respiratory failure and poor feeding are typically present and talipes, thin ribs, and elevated diaphragm are evident. More widespread muscle weakness develops later in life, together with muscle wasting. Myotonia may be observed at this point.

Mental retardation in congenital myotonic dystrophy is typically present, even when anoxia has not been a major concern at birth (58,65). Dilation of cerebral ventricles is common and occlusive hydrocephalus may occur (66). IQ in congenital myotonic dystrophy patients ranges from 50–70, but the cognitive deficit does not seem to deteriorate over time (65). In most patients with the congenital form, cognitive impairment correlates closely with macrocephaly, the degree of ventricular dilatation, hypoplasia of the corpus callosum, and supratentorial white matter hyperintense lesions as seen on brain neuroimaging (67–69). Proton magnetic resonance spectroscopy demonstrates a decrease in *N*-acetyl aspartate, indicating a developmental disorder of neurons in brain (70).

Adult form: Estimates of the incidence of mental retardation (IQ < 75%) or of abnormal scores on measures of general intelligence (in Standard Progressive Matrices, Mini-Mental State Examination) vary from 20% to 80% DM1 (58,59,59a) and have been reported to be associated with an abnormally high CTG repeat size (>1000) (71,72). Abnormal scores on measures of visual and verbal memory have been reported by some authors (73), but not others (74). Estimates of impairment on frontal lobe and perceptual-motor tests range between 50% and 90% (71,75–77). Equivocal results have been found in the neuropsychiatric evaluation of patients with DM1. A high incidence of depressive symptoms has been described by some authors (77–79), which have been ascribed to a reaction to the disabling medical condition rather than being a direct expression of the DM1 protein kinase-related disorder (77,80). However, others have suggested that depressive symptoms are a part of a neurologic apathy syndrome typically present in DM1 patients. Estimates of personality disorders as defined by DSM-IIIR criteria range from 30% to 40% (75,81). A high incidence of dependent tendencies has been observed (77), while others have found a homogeneous personality cluster C profile (avoidant, obsessive–compulsive, passive–aggressive) (81). Inconsistencies may be due to methodological differences in the tests applied and to differences in the patients' neurological profiles.

Correlations between neuropsychological and behavioral disturbances and neuroimaging results have not been clearly evident. Brain MRI studies have shown white matter hyperintense lesions, especially in the anterior portions of the temporal poles, but these do not seem to correlate with the degree of brain dysfunction (82,83). Generalized atrophy has also been observed (82) and dilated convexity Virchow-Robin spaces have been suggested as one of the initial findings on the MRI of patients with adult DM1 (84). Reductions in cerebral blood flow have been demonstrated by H20 PET studies in the orbital and mesial aspects of the frontal poles and in the temporal areas (83).

The relatively few neuropathologic studies available have shown a diffuse loss of myelin in the deep white matter of the brain corresponding to the white matter hyperintensities observed on neuroimaging (78,85). Pathological tau proteins have been found in the hippocampus, the enthorinal cortex, and in most of the temporal areas with a possible relationship to disease severity (86). The pathological tau proteins (hyperphosphorylated) have been shown to aggregate in a characteristic pattern in DM1 brains, where only the shortest tau isoforms aggregate and these correlate positively with the degree of CTG brain expansion (87). A reduced brain expression of DM-associated homeo domain protein (DMAHP) mRNA, the product of a neighboring DMPK gene, has been demonstrated in different brain areas and has been suggested to be responsible for the cognitive impairment in patients with DM1 (88,88a). A possible relationship between a decrease of catecholaminergic neurons in the medullary reticular formation and the presence of alveolar hypoventilation has also been suggested (89). Transgenic mouse models for myotonic dystrophy type 1 have provided evidence that the expansion of the CTGn repeat at the DMPK locus on chromosome 19q determines at the RNA level, a gain-of-function mechanism, with dominant toxic effects of the CUGn repeats containing transcripts (like tau proteins) that is central to the pathophysiology of the disorder. Recent studies have demonstrated that myotonic dystrophy type 1 is associated with nuclear foci of mutant RNA, sequestration of muscleblind proteins and deregulated alternative splicing in neurons. Parallel studies in DM2 have revealed a similar mechanism (89a–89c).

Myotonic Dystrophy Type 2: PROMM/DM2 (Figs. 2 and 3)

Congenital form: No congenital form has been described to date.

Adult form: Hund et al. (90) were the first to describe white matter hyperintense lesions in the brains of nine patients with proximal myotonic myopathy.

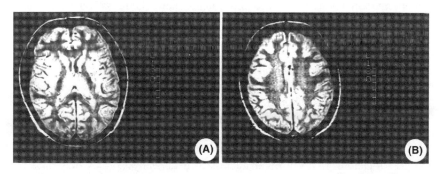

Figure 2 Brain MRI scan of a 56-year-old female patient with myotonic dystrophy type 2 (**A**) and (**B**) having the same, but less severe, abnormalities in cognition and behavior as described for the patient in Figure 1. Note the absence of signs on the scans.

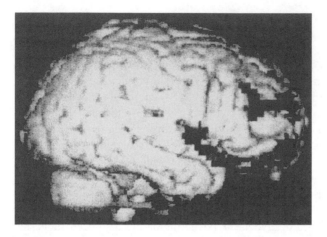

Figure 3 Brain SPECT study of a patient with myotonic dystrophy type 2 with a normal brain MRI scan and the typical abnormalities in frontal lobe function and avoidant personality trait disorder described in the text. Similar but more widespread findings are present in myotonic dystrophy type 1 patients.

These were confluent lesions involving periventricular areas giving rise to an MRI appearance similar to that observed in CADASIL (cerebral autosomal dominant arteriopathy with subcortical infarcts and leukoencephalopathy). The patients described by Hund did not complain of symptoms of mental delay. No neuropsychological studies were performed on these patients so that, although the abnormalities on MRI were striking, no clear correlation between clinical and neuroimaging results could be made. In a more recent study, Meola et al. (83) investigated 20 patients with proximal myotonic myopathy (PROMM), 20 patients with DM1, and 20 age-, sex-, and education-matched controls (85). A selective involvement of visual-spatial functions in DM1 and, to a minor degree, in PROMM, was demonstrated in this study. This cognitive abnormality did not correlate with structural abnormalities demonstrated by brain MRI. In fact, the hyperintense lesions were considered to be non-specific and not responsible for the observed neuropsychological deficits. Conversely, functional neuroimaging with PET demonstrated a common pattern of hypoperfusion in both groups, with regional cerebral blood flow reductions in the ventral and mesial aspects of the frontal lobes (orbitofrontal cortex) and in the temporal poles. Unfortunately, the battery of neuropsychological tests used in this study, which did not include specific measures of frontal lobe function, did not allow a specific correlation with the observed regional cerebral blood flow abnormalities. Moreover, the number of patients with PROMM was limited and the subjects were not fully characterized genetically, so they may have represented a subset of patients with DM2.

More recently, we further investigated cognitive function, specifically frontal lobe function, to determine whether there was a specific and typical cognitive and neuropsychiatric profile in patients with DM1 and DM2/PROMM and to correlate these findings to the degree of (CTG)n and (CCTG)n expansion (submitted paper). Twenty-one patients with moderately severe DM1 (500–700 repeats) and 19 patients with genetically confirmed 3q21 DM2 were included in the study and subjected to a battery of frontal lobe function tests and to a neuropsychiatric assessment and a personality disorder assessment scale. Mini-mental-state-examination (MMSE), in agreement with our previous study (85), was normal in DM1 and DM2/PROMM (score >27 in both groups), although both groups performed worse than controls ($p < 0.01$). Both groups were impaired on frontal lobe function tests. The only significant difference between DM1 and DM2/PROMM in frontal lobe function was on the trail-making test (TMT) where patients with DM2/PROMM had significantly worse scores ($p < 0.001$). This difference was probably not accounted for by the motor impairment in these patients since it was minimal, especially distally. Both groups performed worse than controls on the Tower of London, Stroop and Winsconsin card sorting tests. In general, the neuropsychological pattern appears to be overlapping in DM1 and DM2/PROMM. None of the patients fulfilled DSM-IIIR criteria for axis I or II disorders. Both patients with DM1 and DM2/PROMM showed significant avoidant behavioral trait clustering ($p < 0.05$) compared to control subjects, with the DM2/PROMM patients standing at an intermediate level between DM1 and controls. This is in agreement with the familiar "indifferent" attitude displayed by these patients towards the disease, even when severe manifestations have appeared.

To summarize, the cognitive and neuropsychiatric profile of patients with DM2/PROMM, like DM1, is characterized by a dysexecutive frontal lobe apathy syndrome and by an avoidant personality trait disorder, which is typical of the myotonic dystrophies. The neuropsychological and neuropsychiatric findings cannot be accounted for by depression or anxiety, which were absent in our group of patients.

In agreement with other observations regarding the correlation between degree of expansion and severity of neuromuscular or cardiac involvement (59), there is no clear relationship between degree of leukocyte CTG or CCTG expansion and the scores obtained on neuropsychological and neuropsychiatric testings.

In a previous study investigating brain function in the myotonic dystrophies, we suggested a possible correlation between the selective visual-spatial impairment and the cerebral blood flow reductions observed by H215O and PET (85). The impairment on tests of frontal lobe functions in DM1 and DM2/PROMM fits well with our previous PET findings of rCBF reductions in frontal regions (83,83a). The role of the frontal mesial cortex in executive functions and set shifting behavior is well established (91–93). Furthermore, the finding of avoidant personality trait disorder in DM1 and DM2/PROMM may also be accounted for by the selective frontal lobe dysfunction as revealed by our PET studies. This finding might be in agreement with recent

PET studies of neurotransmission, which showed correlations between dopamine and serotonin receptor binding within the frontal lobe and selective personality traits (94,95).

Specific neurotransmitters may be involved in those brain regions where blood flow is reduced. Impaired executive function, apathy, and impulsivity are hallmarks of frontal–subcortical circuit dysfunction. The elevated number of serotonin (5-HT1A) receptors in the prefrontal cortex and the dopaminergic modulation (D1) of the prefrontal–subcortical circuits suggest that these neurotransmitters may play a role in the modulatory influence of limbic-prefrontal cortex circuits during behavior. Indirectly, recent observations suggest that dysfunction in dopaminergic and serotoninergic signaling in the prefrontal cortex may contribute to impairment of executive frontal lobe functioning, affecting the planning, initiation, and regulation of goal-directed behavior in DM1 and DM2/PROMM. Ongoing studies with specific neurotransmitter ligands may provide support for this hypothesis, further clarify the mechanisms involved in the brain disease that distinctly characterizes patients with myotonic dystrophies, and suggest possible therapies.

Brain Involvement in the Congenital Muscular Dystrophies

Congenital muscular dystrophies (CMDs) are usually autosomal recessive diseases, characterized by very early onset, with hypotonia manifesting in the early years of life. In some, there is prominent brain involvement compared to muscle (96–98). As a group, the CMDs with prominent brain involvement show structural abnormalities of the brain in the form of neuronal migration defects, ocular abnormalities, and variable degrees of mental retardation. The combination of muscle, brain, and ocular involvement gives rise to three main phenotypes in which brain is particularly involved: Fukuyama CMD, muscle-eye-brain disease, and Walker-Warburg syndrome. The white matter abnormalities observed on brain MRI scans are not always associated with cognitive involvement and these cases are sometimes named "occidental type cerebromuscular dystrophy." However, brain necropsy studies of patients with intellectual impairment have revealed a significant decrease in staining of cortical myelin or cortical areas with polymicrogyria, cerebellar neuronal loss, heterotopic nerve cells, degeneration of myelin sheath, cerebellar hypoplasia, and spongy appearance of white matter (99,100). Necropsy neuropathological examination of a case with normal mental development revealed the same gyral abnormalities as in those cases in whom mental involvement is severe, showing overlap between the different groups.

Fukuyama CMD

This form is seen with high frequency in Japan, has recently been localized to chromosome 9q31-33 (101), and the gene (*fukutin*) is known (102). A common retrotransposon insertion is responsible for almost all cases in Japan.

Muscle involvement may be severe with profound muscle weakness and very high CPK. Intellectual impairment is also usually severe and is microscopically associated with neuronal cell migration abnormalities. Ocular involvement may be mild (103–107). Cerebral changes are always present. Type II lissencephaly is the characteristic finding in this disease. Abnormalities of CNS involvement range from cobblestone polymicrogyria to pachygyria to complete agyria due to neuronal migration abnormalities. Dysplasia of the pyramidal tracts is common. Ventricular dilation is mild if present. Delayed myelination is noted on MRI. Cerebellar cysts are common. Seizures occur in 50% of patients (107a). Recent studies have suggested that loss of interaction between alpha-sarcoglycan and its ligands plays a role in the pathogenesis of cortical dysplasia in Fukuyama-type congenital muscular dystrophy (107b,107c).

Muscle-Eye-Brain Disease

This form is seen frequently in Finland and has been localized to chromosome 1p, but the gene is not known yet (108). Muscle involvement varies and is usually associated with high CPK. A deficiency in alpha-dystroglycan has been found (109). Cerebral alterations are more prominent in this form and may be associated with marked cortical atrophy, atrophy of the cerebellar vermis, and the brainstem. Ocular abnormalities are variable.

Walker-Warburg Syndrome

This form is not confined to a particular area. The chromosome involved is yet to be discovered. CPK levels are elevated. It is the most severe form with very marked brain malformations, including type II lissencephaly, ventricular dilatation, and encephalocele. Ocular abnormalities vary. Children usually die before two years of age (110–114). Recently an autosomal recessive limb girdle muscular dystrophy (LGMD2) with mild mental retardation has been shown to be allelic to Walker-Warburg syndrome and is caused by a mutation in the protein O-mannosultransferase (POMT1) gene which affects glycosylation of alpha-sarcoglycan (114a).

Neuropsychological Findings in Motor Neuron Disorders

Motor neuron disease (MND) is typically characterized by muscle atrophy, weakness, and preserved or increased deep tendon reflexes in more than three muscle groups. Diffuse spontaneous limb fasciculations are present. It usually presents in the fourth and fifth decades but can occur at any age in adult life. Both sexes are equally affected. The disease is rapidly progressive in its typical form and death usually occurs on an average of five years from the initial diagnosis. Bulbar involvement, characterized by dysarthria, dysphonia, and dysphagia, is frequently present and is a negative prognostic sign.

Table 2   Forms of Dementia Associated with Motor Neuron Disease

Guam ALS-parkinsonism-dementia complex
ALS associated with dementia and parkinsonism
Alzheimer's disease
Presenile dementia with motor neuron disease of non-Alzheimer type
Aphasic dementia in motor neuron disease
Thalamic dementia
Creutzfeld-Jacob's disease
Gerstmann-Straussler-Scheinker syndrome

Growing evidence of cognitive impairment in MND, in the form of mental delay, has been suggested to support the concept that motor neurons are affected in the cortex as well as in the anterior horn cells of the spinal cord (Table 2).

It is now well accepted that in MND, cognitive impairment occurs in two forms: a progressive dementia and a subclinical cognitive decline. In some cases, MND may manifest largely as a cognitive disorder (115–116a). There is compelling evidence that both direct and indirect glutamate toxicity contribute to the pathogenesis of motor neuron degeneration and that modified function of glutamate channels may be causally linked to the pathogenesis of ALS (116b).

The dementia of MND has been recognized as a form of frontotemporal dementia (117). The association between MND and dementia is more frequent in the familial form (15%) than in the sporadic form (3%). The clinical picture is similar, however, and represents a continuum of pathological changes (118,118a). Neuropsychological studies have demonstrated changes in executive processes, specifically in tests involving problem-solving strategies, like the Winsconsin card sorting test or the computerized version of the Tower of London test (119,120). The presence of a dysexecutive frontal lobe syndrome may complicate the challenges of adjusting to growing physical disability from progression of the disease and may add to the burden for both the patient and caregivers. In addition to the dysexecutive syndrome described previously, dementia in MND may manifest aphasia, apraxia, and behavioral abnormalities of the frontal type (115,121,122).

Dementia in MND can be correlated with bilateral degeneration of the pyramidal tract as observed on brain MRI or with the widened subarachnoid spaces in the frontal and temporal regions. These imaging findings correlate with the neuropathologic findings of atrophy of motor nuclei in the brainstem and anterior horn cells of the cervical spinal cord and with the spongius status in the frontal lobes. Particularly pronounced changes may be observed in Brodman's areas 44 (Broca's area) and 45 in those patients with aphasia and dementia as prominent features (123).

Although the pathological substrate of cognitive decline remains to be defined, the presence of ubiquitin-immunoreactive (Ub+) intraneuronal inclusions in cortical regions has been suggested to be a pathologic marker for the disease process. These inclusions are tau-, synuclein-, and SOD-1 negative. Inclusions were found in four patients with MND and dementia and in four patients with MND and subclinical cognitive impairment (124), although the distribution of the inclusions was more diffuse and widespread in the demented patients. This finding draws parallels between the load of neuronal damage produced by neurofibrillary tangles in Alzheimer's disease and in non-demented middle-aged people, and emphasizes that cognitive impairment in MND is a pathologic continuum underlying a multisystem disorder (124).

Brain Function in the Mitochondrial Encephalomyopathies

Mitochondrial myopathies are a clinically heterogeneous group of disorders caused by biochemical defects affecting one or more of the main steps of substrate oxidation. This may involve substrate transport into mitochondria, the tricarboxylic acid cycle, the electron transport chain, or oxidation/phosphorylation coupling. Mitochondria are ubiquitously distributed so that all tissues may be affected, but those tissues with higher oxidative energy demands, like muscle and brain, are most likely to be clinically affected. The pathogenesis of neurological manifestations in the mitochondrial disorders may also be considered in relation to the possible involvement of free radicals in inducing brain damage (125).

Mental retardation is not typical of these disorders, but in some phenotypes, such as myoclonus epilepsy with ragged red fibers (MERRF), mitochondrial encephalomyopathy, lactic acidosis and stroke-like episodes (MELAS), and Kearns-Sayre syndrome (KSS), cognitive impairment may be present in the later phases of the disease.

MERRF is the result of mitochondrial DNA mutations occurring in the transfer RNA for lysine (tRNA Leu). Some patients with the MELAS mutation, however, have features of MERRF. Typical clinical manifestations are stimulus-sensitive myoclonus, epilepsy in the form of generalized or absence seizures, and the finding of diffuse ragged red fibers on trichrome Gomori stain of muscle biopsy specimens. Progressive neurologic deterioration may include a dementia syndrome or behavioral abnormalities of variable severity in the later stages of the disease (126).

MELAS is the result of point mutations, usually substituting arginine in position 3243 with guanine, in the mitochondrial transfer RNA (tRNA Leu). Cognitive decline and behavioral abnormalities may be present without any clinical evidence of stroke-like episodes (127,128). Progressive dementia with fluctuating symptoms may be the presenting feature of MELAS (129) and may mimic prion-related neurodegenerative disorders (130). Neuropathology of patients with the genetically confirmed MELAS mutation demonstrates widespread cellular disruption, prominent white matter gliosis, cerebellar cortical degeneration of granular cells, and necrotic foci in different cortical regions (131). Alzheimer-type pathology has also been described (132) and is in agreement with the reports of a similar pattern of reduced cerebral blood flow observed by SPECT in brains of patients with MELAS and Alzheimer's disease, both localizing in the parieto-occipital regions (133). A relatively recent report described neuropsychological deficits and cognitive decline in mainly ocular or ocular/myopathic phenotypes, suggesting that cognitive slowing may be present in all forms of mitochondrial disorders (134). An electrophysiological analysis of cognitive slowing, using event-related potentials, has been performed in subjects with chronic progressive ophthalmoplegia. Event-related potentials provide an objective measure of cognitive information processing that is independent of motor response and reflects processes underlying perceptual and cognitive input analysis. In particular, N2 and P3 components reflect processing in the controlled selective attentional stream. They are typically evoked by the active discrimination of target stimuli from other extraneous stimuli. The study (135) demonstrated a significantly increased N2 latency and reduced P3 amplitude on two different tasks of different difficulties, suggesting the presence of an impairment in information processing and resetting of short-term working trace.

Cognitive Function in Neuromyotonia

Neuromyotonia is characterized by stiffness, cramps, myokymia, increased sweating, and occasionally sensory symptoms (136). Pseudomyotonia may be present. It can be associated with a variety of inherited and acquired disorders or it may occur as a paraneoplastic disorder. Thymoma or lung cancer are frequently associated. Most cases are associated with antibodies to glutamic acid decarboxylase, a key enzyme in GABA metabolism. Antibodies against voltage-gated potassium channels (VGKC) have been demonstrated in about 50% of the patients (137).

In some patients with acquired neuromyotonia, behavioral changes have been observed. Poor sleep and hallucinations have been described and may present as limbic encephalitis (138). These neuropsychiatric features may correlate with neuropathological findings of hippocampal degeneration and possibly to the presence of antibodies directed against VGKC in the hippocampus (139).

CONCLUSIONS

It is clear that traditionally considered muscle-restricted diseases are to be viewed more widely as multisystem disorders in which brain function may pose important problems aggravating the muscular disability related to the underlying disorder. The neuropsychological and neuropsychiatric deficits observed in the neuromuscular disorders have important implications for patient management and for planning and implementing support services for patients and their care givers. Although less attention has been given to brain function than to muscle function, slowness in speed of information processing, and impaired capacity for new learning and for problem solving, may impact the patient's everyday life to a similar degree as the limitations caused by the muscle weakness. The dysexecutive deficits may aggravate the patient's dependency separately from their need for physical care. Knowledge of the neuromuscular disorder as a brain disorder as well may help in the management of these patients and could lead to more effective intervention on the part of the patient's care givers. They can be educated in the support required for these patients and in the difficult role of managing behavioral and neuropsychological deficits.

It is clear that studies of brain function in the neuromuscular disorders will not only contribute to understanding the physiology and pathophysiology of the disease process, but will also have practical therapeutic and management implications. Neuropsychological and behavioral measures also need to be considered in the design of potential therapeutic clinical trials in the neuromuscular disorders.

REFERENCES

1. Mehler MF. Brain dystrophin, neurogenetics and mental retardation. Brain Res Rev 2000; 32:277–307.
2. Kneusel I, Zuellig RA, Schaub MC, Fritschy JM. Alterations in dystrophin and utrophin expression parallel the reorganization of GABAergic synapses in a mouse model of temporal lobe epilepsy. Eur J Neurosci 2001; 13:1113–1124.
3. Moukhles H, Carbonetto S. Dystroglycan contributes to the formation of multiple dystrophin-like complexes in the brain. J Neurochem 2001; 78:824–834.
4. Ueda H, Baba T, Terada N, et al. Dystrophin in rod spherules; submembranous dense regions facing bipolar cell processes. Histochem Cell Biol 1997; 108:243–248.
5. Fitzgerald KM, Cibis GW, Gettel AH, et al. ERG phenotype of a dystrophin mutation in heterozygous female carriers of Duchenne muscular dystrophy. J Med Genet 1999; 36:316–322.
6. Pillers DA, Welelber RG, Green DG, et al. Effects of dystrophin isoforms on signal transduction through neural retina: genotype–phenotype analysis of Duchenne muscular dystrophy mouse mutants. Mol Genet Metab 1999; 66:100–110.
7. Pascual Pascual SI, Molano J, Pascual-Castroviejo I. Electroretinogram in Duchenne/Becker muscular dystrophy. Ped Neurol 1998; 18:315–320.
8. Blank M, Koulen P, Blake DJ, Kroger S. Dystrophin and beta-dystroglycan in photoreceptor terminals from normal and mdx3Cv mouse retinae. Eur J Neurosci 1999; 11:2121–2133.
9. Moizard MP, Toutain A, Fournier D, Berret F, Rayndaud M, Billard C, et al. Severe cognitive impairment in DMD: obvious clinical indication for Dp71 isoform point mutation screening. Eur J Hum Genet 2000; 8:552–556.
10. De Stefano ME, Zaccaria ML, Cavaldesi M, et al. Dystrophin and its isoforms in a sympathetic ganglion of normal and dystrophic mdc mice:immunolocalization by electron microscopy and biochemical characterization. Neuroscience 1997; 80: 613–624.
11. Aleman V, Osorio B, Chavez O, Rendon A, Mornet D, Martinez D. Subcellular localization of Dp71 dystrophin isoforms in cultured hippocampal neurons and forebrain astrocytes. Histochem Cell Biol 2001; 115:243–254.
12. Zaccaria ML, Di Tommaso F, Brancaccio A, Paggi P, Petrucci TC. Dystroglycan distribution in adult mouse brain: a light and electron microscopy study. Neuroscience 2001; 104:311–324.

13. Duchenne GBA. Recherches sul la paralysie musculaire pseudohypertrophique, ou paralysie myo-sclerosique. Arc Gen Med 1868; 11:5–25, 179–209, 305–321, 421–443, 552–588.
14. Allen JE, Rogkin DW. Mental retardation in association with progressive dystrophy. Am J Dis Child 1960; 100:208–211.
15. Worden DK, Vignos PJ. Intellectual function in childhood progressive muscular dystrophy. Pediatrics 1962; 29:968–977.
16. Dubowitz V. Intellectual impairment in muscular dystrophy. Arch Dis Child 1965; 40:296–301.
17. Dubowitz V. Involvement of the nervous system in muscular dystrophies in man. Ann NY Acad Sci 1979; 317:431–439.
18. Zellweger H, Niedermeyer E. Central nervous system manifestations in childhood muscular dystrophy (CMD). I. Psychometric and electroencephalographic findings. Ann Pediat 1965; 205:25–42.
19. Zellweger H, Hanson JW. Psychometric studies in muscular dystrophy type 3a (Duchenne). Dev Med Child Neurol 1967; 9:576–581.
20. Cohen HJ, Molnar GE, Taft LT. The genetic relationship of progressive muscular dystrophy (Duchenne type) and mental retardation. Dev Med Child Neurol 1968; 10:754–765.
21. Prosser EJ, Murphy EG, Thompson MW. Intelligence and the gene for Duchenne muscular dystrophy. Arch Dis Child 1969; 44:221–230.
22. Black FW. Intellectual ability as related to age and stage of disease in muscular dystrophy: a brief note. J Psychol 1973; 84:333–334.
23. Marsh GG, Munsat TL. Evidence for early impairment of verbal intelligence in Duchenne muscular dystrophy. Arch Dis Child 1974; 49:118–122.
24. Florek M, Karolak S. Intelligence levels of patients with the Duchenne type of progressive muscular dystrophy (pmd-d). Eur J Pediatr 1977; 126:275–282.
25. Karagan NJ, Zellweger HU. Early verbal disability in children with Duchenne muscular dystrophy. Dev Med Child Neurol 1978; 20:435–441.
26. Karagan NJ. Intellectual functioning in Duchenne muscular dystrophy: a review. [Review]. Psychol Bull 1979; 86:250–259.
27. Leibowitz D, Dubowitz V. Intellect and behavior in Duchenne muscular dystrophy. Dev Med Child Neurol 1981; 23:577–590.
28. Bresolin N, Castelli E, Comi GP, Felisari G, Bardoni A, Perani D, et al. Cognitive impairment in Duchenne muscular dystrophy. Neuromusc Disord 1994; 4:359–369.
29. Hinton VJ, De Vivo DC, Nereo NE, Goldstein E, Stern Y. Poor verbal working memory across intellectual level in boys with Duchenne dystrophy. 2000; 54:2127–2132.
30. Felisari G, Martinelli Boneschi F, Bardoni A, Sironi M, Comi GP, Robotti M, Turconi AC, Lai M, Corrao G, Bresolin N. Neurology 2000; 55:559–564.
31. Bushby KM. Genetic and clinical correlations of Xp21 muscular dystrophy. [Review]. J Inherit Metab Dis 1992; 15:551–564.
32. Lenk U, Hanke R, Thiele H, Speer A. Point mutations at the carboxy terminus of the human dystrophin gene: implications for an association with mental retardation in DMD patients. Hum Mol Genet 1993; 2:1877–1881.
33. Rapaport D, Passos-Bueno MR, Brandao L, Love D, Vainzof M, Zatz M. Apparent association of mental retardation and specific patterns of deletions screened with

probes cf56a and cf23a in Duchenne muscular dystrophy. Am J Med Genet 1991; 39:437–441.

34. Bushby KM, Appleton R, Anderson LV, Welch JL, Kelly P, Gardner-Medwin D. Deletion status and intellectual impairment in Duchenne muscular dystrophy. Dev Med Child Neurol 1995; 37:260–269.

34a. Haenggi T, Sootornmalai A, Schaub MC, Fritschy JM. The role of utrophin and Dp71 for assembly of different dystrophin-associated protein complexes (DPCs) in the choroid plexus and microvasculature of the brain. Neuroscience 2004; 129: 403–413.

34b. Zaccaria ML, Di Tommaso F, Brancaccio A, Paggi P, Petrucci TC. Dystroglycan distribution in adult mouse brain: a light and electron microscopy study. Neuroscience 2001; 104:311–324.

34c. Jancsik V, Hajos F. The demonstration of immunoreactive dystrophin and its developmental expression in perivascular astrocytes. Brain Res 1999; 831:200–205.

34d. Nico B, Roncali L, Mangieri D, Ribatti D. Blood-brain barrier alterations in MDX mouse, an animal model of the Duchenne muscular dystrophy. Neurovasc Res 2005; 2:47–54.

35. Nicchia GP, Nico B, Camassa LM, Mola MG, Loh N, Dermietzel R, Spray DC, Svelto M, Frigeri A. The role of aquaporin-4 in the blood-brain barrier development and integrity: studies in animal and cell culture models. Neuroscience 2004; 129:935–945.

36. Nicchia GP, Srinivas M, Li W, Brosnan CF, Frigeri A, Spray DC. New possible roles for aquaporin-4 in astrocytes: cell cytoskeleton and functional relationship with connexin43. FASEB J 2005; 19:1674–1676.

37. Sesay AK, Errington ML, Levita L, Bliss TV. Spatial learning and hippocampal long-term potentiation are not impaired in mdx mice. Neurosci Lett 1996; 211:207–210.

37a. Vaillend C, Billard JM, Laroche S. Impaired long-term spatial and recognition memory and enhanced CA1 hippocampal LTP in the dystrophin-deficient Dmd (mdx) mouse. Neurobiol Dis 2004; 17:10–20.

38. Di Lazzaro V, Restuccia D, Servidei S, Nardone R, Oliviero A, Profice P, et al. Functional involvement of cerebral cortex in Duchenne muscular dystrophy. Muscle & Nerve 1998; 21:662–664.

39. Dubowitz V, Crome L. The central nervous system in Duchenne muscular dystrophy. Brain 1969; 92:805–808.

40. Rosman NP, Kakulas BA. Mental deficiency associated with muscular dystrophy. A neuropathological study. Brain 1966; 89.769–788.

41. Rosman NP. The cerebral defect and myopathy in Duchenne muscular dystrophy. A comparative and clinicopathological study. Neurology 1970; 20:329–335.

42. Jagadha V, Becker LE. Brain morphology in Duchenne muscular dystrophy: a Golgi study. Pediatr Neurol 1988; 4:87–92.

43. Rae C, Scott RB, Thompson CH, Dixon RM, Dumughn I, Kemp GJ, et al. Brain biochemistry in Duchenne muscular dystrophy: a 1H magnetic resonance and neuropsychological study. J Neurol Sci 1998; 160:148–157.

44. Itoh K, Jinnai K, Tada K, Hara K, Itoh H, Takahashi K. Multifocal glial nodules in a case of Duchenne muscular dystrophy with severe mental retardation. Neuropathology 1999; 19:322–327.

45. Yoshioka M, Okuna T, Honda Y, Nakano Y. Central nervous system involvement in progressive muscular dystrophy. Arch Dis Child 1980; 55:589–594.

46. Tracey I, Scott RB, Thompson CH, Dunn JF, Barnes PR, Styles P, et al. Brain abnormalities in Duchenne muscular dystrophy: phosphorus-31 magnetic resonance spectroscopy and neuropsychological study. Lancet 1995; 345:1260–1264.

47. Desmond JE, Gabrieli JD, Wagner AD, Ginier BL, Glover GH. Lobular patterns of cerebellar activation in verbal working-memory and fiber-tapping tasks as revealed by functional MRI. J Neurosci 1997; 17:9675–9685.

48. Thornton CA, Griggs RC, Moxley RT. Myotonic dystrophy with no trinucleotide repeat expansion. Ann Neurol 1994; 35:269–272.

49. Ricker K, Koch MC, Lehmann-Horn F, Pongratz D, Otto M, Heine R, Moxley RT III. Proximal myotonic myopathy: a new dominant disorder with myotonia, muscle weakness, and cataracts. Neurology 1994; 44:1448–1452.

50. Ricker K, Koch MC, Lehmann-Horn F, Pongratz D, Speich N, Reiners K, et al. Proximal myotonic myopathy. Clinical features of a multisystem disorder similar to myotonic dystrophy. Arch Neurol 1995; 52:25–31.

51. Meola G, Moxley RT. Myotonic disorders: myotonic dystrophy and proximal myotonic myopathy. In: Schapira AHV, Griggs RC eds. Muscle Disorders. Boston: Butterworth-Heinemann 1999: Chapter 5, 115–134.

52. Meola G. Clinical and genetic heterogeneity in myotonic dystrophies. Muscle & Nerve 2002; 23:1789–1799.

53. Meola G. Myotonic dystrophies. Curr Opin Neurol 2000b; 2000; 13:519–525.

54. Moxley RT. Proximal myotonic myopathy: mini-review of a recently delineated clinical disorder. Neuromusc Disord 1996; 6:87–93.

55. Moxley RT, Meola G, Udd B, Ricker K. 84th ENMC International Workshop: PROMM (Proximal Myotonic Myopathy) and other Proximal Myotonic Syndromes—Workshop Report: Neuromusc Disord 2002; 12:306–317.

56. Buxton J, Shelbourne P, Davies J, Jones C, Van Tongeret T, Aslanidis C, et al. Detection of an unstable fragment of DNA specific to individuals with myotonic dystrophy. Nature 1992; 355:547–548.

57. Harley HG, Brook JD, Rundle SA, Crow S, Reardon W, Buckler AJ, et al. Expansion of an unstable DNA region and phenotypic variation in myotonic dystrophy. Nature 1992; 355:545–546.

58. Harper PS. Myotonic Dystrophy, 3rd ed. London: WB Saunders Co., 2001.

59. Modoni A, Silvestri G, Pomponi MG, Mangiola F, Tonali PA, Marra C. Characterization of the pattern of cognitive impairment in myotonic dystrophy type 1. Arch Neurol 2004; 61:1943–1947.

59a. Winblad S, Lindberg C, Hansen S. Temperament and character in patients with classical myotonic dystrophy type 1 (DM1). Neuromusc Disord 2005; 15:287–292.

60. Mahadevan M, Tsilfidis C, Sabourin L, Shutler G, Amemiya C, Jansen G, et al. Myotonic dystrophy mutation: an unstable CTG repeat in the 3′ untranslated region of the gene. Science 1992; 255:1253–1255.

61. Ranum LPW, Rasmussen PF, Benzow KA, Koob MD, Day JW. Genetic mapping of a second myotonic dystrophy locus. Nature Gen 1998; 19:196–198.

62. Day JW, Roelofs R, Leroy B, Pech I, Benzow R, Ranum LP. Clinical and genetic characteristics of a five-generation family with a novel form of myotonic dystrophy (DM2). Neuromusc Disord 1999; 9:19–24.

62a. Liquori CL, Ricker K, Moseley M, Jacobsen JF, Kress W, Naylor SL, Day JW, Ranum LP. Myotonic dystrophy type 2 caused by a CCTG expansion in intron 1 of ZNF9. Science 2001; 293:864–867.

62b. Schoser BG, Kress W, Walter MC, Halliger-Keller B, Lochmuller H, Ricker K. Homozygosity for CCTG mutation in myotonic dystrophy type 2. Brain 2004; 127:1868–1877.

62c. Day JW, Ricker K, Jacobsen JF, Rasmussen LJ, Dick KA, Kress W, Schneider C, Koch MC, Beilman GJ, Harrison AR, Dalton JC, Ranum LP. Myotonic dystrophy type 2: molecular, diagnostic and clinical spectrum. Neurology 2003; 60:657–664.

63. Ashizawa T. Myotonic dystrophy as a brain disorder. Arch Neurol 1998; 55: 305–311.

64. Tanaka Y, Suzuki Y, Shimozawa N, Nanba E, Kondo N. Congenital myotonic dystrophy: report of paternal transmission. Brain Dev 2000; 22:132–134.

65. Tanabe Y, Iai M, Tamai K, Fujimoto N, Sugita K. Neuroradiological findings in children with congenital myotonic dystrophy. Acta Paediatr 1992; 81:613–617.

66. Rettwitz-Volk, Wiilkstroem M, Flodmark O. Occulsive hydrocephalus in congenital myotonic dystrophy. Brain Dev 2001; 23:122–124.

67. Martinello F, Piazza A, Pastorello E, Angelini C, Trevisan CP. Clinical and neuro-imaging study of central nervous system in congenital myotonic dystrophy. J Neurol 1999; 246:186–192.

68. Rogev R, de Vries LS, Heckmatt JZ, Dubowitz V. Cerebral ventricular dilation in congenital myotonic dystrophy. J Paediatr 1987; 111:372–376.

69. Garcia-Alix A, Cabanas F, Morales C, Pellicer A, Echevarria J, Paisan L, Quero J. Cerebral abnormalities in congenital myotonic dystrophy. Pediatr Neurol 1991; 7:28–32.

70. Hashimoto T, Tayama M, Yoshimoto T, Miyazaki M, Harada M, Miyoshi H, Tanouchi M, Kuroda Y. Proton magnetic spectroscopy of brain in congenital myotonic dystrophy. Pediatr Neurol 1995; 12:335–340.

71. Rubinsztein JS, Rubinsztein DC, McKenna PJ, Goodburn S, Holland AJ. Mild myotonic dystrophy is associated with memory impairment in the context of normal intelligence. J Med Genet 1997; 34:229–233.

72. Damian MS, Bachmann G, Koch MC, Schilling G, Stoppler S, Dondorf W. Brain disease and molecular analysis in myotonic dystrophy. Neuroreport 1994; 5:2549–2552.

73. Chang L, Anderson T, Migneco OA, Boone K, Mehringer CM, Villanueva-Meyer J, Berman N, Mena I. Cerebral abnormalities in myotonic dystrophy. Cerebral blood flow, magnetic resonance imaging, and neuropsychological tests. Arch Neurol 1993; 50:917–923.

74. Portwood MM, Wicks JJ, Lieberman JAS, Duveneck MI. Intellectual and cognitive function in adults with myotonic muscular dystrophy. Arch Phys Med Rehabil 1986; 67:299–303.

75. Bird T, Follet C, Griep E. Cognitive and personality function in myotonic muscular dystrophy. J Neurol Neurosurg Psych 1983; 46:971–980.

76. Van Spaendonck KPM, Bruggen TJP, Banningh WEWA, et al. Cognitive function in early-adult and adult onset myotonic dystrophy. Acta Neurol Scand 1995; 91:456–461.

77. Palmer B, Brauer Boone KI, Chang L, Lee A, Black S. Cognitive deficits and person-ality patterns in maternally versus paternally inherited myotonic dystrophy. J Clin Exp Neuropsychol 1994; 16:784–795.

78. Abe K, Fujimura H, Toyooka K, et al. Involvement of the central nervous system in myotonic dystrophy. J Neurol Sci 1994; 127:179–185.

79. Huber SJ, Kissel JT, Shuttleworth EC, et al. Magnetic resonance imaging and clinical correlates of intellectual impairment in myotonic dystrophy. Arch Neurol 1989; 46:536–540.

80. Brumback RA, Wilson H. Cognitive and personality function in myotonic muscular dystrophy. J Neurol Neurosurg Psych 1984; 47:888–890.

81. Delaporte C. Personality patterns in patients with myotonic dystrophy. Arch Neurol 1998; 55:635–640.

82. Damian MS, Schilling G, Bachmann G, Simon C, Stopper S, Donrdorf W. White matter lesions and cognitive deficits: relevance of lesion pattern? Acta Neurol Scand 1994; 90:430–436.

83. Meola G, Sansone V, Perani D, Colleluori A, Cappa S, Cotelli M, et al. Reduced cerebral blood flow and impaired visual-spatial function in proximal myotonic myopathy. Neurology 1999; 53:1042–1050.

83a. Meola G, Sansone V, Perani D, Scarone S, Cappa S, Dragoni C, Cattaneo E, Cotelli M, Gobbo C, Fazio F, Siciliano G, Mancuso M, Vitelli E, Zhang S, Krhae R, Moxley RT. Executive dysfunction and avoidant personality trait in myotonic dystrophy type 1 (DM1) and in proximal myotonic myopathy (DM2/PROMM). Neuromusc Disord 2003; 13:813–821.

84. Di Costanzo A, Di Salle F, Santoro L, Bonavita V, Tedeschi G. Dilated Virchow-Robin spaces in myotonic dystrophy: frequency, extent and significance. Eur Neurol 2001; 46:131–139.

85. Ogata A, Terae S, Fujita M, Tashiro K. Anterior temporal white matter lesions in myotonic dystrophy with intellectual impairment: an MRI and neuropathological study. Neuroradiology 1998; 40:411–415.

86. Vermersch P, Sergeant N, Ruchoux MM, et al. Specific tau variants in the brains of patients with myotonic dystrophy. Neurology 1996; 47:711–717.

87. Sergeant N, Sablonniere B, Schraen-Maschke S, Ghestem A, Maurage CA, Wattez A, Vermersch P, Delacourte A. Dysregulation of human brain microtubule associated tau mRNA maturation in myotonic dystrophy type 1. Hum Mol Genet 2001; 10:2143–2155.

88. Gennarelli M, Pavoni M, Amicucci P, Angelini C, Menegazzo E, Zelano G, Novelli G, Dallapiccola B. Reduction of the DM-associated homeo domain protein (DMAHP) mRNA in different brain areas of myotonic dystrophy patients. Neuromusc Disord 1999; 9:215–219.

88a. Westerlaken JH, Vam der Zee CE, Peters W, Wieringa B. The DMWD protein from the myotonic dystrophy (DM1) gene region is developmentally regulated and is present most prominently in synapse-dense brain areas. Brain Res 2003; 971:116–127.

89. Ono S, Takahashi K, Jinnai K, et al. Loss of catecholaminergic neurons in the medullary reticular formation in myotonic dystrophy. Neurology 1998; 51:1121–1124.

89a. Wansink DG, Wieringa B. Transgenic mouse models for myotonic dystrophy type 1 (DM1). Cytogenet Genome Res 2003; 100:230–242.

89b. Jiang H, Mankodi A, Swanson MS, Moxley RT, Thornton CA. Myotonic dystrophy type 1 is associated with nuclear foci of mutant RNA, sequestration of muscleblind proteins and deregulated alternative splicing in neurons. Hum Mol Genet 2004; 13:3079–3088.

89c. Machuca-Tzili L, Brook D, Hilton-Jones D. Clinical and molecular aspects of the myotonic dystrophies: a review. Musce & Nerve 2005; 32:1–18.

90. Hund E, Jansen O, Koch MC, et al. Proximal myotonic myopathy with MRI white matter abnormalities of the brain. Neurology 1997; 48:33–37.

91. Bechara A, Damasio H, Tranel D, Anderson SW. Dissociation of working memory from decision making within the human prefrontal cortex. J Neurosci 1998; 18:428–437.

92. Andres P, Van der Linden M. Are central executive functions working in patients with focal frontal lesions? Neuropsychologia 2002; 40:835–845.

93. Chayer C, Freedman M. Frontal lobe functions. Curr Neurol Neurosci 2001; Rep.1:547–552. Review.

94. Farde L. Brain imaging of schizophrenia—the dopamine hypothesis. Schizophr Res. 1997; 28:157–162.

95. Breier A, Kestler L, Adler C, Elman I, Wiesenfeld N, Malhotra A, Pickar D. Dopamine D2 receptor density and personal detachment in healthy subjects. Am J Psych 1998; 155:1440–1442.

96. Topaloglu H, Kale G, Yalnizoglu D, Tasdemir AH, Karaduman A, Topcu M, Kotiloglu E. Analysis of 'pure' congenital muscular dystrophies in thirty-eight cases. How different is the classical type 1 from the occidental type cerebromuscular dystrophy? Neuropediatrics 1994; 25:94–100.

97. Olive M, Sirvent J, Ferrer I. Congenital muscular dystrophy with distinct CNS involvement. Neuropediatrics 1994; 25:48–50.

98. Tanaka J, Mimaki T, Okada Sh, Fujimura H. Changes in cerebral white matter in a case of congenital muscular dystrophy (non-Fukuyama type). Neuropediatrics 1990; 21:183–186.

99. Egger J, BE Kendall, M Erdohazi, BD Lake, Wilson J, Brett EM. Involvement of the central nervous system in congenital muscular dystrophies. Dev Med Child Neurol 1983; 25:32–42.

100. Malik S, Cruse P, Chou SM, Chafel T. Non-Fukuyama congenital muscular dystrophy with central nervous system involvement: clinical, radiographic and pathological correlates (abstract). Ann Neurol 1990; 28:430.

101. Toda T, Segawa M, Nomura Y, Nonaka I, Masuda K, Ishiara T, et al. Localization of a gene for Fukuyama type congenital muscular dystrophy to chromosome 9q31-33. Nature Genetics 1993; 5:283.

102. Kobayashi K, Nakahori Y, Miyake M, et al. An ancient retrotransposol insertion causes Fukuyama-type congenital muscular dystrophy. Nature 1998; 394:388–392.

103. Sunada Y, Saito F, Higuchi I, Matsumara K, Shimizu T. Deficiency of a 180-kDa extracellular matrix protein in Fukuyama type congenital muscular dystrophy skeletal muscle. Neuromuscul Disord 2002; 12:117–120.

104. Brockington M, Blake DJ, Prandini P, Brown SC, Torelli S, Benson MA, Ponting CP, Estournet B, Romero NB, Mercuri E, Voit T, Sewry CA, Guicheney P, Muntoni F. Mutations in the fukutin-related protein gene (FKRP) cause a form of congenital muscular dystrophy with secondary laminin alpha2 deficiency and abnormal glycosylation of alpha-dystroglycan. Am J Hum Genet 2001; 69:1198–1209.

105. Ruggieri V, Lubieniecki F, Meli F, Diaz D, Ferragut E, Saito K, Brockington M, Muntoni F, Fukuyama Y, Taratuto AL. Merosin-positive congenital muscular dystrophy with mental retardation, microcephaly and central nervous system abnormalities unlinked to the Fukuyama muscular dystrophy and muscular-eye-brain loci: report of three siblings. Neuromuscul Disord 2001; 11:570–578.

106. Tachi N, Chiba S, Matsuo M, Matsumura K, Saito K. Fukuyama muscular dystrophy associated with lack of C-terminal domain of dystrophin. Pediatr Neurol 2001; 24:373–378.

107. Cao H, Yuen J, Hegele RA. Single nucleotide polymorphisms of the fukutin gene. J Hum Genet 2001; 46:487–489.

107a. Muntoni F, Voit T. The congenital muscular dystrophies in 2004: a century of exciting discoveries. Neuromusc Disord 2004; 14:635–649.

107b. Chiyonobu T, Sasaki J, Nagai Y, Takeda S, Funakoshi H, Nakamura T, Sugimoto T, Toda T. Effects of fukutin deficiency in the developing mouse brain. Neuromusc Disord 2005; 15:416–426.

107c. Brancaccio A. Alpha-dystroglycan, the usual suspect? Neuromusc Disord 2005; 15:825–828.

108. Yoshida A, Kobayashi K, Manya H, Taniguchi K, Kano H, Mizuno M, Inazu T, Mitsuhashi H, Takahashi S, Takeuchi M, Herrmann R, Straub V, Talim B, Voit T, Topaloglu H, Toda T, Endo T. Muscular dystrophy and neuronal migration disorder caused by mutations in a glycosyltransferase, POMGnT1 Dev Cell 2001; 1:717–724.

109. Kano H, Kobayashi K, Herrmann R, Tachikawa M, Manya H, Nishino I, Nonaka I, Straub V, Talim B, Voit T, Topaloglu H, Endo T, Yoshikawa H, Toda T. Deficiency of alpha-dystroglycan in muscle-eye-brain disease. Biochem Biophys Res Commun 2002; 291:1283–1286.

110. Cormand B, Pihko H, Bayes M, Valanne L, Santavuori P, Talim B, Gershoni-Baruch R, Ahmad A, van Bokhoven H, Brunner HG, Voit T, Topaloglu H, Dobyns WB, Lehesjoki AE. Clinical and genetic distinction between Walker-Warburg syndrome and muscle-eye-brain disease. Neurology 2001; 56:1059–1069.

111. Villanova M, Mercuri E, Bertini E, Sabatelli P, Morandi L, Mora M, Sewry C, Brockington M, Brown SC, Ferreiro A, Maraldi NM, Toda T, Guicheney P, Merlini L, Muntoni F. Congenital muscular dystrophy associated with calf hypertrophy, microcephaly and severe mental retardation in three Italian families: evidence for a novel CMD syndrome. Neuromuscul Disord 2000; 10:541–547.

112. Karadeniz N, Zenciroglu A, Gurer YK, Senbil N, Karadeniz Y, Topalolu H. De novo translocation t(5;6)(q35;q21) in an infant with Walker-Warburg syndrome. Am J Med Genet 2002; 109:67–69.

113. Chadani Y, Kondoh T, Kamimura N, Matsumoto T, Matsuzaka T, Kobayashi O, Kondo-Iida E, Kobayashi K, Nonaka I, Toda T. Walker-Warburg syndrome is genetically distinct from Fukuyama type congenital muscular dystrophy. J Neurol Sci 2000; 177:150–153.

114. Saito K, Osawa M, Wang ZP, Ikeya K, Fukuyama Y, Kondo-Iida E, Toda T, Ohashi H, Kurosawa K, Wakai S, Kaneko K. Haplotype-phenotype correlation in Fukuyama congenital muscular dystrophy. Am J Med Genet 2000; 92:184–190.

114a. Balci B, Uyanik G, Dincer P, Gross C, Willer T, Talim B, Haliloglu G, Kale G, Hehr U, Winkler J, Topaloglu H. An autosomal recessive limb-girdle muscular dystrophy (LGMD2) with mild mental retardation is allelic to Walker-Warburg syndrome (WWS) caused by a mutation in the POMT1 gene. Neuromusc Disord 2005; 15:271–275.

115. Hazouard E, Bergemer-Fouquet AM, Hommet C, Corcia P, Cottier JP, Beauchamp D, Baulieu JL, de Toffol B. Amyotrophic lateral sclerosis manifesting as cognitive

disorders. Value of brain perfusion scintigraphic tomography in intensive care. Presse Med 2000; 29:299–302.

116. Abe K, Fujimura H, Toyooka K, Sakoda S, Yorifuji S, Yanagihara T. Cognitive function in amyotrophic lateral sclerosis. J Neurol Sci 1997; 148:95–100.

116a. Ringholz GM, Appel SH, Bradshaw M, Cooke NA, Mosnik DM, Schulx PE. Prevalence and patterns of cognitive impairment in sporadic ALS. Neurology 2005; 65:586–590.

116b. Kuner R, Groom AJ, Muller G, Kornau HC, Stefovska V, Biesink I, Hartmann B, Tschauner K, Waibel S, Ludolph AC, Ikonomidou C, Seeburg PH, Turski L. Mechanisms of disease: motoneuron disease aggravated by transgenic expression of functionally modified AMPA receptor subunit. Ann N Y Acad Sci 2005; 1053:269–286.

117. Brun A, Gustafson L, Mann DMA, Neary D, Snowden JS. Clinical and neuropathological criteria for frontotemporal dementia. J Neurol Neurosurg Psych 1994; 57:416–418.

118. Talbot PR, Goulding PJ, Lloyd JJ, Snowden JS, Neary D, Testa HJ. Inter-relation between 'classic' motor neuron disease and frontotemporal dementia: neuropsychological and single photon emission computed tomography study. J Neurol Neurosurg Psych 1995; 58:541–547.

118a. Annesi G, Savettieri G, Pugliese P, D'Amelio M, Tarantino P, Ragonese P, La Bella V, Piccoli T, Civitelli D, Annesi F, Fierro B, Piccoli F, Arabia G, Caracciolo M, Ciro Candiano IC, Quattrone A. DJ-1 mutations and parkinsonism-dementia-amyotrophic lateral sclerosis complex. Ann Neurol 2005; 58:803–807.

119. Neary D, Snowden JS, Mann DMA, Northen B, Goulding PJ, Macdermott N. Frontal lobe dementia and motor neuron disease. J Neurol Neurosurg Psych 1990; 53:23–32.

120. Peavy G, Herzog AG, Rubin NP, Mesulam MM. Neuropsychological aspects of dementia of motor neuron disease: a report of two cases. Neurology 1992; 42:1004–1008.

121. Tsuchiya K, Ozawa E, Fukushima J, Yasui H, Kondo H, Nakano I, Ikeda K. Rapidly progressive aphasia and motor neuron disease: a clinical, radiological, and pathological study of an autopsy case with circumscribed lobar atrophy. Acta Neuropathol 2000; 99:81–87.

122. Gentileschi V, Muggia S, Poloni M, Spinnler H. Fronto-temporal dementia and motor neuron disease: a neuropsychological study. Acta Neurol Scand 1999; 100:341–349.

123. Dak TH, O'Donovan DG, Xuчieb JH, Boniface S, Hodges JR. Selectvie impairment of verb processing associated with pathological changes in Brodmann areas 44 and 45 in the motor neurone disease-dementia-aphasia syndrome. Brain 2001; 124:103–120.

124. Wilson CM, Grace GM, Munoz DG, He BP, Strong MJ. Cognitive impairment in sporadic ALS. A pathologic continuum underlying a multisystem disorder. Neurology 2001; 57:651–657.

125. Seyama K, Suzuki K, Mizuno Y, Yoshida M, Tanaka M, Ozawa T. Mitochondrial encephalomyopathy with lactic acidosis and stroke-like episodes with special reference to the mechanism of cerebral manifestations. Acta Neurol Scand 1989; 80:561–568.

126. Jaksch M, Lochmuller H, Schmitt F, Vopel B, Obermaier-Kusser B, Horvath R. A mutation in mt tRNALeu (UUR) causing a neuropsychiatric syndrome with depression and cataract. Neurology 2001; 57:1930–1931.

127. Thomeer EC, Verhoeven WM, van de Vlasakker CJ, Klompenhouwer JL. Psychiatric symptoms in MELAS: a case report. J Neurol Neurosurg Psych 1998; 64:692–693.

128. Mizukami K, Sasaki M, Suzuki T, Shiraishi H, Koizumi J, Ohkoshi N, Ogata T, Mori N, Ban S, Kosaka K. Central nervous system changes in mitochondrial encephalomyopathy: light and electron microscopic study. Acta Neuropathol 1992; 83:449–452.

129. Pachalska M, DiMauro S, MacQueen BD, Tlokinski W, Jelenska-Szygula I. Pathomechanism and clinical presentation of neurobehavioral disturbances in a patient with MELAS syndrome. Neurol Neurochir Pol 2001; 35:681–693.

130. Isozumi K, Fukuuchi Y, Tanaka K, Nogawa S, Ishihara T, Sakuta R. A MELAS (Mitochondrial myopathy, encephalopathy, lactic acidosis and stroke-like episodes.) mtDNA mutation that induces subacute dementia which mimicks Creutzfeld-Jakod disease. Intern Med 1994; 33:543–546.

131. Tsuchiya K, Miyazaki H, Akabane H, Yamamoto M, Kondo H, Mizusawa H, Ikeda K. MELAS with prominent white matter gliosis and atrophy of the cerebellare granular layer: a clinical, genetic, and pathologic study. Acta Neuropathol 1999; 97:520–524.

132. Kaido M, Fujimura H, Soga F, Toyooka K, Yoshikawa H, Nishimura T, Higashi T, Inui K, Imanishi H, Yorifuji S, Yanagihara T. Alzheimer-type pathology in a patient with mitochondrial myopathy, encepahlopathy, lactic acidosis and stroke-like episodes (MELAS). Acta Neuropathol 1996; 92:312–318.

133. Grunwald F, Zierz S, Broich K, Schumacher S, Bockisch A, Biersack HJ. HMPAO-SPECT imaging resembling Alzheimer-type dementia in mitochondrial myopathy, encephalopathy, lactic acidosis and stroke-like episodes (MELAS). J Nucl Med 1990; 31:1740–1742.

134. Turconi AC, Benti R, Castelli E, Pochintesta S, Felisari G, Comi G, et al. Focal cognitive impairment in mitochondrial encephalomyopathies: a neuropsychological and neuroimaging study. J Neurol Sci 1999; 170:57–63.

135. Montirusso R, Brambilla D, Felisari G, Sclaunich F, Filipponi E, Pozzoli U, Bresolin N. Electrophysiological analysis of cognitive slowing in subjects with mitochondrial encephalomyopathy. J Neurol Sci 2002; 194:3–9.

136. Newsom-Davies J, Mills KR. Immunological association of acquired neuromyotonia (Isaac's syndrome): report of 5 cases and literature review. Brain 1993; 116:453–469.

137. Hart IK. Waters C, Vincent A, Newland C, Beeson D, Oongs O, Morris C, Newsom-Davis J. Autoantibodies detected to expressed K+ channels are implicated in neuromyotonia. Ann Neurol 1997; 41:238–246.

138. Buckley C, Oger J, Clover L, Tuzun E, Carpenter K, Jackson M, Vincent A. Potassium channel antibodies in two patients with reversible limbic encephalitis. Ann Neurol 2001; 50:73–78.

139. Liguori R, Vincent A, Clover L, Avoni P, Plazzi G, Cortelli P, Baruzzi A, Carey T, Gambetti P, Lugaresi E, Montagna P. Morvan's syndrome: peripheral and central nervous system and cardiac involvement with antibodies to voltage-gated potassium channels. Brain 2001; 124:2417–2426.

10

Dementia in Metabolic Disorders of Children and Adults

William D. Graf

Section of Neurology, Children's Mercy Hospitals and Clinics, University of Missouri-Kansas City, Kansas City, Missouri and Department of Neurology, University of Kansas School of Medicine, Kansas City, Kansas, U.S.A.

INTRODUCTION

Dementia is a clinically defined syndrome of significant decline in memory and other cognitive functions. Clinical dementia secondary to discrete metabolic disorders may originate at any time along the human life span (Fig. 1). Such metabolic disorders include hundreds of nutritional imbalances, toxic disturbances, genetic susceptibility states, and consequences of systemic illness, all of which can present within a broad range of chronicity and severity.[a] Practicing physicians know the importance of recognizing acquired metabolic encephalopathies because of the potential to treat these life-altering disorders with nutritional supplements, detoxification, or other medical interventions. However, it is often challenging for physicians to diagnose and reverse these conditions for a number of reasons.

First, almost all degenerative dementias are associated with abnormal protein metabolism, which may make the exact distinction between primary

---

[a]Patients referred for the initial evaluation of acquired cognitive deficits may not have primary dementia or even an isolated neurological disorder. Prevalent definitions of *primary dementia* exclude the ultimate diagnosis of specific neurological and systemic diseases, including specific metabolic disorders. Conversely, many biologically defined diseases may include a non-specific dementia-like symptom complex and a part of the clinical phenotype.

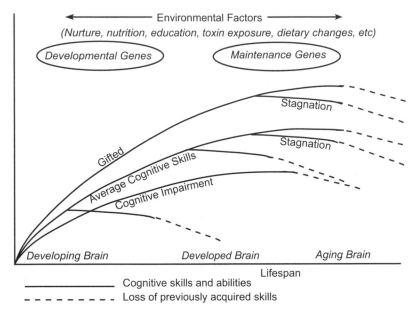

Figure 1 The variable ranges of cognitive ability and performance (*vertical axis*) relative to time (*horizontal axis*), developmental stages, and education. Loss of previously acquired skills can occur at any time along the average human life span regardless of the previous level of relative ability or accomplishment.

and secondary dementia difficult. Focusing strictly on causation, metabolic dementias can stem from *primary* genetically defined conditions; *secondary* nutritional deficiencies, toxic perturbations, or hormonal imbalances; or combined *ecogenetic* susceptibility states, where complex genetic risk factors interact with environmental stressors to cause subtle metabolic derangements. The abnormalities of just three proteins (amyloid-beta, alpha-synuclein, and hyperphosphorylated tau protein) account for the great majority of *primary* adult-onset degenerative dementias. *Secondary* deficits in essential components of individual metabolic pathways may alter other pathways or induce regulatory systems to produce cerebral dysfunction. Thus, for the individual patient under evaluation, additional laboratory testing is usually necessary to explain whether a clinically defined dementia results from a primary metabolic error or from a secondary decompensation of neural systems sharing vulnerabilities from multiple causes.

Second, the number of potential metabolic disorders is large. Specific metabolic disorders can be organized into groups or categories (e.g., cofactor deficiency states, small molecule disorders, peroxisomal disorders, etc.); however, nosological sub-classification or an alternative classification may lead to changes in the way clinicians consider these conditions (e.g., certain white matter disorders could also be classified as long-chain fatty acid disorders or peroxiso-mal disorders).

Third, some metabolic disorders produce dementia only in the advanced stages of the disorder. Paradoxically, certain therapies may be beneficial only if they are offered during early stages of the condition when recognition is most difficult. Thus, the challenge for the clinician is to know when to order appropriate screening tests for metabolic disorders in patients presenting with altered mental status or mild cognitive impairment in these early stages of their illness.

Fourth, metabolic disorders leading to dementia can differ in the developing brain, the developed brain, and the aging brain due to the diversity in risk factors and genetic etiologies in the pediatric, adult, and geriatric populations (1,2). Differential diagnostic considerations depend on the clinician's ability to recognize metabolic patterns in particular age groups.

Lower limits of age in the diagnostic designation of dementia vary in clinical practice. In pediatrics, terms such as *mental retardation* and *intellectual disability* refer to a significant intellectual deficit present from birth or at an early age. However, the concept of intellectual disability, which has been adopted by the World Health Organization (WHO) and the American Association on Mental Retardation (AAMR), describes functional outcome rather than causation. Other age-related terms, such as developmental disability, fail to distinguish etiologic subgroups or specific neurological deficits. Irrespective of age, evidence-based research into cognitive dysfunction calls for clear definitions that are widely regarded across the disciplines of education, psychology, medicine, and neuroscience. For the purposes of this review of acquired cognitive impairment secondary to metabolic disorders across the lifespan, the term *dementia* will broadly include pediatric, adult, and geriatric age groups and will refer to any individual with progressive intellectual decline in two or more spheres of function severe enough to impair daily social and educational/vocational performance from a previous level of function (1).

There are no "cookbook" approaches to complex disorders such as dementia. General guidelines for basic metabolic screening will never be the same as the focused work-up of an individual patient. Decisions about whether to pursue additional metabolic or genetic testing depend upon multiple factors, such as the nature of the clinical findings, the experience of the physician, the perceived diagnostic yield of specific tests beyond general practice parameters (3), or the interpretation of their cost/benefit ratio. New discoveries in medical science create new ethical issues for physicians and patients. The expansion of diagnostic testing in pre-symptomatic, at-risk individuals, especially where effective therapy is lacking, raises concern about the suitability of the new diagnostic process. These dilemmas about when to limit or expand the diagnostic evaluation will continue for practicing physicians even with contemporary guidelines derived from evidence-based medicine, advances from Internet-based consumer education resources, legal assurances for strict confidentiality, and appropriate patient counseling before, during, and after testing.

This chapter is organized according to an outline that makes use of the mnemonic acronym "M.E.T.A.B.O.L.I.C. D.E.M.E.N.T.I.A.S." (from the Macronutrient Deficiency section to Systemic Illness section and Table 1) as one approach to this broad topic. Each subsection emphasizes anticipated metabolic differences and a model metabolic disorder for each stage of human life.

MODES OF PRESENTATION AND GENERAL DIAGNOSTIC CONSIDERATIONS IN METABOLIC DEMENTIAS

In assessing a patient with possible dementia, clinicians compile clues about the etiology of metabolic dementia through medical history and physical examination with special attention to higher cortical function. Simultaneously, the experienced physician recognizes general patterns that may suggest a metabolic disorder, such as:

- *Onset and progression of symptoms and signs.* The temporal profile of cognitive disorders is the single best piece of historical information in narrowing the diagnostic possibilities. The "rapidly progressive dementias" are disorders of cognitive change that have been present for days to months before the initial medical assessment. In the clinical evaluation of these dementias, broad laboratory screening for treatable metabolic and toxic disorders is critical (4).
- *Disturbances in consciousness.* Except for possible changes in sleep regulation, patients with dementia usually have normal states of consciousness. Altered consciousness is more likely to result from a metabolic disorder than a primary dementia. By definition, delirium and other types of acute alteration of consciousness, especially those related to transient or reversible metabolic derangements, must be excluded from the differential diagnosis.
- *Salient individual findings.* Pertinent historical or physical findings, such as dietary changes, weight loss, hepatomegaly, ataxia, seizures, headaches, movement disorders, or certain behavioral changes, may prompt the physician to pursue particular diagnostic hypotheses. For example, in addition to signs of dementia, disorders of small-molecule metabolism may present with seizures, protein intolerance, failure to thrive, acidosis, hypoglycemia, or hyperammonemia; disorders of hormone function may present with weight gain/loss or amenorrhea; and disorders of large-molecule metabolism are likely to have MRI signs of neurodegeneration, hepatomegaly, or skin changes.

Neuroimaging studies (CT, MRI, MRA) are helpful in the workup of suspected metabolic disorders. The subsequent diagnostic evaluation can be guided by either the presence or the absence of certain morphological findings, such as basal ganglia calcifications, white matter changes, cortical malformations, focal lesions or diffuse parenchymal volume loss.

Table 1 A Classification of Major Metabolic Causes of Secondary Dementia Along the Life Span

Metabolic disorder category	Model disorder and secondary dementia by age group		
	The developing brain	The developed brain	The aging brain
Macronutrient deficiency	Choline deficiency	Mild malnutrition in childhood	Malnutrition in the elderly
Environmental toxins	Methylmercury toxicity	Lead toxicity	Aluminum toxicity
Thyroid disorders	Iodine deficiency	Autoimmune thyroid disease	Subclinical hypothyroidism in the elderly
Amino acid metabolism disorders	Maternal hyperphenylalaninemia (prenatal phenylalanine toxicity)	Severe hyperhomocysteinemia (secondary to CBS deficiency)	Mild hyperhomocysteinemia (secondary to MTHFR deficiency)
B_{12} deficiencies	Infant cobalamin deficiency	Cobalamin deficiency in vegan diets	Pernicious anemia in the elderly
Other B-vitamin deficiencies	Folic acid dependency	Thiamine deficiency	Pyridoxine dependency, Niacin deficiency
Lipid disorders	Niemann-Pick type C	HIV-associated dementia in young adults	Cholestanol lipidosis (cerebrotendinous xanthomatosis)
Iron metabolism disorders	Iron deficiency anemia in infants	Iron deficiency anemia in adolescents	Aceruloplasminemia
Carbohydrate metabolism disorders	Glycogen storage diseases	Diabetic encephalopathy (Type I diabetes mellitus)	Diabetic encephalopathy (Type II diabetes mellitus)
Drugs	Teratogenic effects of illicit drugs	Marijuana abuse	Prescription drugs (see chapter 11)
Energy metabolism disorders	GLUT deficiency syndromes	Biologically defined mitochondrial disorders	Mitochondrial oxidative deficiency in the elderly

(Continued)

Table 1 A Classification of Major Metabolic Causes of Secondary Dementia Along the Life Span (*Continued*)

Metabolic disorder category	Model disorder and secondary dementia by age group		
	The developing brain	The developed brain	The aging brain
Micronutrient and trace element deficiency states	Chloride deficiency	Zinc deficiency	Magnesium deficiency, Selenium deficiency
Endocrine disorders (other than thyroid)	Persistent hyperinsulinemic hypoglycemia of infancy	PHP	HRT and cognition performance in elderly women
Neurotransmitter deficiency disorders	Creatine deficiency syndromes	Serotonin deficiency syndromes	Acetylcholine deficiency syndromes
Trace element disorders	Molybdenum cofactor disorders	Wilson disease	Chronic trace element accumulation and depletion in the elderly
Immune response disorders	Pediatric AIDS–dementia complex	Celiac disease	Limbic encephalitis
Alcohol-related dementia	Fetal alcohol spectrum disorders	Wernicke-Korsakoff syndrome	Alcohol-related dementia in the elderly
Systematic illness (other)	Other inborn errors of metabolism	Uremia and metabolic effects of renal insufficiency	Chronic hypoxemia, sleep apnea, and effects of cardiopulmonary failure

Note: Systematic searches for treatable metabolic disorders rely on organizing disorders into various categories based on clinical symptoms, laboratory tests, role in cell function, nutrient type, molecule etiology or other factors. Here, the mnemonic acronym "M.E.T.A.B.O.L.I.C. D.E.M.E.N.T.I.A.S." is used as one such approach. The model disorders listed here exemplify the broad range of conditions that can lead to functional cognitive impairment and neuropsychiatric changes.
Abbreviations: GLUT, glucose transporter; PHP, primary hyperparathyroidism; HRT, hormone replacement therapy.

General diagnostic laboratory tests to screen for broad categories of illness are outlined in practice parameter guidelines (3). Such tests include complete blood count, serum electrolytes, calcium, glucose, blood urea nitrogen, creatinine, aspartate aminotransferase (AST), thyroid function tests (thyroid-stimulating hormone and free thyroid index), and serum vitamin B_{12} concentration. Additional blood, urine or CSF metabolic tests, nutritional panels or toxicology screens may be indicated based on the mode of clinical presentation and age group. Screening for syphilis in patients with dementia is not justified unless clinical suspicion for neurosyphilis is present.

Nuclear magnetic resonance spectroscopy (MRS) can provide a non-invasive, in vivo evaluation of proton-containing metabolites and can lead to the diagnosis of certain rare, but potentially treatable, neurometabolic disorders (5). The various cerebral metabolites of particular interest to specific neuronal and glial metabolic pathways, membrane constituents, and energy metabolism include *N*-acetyl-aspartate and *N*-acetyl-aspartyl-glutamate, trimethylamines, creatine and creatine phosphate, inositol, glutamate, and lactate (6). Dementias detected by MRS during early childhood, such as guanidino acetate methyl-tranferase (GAMT) deficiency (decreased creatine in proton MR spectra) and succinic semialdehyde dehydrogenase (SSADH) deficiency (elevated gamma-hydroxybutyric acid), are examples of treatable metabolic disorders that may have been diagnosed as primary mental retardation in the past. MRS can also potentially monitor neurochemical changes during therapy (e.g., creatine-monohydrate in GAMT deficiency or a gamma-aminobutyric acid (GABA) transaminase inhibitor in SSADH) (7,8).

Cerebrospinal fluid (CSF) may be helpful in the evaluation of certain metabolic disorders; however, a lumbar puncture is usually considered only after the findings of neuroimaging studies and basic blood and urine analyses have been carefully evaluated. Common CSF studies include cells (to rule out inflammatory disorders), glucose (plus plasma glucose to evaluate for blood–brain barrier or glucose transporter disorders), lactate (as a marker of energy metabolism or mitochondrial disorders), total protein, and quantitative amino acids. Additional studies to evaluate for amine neurotransmitter metabolites, individual pterin species, 5-methyltetrahydrofolate, or free GABA require appropriate CSF protocols with immediate placement in dry ice or liquid nitrogen, consistent timing of the samples (because of diurnal CSF variations), and collection of adequate CSF volume (because of variable CSF distribution gradients) (9).

General Diagnostic Considerations in Metabolic Dementia of the Developing Brain

Especially during the developmental period of life, physicians strive to make fundamental distinctions between *primary-genetic* and *secondary-induced* disorders. Historical observations of homogeneous groups of persons with familial syndromes of cognitive impairment have led to the identification of numerous clinically recognizable neurodevelopmental disorders. The etiology of cognitive impairment is often the result of structural CNS changes beginning in fetal life, potentially secondary to genetic or metabolic determinants, or both. Persons with non-specific mental retardation syndromes should be assessed by standard cytogenetic analyses with at least a 500-band resolution, and if necessary, by multiplex fluorescent in situ hybridization studies to test for known microdeletion syndromes, gene expansion syndromes, and subtle unbalanced subtelomeric or other interstitial chromosome rearrangements (10–12).

"Inborn errors" of metabolism (see the subsection Systemic Illness and Metabolic Dementia in the Developing Brain) that present during the first few days and weeks of life include urea cycle disorders and protein synthesis or degradation disorders. The relative immaturity of the newborn brain limits the presentation of these metabolic illnesses to non-specific physical signs, such as lethargy, hypotonia, vomiting, apnea, and seizures. As the infant matures, signs of inborn errors of metabolism also may include paroxysmal stupor, failure to thrive, or organomegaly. Essential laboratory investigations for the infant with a suspected metabolic disorder are venous blood gas and serum lactate (to test for metabolic acidosis with or without lactic acidosis), serum ammonia and beta-hydroxybutyrate (for hyperammonemia with or without ketoacidosis), fasting glucose (particularly for hypoglycemia in infants), urine or plasma quantitative amino acid profiles, and urine for organic acids. Infants and children presenting with acute metabolic decompensation precipitated by periods of prolonged fasting are candidates for expanded neonatal screening programs that use electrospray ionization-tandem mass spectrometry (MS/MS), a technology based on the fragmentation of ions based on their mass-to-charge ratio. The MS/MS analysis of ion spectra allows accurate detection of certain organic acid disorders and fatty acid disorders (Table 2, Fig. 2). MS/MS also can detect novel markers of oxidative injury, such as certain isoprostanes (e.g., 8,12-iso iPF2a-VI), which are generated by the free radical-mediated peroxidation of arachidonic acid (13,14). Thus, MS/MS technology may have future application in tracking biomarkers of adult-onset dementia (15).

Consistent features of metabolic dementias in toddlers and preschool children include stagnation or loss of cognitive milestones, loss of expressive language skills, progressive deficits in attention, focus, concentration, and other behavioral changes. Neurological findings of neurometabolic disorders are acquired relative macrocephaly or microcephaly (CNS storage or CNS atrophy), hypotonia, hypertonia/spasticity, or other movement disorders. General non-neural manifestations of neurometabolic disorders include skeletal abnormalities and coarse facial features (mucopolysaccharidoses), macular or retinal changes (leukodystrophies, poliodystrophies, or mitochondrial disorders), corneal clouding (e.g., galactosemia), skin changes (e.g., angiokeratomas in Fabry disease), or hepatosplenomegaly (Table 3).

Table 2 Inborn Errors of Metabolism Typically Detected or Not Detected/Reported by Tandem Mass Spectroscopy (MS/MS)[a]

Generally detected[b]	Generally NOT detected/reported[c]
Amino acid disorders	
Homocystinuria	Cystinosis
Hypermethioninemia	Cystinuria
Hyperphenylalaninemia	Dibasic aminoaciduria
PKU	Hartnup disorder
Biopterin cofactor	Hyperornithinemia with gyrate atrophy
deficiencies	Hypophosphatasia
MSUD	Non-ketotic hyperglycinemia
Tyrosinemia	5-Oxoprolinuria (pyroglutamic aciduria)
Tyrosinemia Type II	Tyrosinemia Type I
Tyrosimenia Type III	
Urea cycle defects/inherited hyperammonemias	
Argininemia	CPS deficiency
Argininosuccinic aciduria	HHH
Citrullinemia Type I (ASA	LPI
synthetase) deficiency	NAG deficiency
	OTC deficiency
Organic acids disorders	
HMG-CoA lyase deficiency	2-Hydroxyglutaric aciduria
GA I	2-Ketoadipic aciduria
IVA	2-Ketoglutaric aciduria
3MCC deficiency	2-Methylbutryl-CoA
Methylmalonic acidemias	dehydrogenase deficiency
Mitochondrial acetoacetyl-CoA	3-Methylglutaconyl-CoA
thiolase (3-Ketothiolase)	hydratase deficiency
deficiency	Alkaptonuria
PA	Biotinidase deficiency
Multiple-CoA carboxylase	Fumarase deficiency
deficiency	Glyceric aciduria
	Hawkinsinuria
	Hyperoxaluria
	Isobutyryl-CoA dehydrogenase
	deficiency
	Lactic acidemia
	Canavan disease
	Malonic aciduria
	Mevalonic aciduria
	Succinic semialdehyde dehydrogenase
	deficiency (4-hydroxy butyric aciduria)

(Continued)

Table 2   Inborn Errors of Metabolism Typically Detected or Not Detected/Reported by Tandem Mass Spectroscopy (MS/MS)[a] (*Continued*)

Generally detected[b]	Generally NOT detected/reported[c]
Fatty acid oxidation disorders	
Carnitine/acylcarnitine translocase (translocase) deficiency	2,4-Dienoyl-CoA reductase deficiency
	Carnitine transporter defect
	SCHAD deficiency
CPT-I deficiency	MCKAT
LCHAD deficiency	Peroxisomal fatty acids oxidation defects
MCAD deficiency	
Multiple acyl-CoA dehydrogenase (MADD or glutaric acidemia-type II) deficiency	
Neonatal carnitine palmitoyl transferase-type II (CPT-II) deficiency	
SCAD deficiency	
TFP deficiency	
VLCAD deficiency	

[a]A partial list.
[b]This list represents a constantly growing field with variation between states and laboratories.
[c]Disorders listed under NOT detected/reported are either not reliably detected or not reported due to: (i) high false positive rates, (ii) high false negative rates, or (iii) limitation of technology. Disorders that are typically not detected/reported include disorders of glycogen metabolism, purine, pyrimidine and bile acid synthesis, muccopolysaccharidoses, and oligosaccharidoses.
Abbreviations: PKU, phenylketonuria; MSUD, maple syrup urine disease; CPS, carbamoylphosphate synthase; HMG, 3-Hydroxy-3-methylglutaryl; GA I, glutaric acidemia type I; IVA, Isovaleric acidemia; 3MCC, 3-Methylcrotonyl-CoA carboxylase; PA, Propionic acidemia; HHH, Hyperammonemia, hyperonithinemia, homocitrullinemia; LPI, Lysinuric protein intolerance; NAG, *N*-Acetylglutamate synthase; OTC, Ornithine transcarbamoylase; CPT-I, Carnitine palmitoy transferase type I; LCHAD, 3-Hydroxy long chain acyl-CoA dehydrogenase; MCAD, Medium chain acyl-CoA dehydrogenase; SCAD, short chain acyl-CoA dehydrogenase; TFP, Trifnctional protein; VLCAD, very long-chain acyl-CoA dehydrogenase; SCHAD, short chain hydroxy acyl CoA dehydrogenase; MCKAT, medium chain 3-ketoacyl CoA thiolase deficiency.

General Diagnostic Considerations in Metabolic Dementia of the Developed Brain

School age children, adolescents, and young adults with metabolic disorders can present along a chronological spectrum ranging from acute encephalopathy in children with previously normal neurological function to chronic progressive deterioration of academic performance after a period of apparent stagnation. Coincidental environmental factors, such as psychosocial stress, hunger, concurrent infections, mild trauma, drugs, or toxic agents often divert attention from the ultimate diagnosis of an unexpected, rare metabolic disorder.

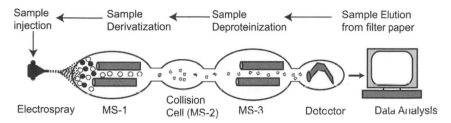

Figure 2 A process of sample preparation from blood or screening filter paper spot and analysis by electrospray ionization-tandem mass spectrometry (MS/MS). The sample is prepared and injected in MS/MS. In MS-1, ions are separated based on their mass-to-charge ratio. The selected ions enter the collision cell (another mass spectrometer having inert gas for collision), where fragmentation of selected ions takes place. The MS-3 separates fragmented ions and presents to the detector. Data analysis involves comparing unknown spectra with known spectra and flagging abnormal results.

A distinction between genetically determined disorders from secondary metabolic disorders, particularly in the early stages of the disorder, often depends upon the detailed clinical and family history, the presence of certain findings on physical examination, and the results of initial laboratory tests. Potentially helpful general laboratory screens may include erythrocyte sedimentation rate, urinalysis, urine toxicology screen, and 24-hour urine collection for quantitative measurement of heavy metals, blood lead concentrations, or free erythrocyte protoporphyrin. Electron microscopic evaluation of a skin biopsy is a highly sensitive screening tool that provides valuable clues based on the morphologic appearance of stored membrane material or ultrastructural organelle changes. Skin biopsy analysis can be performed prior to individual gene tests or specific enzyme assays and is often a more cost-effective diagnostic approach (16).

General Diagnostic Considerations in Metabolic Dementia of the Aging Brain

In the clinical evaluation of patients with possible dementia, as well as in formal dementia research, there is considerable discussion about the range of cognitive changes associated with the natural aging process. Memory aging may naturally begin in early adulthood despite overlap with other aspects of cognitive stimulation and cognitive aging (17). Progressive, gender-related regional cerebral volume changes are observed in longitudinal MRI studies (18,19), and relative differences in frontal and hippocampus metabolism are observed during positron emission tomography (PET) studies in younger and older individuals performing visual or verbal tasks (20,21), Specific disorders and categories of disorders that may distinguish secondary metabolic dementias from the general cognitive changes of aging will be illustrated in various sections of this chapter.

(*Text continues on p. 221*)

Table 3 Associations Between Organ System Manifestations and Characteristic Metabolic Disorders That Are Not Reliably Detected by Electrospray Ionization-Tandem Mass Spectrometry MS/MS[a]

CNS/nerve	Skin/eye	Muscle/bone/kidney	Other (systemic)
ACC	Alopecia	Arthrosis	Bleeding disorder
ACTH deficiency	Biotin deficiency	Alkaptonuria	Abetalipoproteinemia
Aicardi syndrome	Multiple carboxylase deficiency (e.g., HCS and biotinidase deficiencies)	Farber disease	α1-Antitrypsin deficiency
Mitochondrial disorders (e.g., PDHC deficiency)	Trichorrhexis nodosa-arginosuccinic aciduria	Gaucher type I	CDG
Nonketotic hyperglycinemia	Angiokeratomas	Gout-2° to HPRT deficiency (Lesch-Nyhan disease); or PRPPS overactivity	Chediak-Higasbi syndrome
Peroxisomal disorders	Fabry disease	I-cell disease (mucolipidosis II)	Fructose intolerance
	Fucosidosis	Lesch-Nyhan disease	Gaucher disease
	Galactosialidosis	Mucolipidosis III	Glucogenoses types I & IV
	GM1 gangliosidosis	MPS IS (Hurler) or IIS (Scheie)	Hepatorenal tyrosinemia (type I)
	Sialidosis		
Cerebral calcifications	Dermatosis	Cardiomyopathy	Enteropathy/diarrhea
Adrenoleukodystrophy	Acrodermatitis enteropathica	Fatty acid oxidation disorders	Abetalipoproteinemia
Aicardi-Goutiere syndrome	Biotinidase deficiency	ETC disorders	Acrodermatitis enteropathica
Biopterin abnormalities	HCS deficiency	Glycogenosis type III	ETC disorders
		Hemochromatosis	(e.g., Pearson syndrome)

Cockayne syndrome	Xanthomas	D-2-Hydroxyglutaric aciduria	Enterokinase deficiency
G_{M2} gangliosidosis	Cerebrotendinous xanthomatosis	3-Methylglutaconic aciduria (Barth syndrome)	Lactase deficiency
L-2-Hydroxyglutaric aciduria	Familial hypercholesterolemia	Mucopolysaccharidoses	Lysinuric protein intolerance
Mitochondrial disorders	Lipoprotein lipase deficiency	Pompe disease	Shwachman-Diamond syndrome
	Niemann-Pick disease (types A+B)		Sucrase deficiency
			Wolman disease

↑ CSF protein	Ichthyosis	Dysostosis multiplex	Hemolytic anemia
CDG	Gaucher disease	Galactosialidosis	Glycolysis disorders
L-2-Hydroxyglutaric aciduria	Krabbe disease	Generalized GM1 gangliosidosis	5-Oxoprolinuria
Kearns-Sayre syndrome	Multiple sulfatase deficiency	Hunter disease (MPS II)	Purine and pyrimidine disorders
Krabbe disease	Refsum disease	Hurler disease, Hurler-Scheie disease (MPS I)	Wilson disease
Mitochondrial disorders (e.g., MELAS or MERRF)	Sjögren-Larsson syndrome	Maroteaux-Lamy syndrome (MPS VI)	Megaloblastic Anemia
Metachromatic leukodystrophy	X-linked ichthyosis (steroid sulfatase deficiency)	I-cell disease (mucolipidosis II)	Abnormalities of folate metabolism
Multiple sulfatase deficiency		Mucolipidosis III	Mevalonic aciduria
Neonatal adrenoleukodystrophy		Multiple sulfatase deficiency	Orotic aciduria
Refsum disease		Sanfilippo disease (MPS III)	Pearson syndrome
		Sly disease (MPS VII)	Transcobalamin II deficiency

(Continued)

Table 3   Associations Between Organ System Manifestations and Characteristic Metabolic Disorders That Are Not Reliably Detected by Electrospray Ionization-Tandem Mass Spectrometry MS/MS[a] (*Continued*)

CNS/nerve	Skin/eye	Muscle/bone/kidney	Other (systemic)
	Refoum disease (*contd.*)	Exercise intolerance	Recurrent emesis
	Lens dislocation (ectopia lentis)	Glycogenolysis disorders	Galactosemia
	Marfan syndrome	Fatty acid oxidation disorders	D-2-Hydroxyglutaric aciduria
	MCD or SOD	Mitochondrial disorders	3-Oxothiolase deficiency
	Optic atrophy	Myoadenylate deaminase deficiency	
	Peroxisomal disorders	Lipoamide dehydrogenase deficiency	
Macrocephaly	Upward gaze paralysis	Hypophosphatemia	Hypouricemia
Canavan disease	Leigh and Kearns-Sayre syndromes	Fanconi syndrome (cystinosis)	Fanconi syndrome (cystinosis)
Hurler disease (MPS I)	Niemann-Pick type C disease	MELAS	MCD
4-Hydroxybutyric aciduria		Pearson syndrome	Purine nucleoside phosphorylase deficiency
D-2-Hydroxyglutaric aciduria	Cherry red macula	X-linked hypophosphatemic rickets	Wilson disease
L-2-Hydroxyglutaric aciduria	Galactosialidosis	Muscle spasticity	Xanthine oxidase deficiency
HMG-CoA lyase deficiency	GM1 gangliosidosis	Biotinidase deficiency	
Krabbe disease	Mucolipidosis I	HHH syndrome	
Mannosidosis	Multiple sulfatase deficiency	Metachromatic leukodystrophy	
Multiple sulfatase deficiency	Niemann-Pick disease (types A+B)	Pyroglutamic aciduria	
		Sjogren-Larsson syndrome	

Encephalopathy (rapidly progressive)
Adenylosuccinase deficiency
Atypical PKU (pterin defects)
MCD or SOD

Subacute necrotizing encephalomyelitis (Leigh syndrome)
Biotinidase deficiency
Complex I deficiency (electron transport chain disorders)
Fumarase deficiency
3-Methylglutaconic aciduria
Pyruvate carboxylase deficiency
PDHC deficiency
MCD or SOD

Cataracts—Lenticular
Cerebrotendinous xanthomatosis
ETC disorders
Fabry disease
Galactokinase deficiency
Galactosemia (GALT deficiency)
Hyperornithinemia (ornithine aminotransferase deficiency)
Lowe syndrome
Lysinuric protein intolerance
Mannosidosis
Mevalonic aciduria
Multiple sulfatase deficiency
Peroxisomal disorders

Ragged red fibers
Mitochondrial disorders
Menkes disease
Myocardial infarction-cerebral vascular disease
Familial hypocholesterolemia
Fabry disease
Menkes disease
MTHFR deficiency

Hydrops fetalis
CDG
Galactosialidosis
Gaucher disease
GM1 gangliosidosis
Mucolipidosis II (one-cell disease)
Neonatal hemochromatosis
Niemann-Pick disease (types A+B)
Niemann-Pick type C disease
Pearson syndrome (anemia)
Sialidosis
Sly syndrome (MPS VII)
Wolman disease

(Continued)

Table 3 Associations Between Organ System Manifestations and Characteristic Metabolic Disorders That Are Not Reliably Detected by Electrospray Ionization-Tandem Mass Spectrometry MS/MS[a] (*Continued*)

CNS/nerve	Skin/eye	Muscle/bone/kidney	Other (systemic)
Acute encephalopathy	Hair abnormalities	Osteoporosis and fractures	Hepatic cirrhosis
CPS deficiency	Menkes disease (pili torti, trichorrhexis nodosa, monilethrix)	Adenosine deaminase deficiency	α1-Antitrypsin deficiency
Mitochondrial disorders	Inverted nipples	Gaucher disease	Cholesteryl ester storage disease
Acute stroke	BH4 synthesis disorders	Glycogenosis I	Cystic fibrosis
CDG	CDG	I-cell disease (mucolipidosis II)	ETC disorders (e.g. mitochondrial DNA depletion syndromes)
Fabry disease	Menkes disease	Infantile Refsum disease	Fructose intolerance
Menkes disease		Lysinuric protein intolerance	Galactosemia
MTHFR deficiency		Menkes disease	Gaucher disease
Stroke-like episodes			Glycogenosis type IV
CPS deficiency			Hemochromatosis
Chédiak-Higashi syndrome			Hepatorenal tyrosinemia (type I)
CDG			Hypermethioninemia
MELAS			Niemann-Pick disease (types A+B)
OTC deficiency			Phosphoenolpyruvate carboxykinase deficiency
			Wilson disease
			Wolman disease

Neonatal adrenoleukodystrophy
Pyruvate carboxylase deficiency
Tay-Sachs disease

Sandhoff disease
Sialidosis
Tay-Sachs disease

Peripheralneuropatiiy
CDG
Metachromatic leukodystrophy
MTHFR deficiency
Mitochondrial disorders
Refsum disease
Vitamin E deficiency
Sensorineuronal Deafness
Biotinidase deficiency
Canavan disease
Kearns-Sayre syndrome (and other ETC disorders)
Peroxisomal disorders
PRPPS synthetase abnormality

Corneal opacity
Cystinosis
Fabry disease
Galactosialidosis
GM1 gangliosidosis
Hurler disease (MPS I)
I-cell disease
Mannosidosis
Mucolipidosis III
Multiple sulfatase deficiency

Renal fanconi syndrome
Cystinosis
ETC disorders
Galactosemia
Hepatorenal tyrosinemia (type I)
Lysinuric protein intolerance
Wilson disease
Lowe syndrome
Glycogenosis I and III
Renal calculi
APRT deficiency
Cystinuria
HPRT deficieny (Lesch-Nyhan disease)
Oxaluria

Leukopenia, thrombopenia and anemia
Abnormalities of folate metabolism
Johanson-Blizzard syndrome
3-Oxcthiolase deficiency
Pearson syndrome
Shwachman-Diamond syndrome
Transcobalamin II deficiency
Pancreatitis
Cytochrome C oxidase deficiency
Glycogenosis type I

(Continued)

Table 3   Associations Between Organ System Manifestations and Characteristic Metabolic Disorders That Are Not Reliably Detected by Electrospray Ionization-Tandem Mass Spectrometry MS/MS[a] (*Continued*)

CNS/nerve	Skin/eye	Muscle/bone/kidney	Other (systemic)
Refsum disease		PRPPS synthetase abnormalities Wilson disease Xanthine oxidase deficiency	Hyperlipoproteinemia types I and IV Lipoprotein lipase deficiency Lysinuric protein intolerance MELAS Pearson syndrome

[a]Reliable determination of certain metabolic disorders varies between laboratories.

Abbreviations: ACC, agenesis of the corpus callosum; ACTH, adrenocorticotrophic hormone; APRT, adeninephosphoribosyltransferase; BH4, tetrahydrobiopterin; CDG, congenital disorders of glycosylation; CPS carbamyl phosphate synthetase; CSF, cerebrospinal fluid, ETC, electron transport chain; GALT, galactose-1-phosphate uridyl transferase; HCS, holocarboxylase synthetase; HHH, hyperammonemia, hyperornithinemia, homocitrullinuria; HMG, 3-hydroxy-3-methylglutaryl; HPRT, hypoxanthine-guanine phosphoribosyl transferase; MCD, molybdenum cofactor deficiency; MELAS, mitochondrial encephalomyopathy, lactic acidemia, and stroke-like episodes; MERRF, myoclonic epilepsy with ragged-red fibers; MTHFR, methylene tetrahydrofolate reductase; MMA, methylmalonic aciduria; MPS, mucopolysaccharidosis; OTC, ornithine transcarbamylase; PDHC, pyruvate dehydrogenase complex; PKU, phenylketonuria; PRPPS, phosphoribosylprophosphate synthetase; SOD, sulfite oxidase deficiency.

MACRONUTRIENT DEFICIENCY

Macronutrient deficiency secondary to malnutrition, especially in infants and children, deserves highest mention in the "M.E.T.A.B.O.L.I.C. D.E.M.E.N.T.I.A.S." acronym because of its high incidence worldwide. According to the WHO, malnutrition affects approximately 792 million people and can include a lack of food, too much food, malabsorption of nutrients due to a secondary infection, or the body's inability to use nutrients to maintain health.

Although diet plays a vital role in cognitive function, the best nutrition for optimal brain development and function has not been determined. A multitude of genetic and environmental influences are required for ideal cerebral growth and maintenance of function. Brain disorders that are associated with malnutrition include non-specific intellectual disability, cerebral atrophy, marasmus, depression, cerebrovascular disease, optic neuropathy, and protein-calorie malnutrition (Kwashiorkor). Well-defined nutritional deficiency states, such as iodine deficiency, are still leading causes of clinically recognizable dementia throughout the world. Cognition-related disorders, such as visual impairment or blindness, may result from malnourishment involving vitamin A deficiency.

Most neurological disorders have few standard dietary treatment regimens or modes of nutritional prophylaxis when compared with the disorders of other organ systems. Specific dietary measures directed at neurometabolic disorders or at disorders with risk factors for neurological diseases have been studied extensively. Unless the exact metabolic defect and its mechanisms are known, precise dietary or pharmacologic interventions to reverse the disturbance may not be possible. In general, beyond a diet consisting of sufficient calories and protein with adequate sources of leafy vegetables and fruits, no additional nutritional supplement has consistently resulted in the improvement of memory impairment in otherwise healthy subjects.

Macronutrient Deficiency and Impairment of Intellectual Function in the Developing Brain

Many children born of malnourished mothers have relatively low IQs. Malnutrition plays a direct role in shaping cognitive function, but its exact biological effects are difficult to establish because of the overlapping environmental alterations that invariably accompany malnutrition (22,23).

Certain essential nutrients, such as fatty acids, are needed to complete cell membrane formation (24). In animals, maternal malnutrition causes a reduced rate of neuronal cell division and reduced learning ability that may persist throughout life (25). In humans, glial cell division continues until at least six months of age, and thus, early postnatal life represents a time of particular vulnerability to malnutrition. Sufficient calories but deficient protein intake (Kwashiorkor) also diminishes the rate of brain development and growth of intelligence (26), especially if treatment is delayed until after brain cell division has ceased (27). When compared with well-nourished peers, these children tend to have smaller brains with decreased head circumferences (28,29). If malnutrition is corrected in early postnatal life, successful catch-up growth of head circumference and development can occur (30).

Model Disorder: Choline Deficiency in Infancy

Better cognition and visual function is noted in breast-fed infants compared with formula-fed infants (31–33). Breast milk contains both docosahexaenoic acid and arachidonic acid, which are essential for normal brain development and are often absent or reduced in formula feeds (34). Choline is a required nutrient for human brain development with recommended daily intake amounts during pregnancy and lactation. Choline is a precursor to betaine and other metabolites, which are necessary for DNA methylation, neurotransmitter metabolism, lipid transport, and cell signaling (35,36).

Macronutrient Deficiency and Metabolic Dementia in the Developed Brain

Up to 10% of the world's children still endure protein and macronutrient energy malnutrition resulting in growth failure and adverse neurodevelopmental sequelae (37,38). Because most malnourished children are raised in profound poverty, it is often not possible to distinguish primary causes of intellectual disability from secondary causes, such as malnutrition, deprivation, or sociocultural influences. Early research suggested that malnourished laboratory animals lack the energy to interact with their environment and thus perform poorly on tests of mental ability. Similarly, malnourished infants and children are less vigorously able to compete in educational programs, and conversely, children who are intellectually impaired for reasons other than malnutrition may compete less effectively for food and are more likely to be malnourished. Recent research shows that malnutrition in childhood not only impairs intellectual function in more ways than previously recognized, but also that some of the injury to the brain caused by malnutrition may be reversed (39). Malnourished children particularly tend to have inadequate language development and low motivation, but these discrepancies last far longer if the child continues to live in a poverty environment. Subsequent nutritional, social, and educational intervention may lessen the cognitive deficits caused by severe malnutrition (40,41). While enriched educational programs can ameliorate some of the problems associated with malnutrition, poor children rarely live where such programs are available (40).

Model Disorder: Malnutrition in Early Childhood and Lower IQ in Later Childhood

Mild malnutrition is far more common than starvation, but its negative effects on intellectual development are evident in many studies. Neurodevelopmental follow-up of infants who suffered significant non-organic growth retardation because of nutritional neglect had evidence of decreased physical stature and more limited quantitative and memory skills than comparable children at six years of age; however, maternal IQ was a greater predictor of performance on all indices of child cognitive abilities (42).

Prospective longitudinal studies, controlled for multiple indicators of psychosocial adversity, have measured several malnutrition indicators, cognitive measures across time, and a response relationship between malnutrition and cognition. Results show that children with malnutrition in infancy and early childhood have lower verbal and spatial cognitive abilities, which are measurable at three years of age and subsequently at 11 years of age (22). A dose–response relationship is observed between malnutrition and cognition. Children with moderate-to-severe malnutrition can have a 15-point deficit in IQ by early adolescence (22,43).

Children at nutritional risk who participate in a free school breakfast program show improvements in nutrient intake, less hunger, and significant improvements in academic performance (44). Other studies show that food supplements alone are less effective than cognitive stimulation in improving young children's test performances (45).

Macronutrient Deficiency and Metabolic Dementia in the Aging Brain

Various studies show an association between nutritional status and cognitive function in the elderly. For those elderly persons who live independently, poor nutrition and cognitive impairment overlapping with forgetfulness can lead to an inability to prepare proper meals. As dementia progresses, information on dietary patterns is often difficult to attain because of deteriorating cognition, recall bias, and the development of cachexia. Thus, it is not known whether a healthier diet is directly protective for dementia or whether it is just a marker for other lifestyle patterns promoting general health. Whether modification of dietary patterns to protect from dementia and the number of other chronic conditions linked to diet requires a lifetime of discipline or can be instituted later in life is not known. An open pilot study suggests that oral nutritional supplements can improve cognitive function in certain patients (46).

Patients with intestinal failure and small bowel resection who are on long-term parenteral therapy may develop various neurological disorders, the most common being cerebral atrophy, which may be due to inadequate intake of essential nutrients in the parenteral nutrition (47). High tofu consumption has been independently associated with cognitive impairment and brain atrophy in late life (48).

Model Disorder: Malnutrition and the Role of Dietary Supplements to Improve Memory Deficits in the Elderly

Several widely marketed non-prescription "brain-specific" nutrients claim to be memory enhancers and treatments for age-related memory decline (49).

Popular compounds include phosphatidylserine, phosphatidylcholine, citicoline, piracetam, vinpocetine, and acetyl-L-carnitine. Few if any effects have been found for these supplements when based on controlled, standard psychometric memory assessments (50). Studies of antioxidants, such as vitamin E and selegiline, which have been proposed to retard or reverse the damaging effects of free radicals on neurons, have shown either no benefit or minimal benefits in the delay of memory loss for patients with memory impairment (51–53). High-dosage vitamin E supplementation (>400 IU/day) is associated with higher all-cause mortality and probably should be discouraged (54).

Alzheimer dementia (AD) has long been referred to as a cholinergic syndrome (55). Decreased activities of cholinergic enzymes due to early loss of cholinergic neurons and increased activity of acetylcholine esterase (AChE) was suggested as an explanation of the early memory deficits of Alzheimer dementia. Randomized trials of oral choline and lecithin, dietary precursors of CNS acetylcholine, have failed to improve the synthesis and release of acetylcholine or influence cognitive function in patients with dementia (56). There is some evidence that citicoline (cytidine diphosphate choline) may have a positive short-term effect on memory and behavior, especially in patients with cognitive impairment secondary to cerebrovascular disorders (57). Long-term benefits of CDP-choline have not been shown, possibly because of the chronic and irreversible nature of such disorders (58).

Overall, current evidence does not support a strong benefit from instituting dietary modification after dementia onset. However, consumers are likely to remain the target of commercial drives for nutritional supplements as long as the industry of dietary products for memory enhancement remains unregulated.

ENVIRONMENTAL TOXINS

Several environmental toxins can affect cognitive function. Neurotoxic actions can be expressed either as developmental disorders or as an increased risk of neurodegenerative diseases in later life. The major metals and minerals that are considered to be toxic include lead, mercury, aluminum, arsenic, and cadmium. No clear beneficial biochemical effect of these metals in humans is known. Environmental toxins associated with cognitive and neurobehavioral disorders include perchlorethylene, toluene, carbon tetrachloride, ethylene glycol, methyl alcohol, organophosphates, formaldehyde, and carbon monoxide.

Environmental toxins can affect the nervous system by alteration of membrane permeability and axonal transport, by inactivation of specific enzymes in cell respiration and protein synthesis, and by interference with neurotransmitters or their receptors. The clinical manifestations of exposure to a neurotoxicant can be reversible or irreversible depending on many factors including the particular neurotoxic chemical, the quantity of toxic exposure, and the age of the individual at the time of exposure.

Neurotoxicants can be categorized by the basis of their metabolic activation. Metabolic activation of some xenobiotic chemicals is mediated by cytochrome P450 enzymes (e.g., CYP-2E1), and other enzymes including gluta-thione-S-transferase. The cytochrome P450 enzymes are involved in phase I of the detoxification process. These enzymes add an oxygen atom to the parent molecule, thereby permitting the formation of an epoxide or ketone. Phase II enzymes then form conjugates with glutathione or other materials for excretion in the urine. The epoxide or ketone also can react with cellular macromolecules, which results in neurotoxic effects. Neurotoxic chemicals that require metabolic activation to induce effects include *n*-hexane, methyl *n*-butyl ketone, styrene, tri-chloroethylene, and perchloroethylene. Neurotoxicants that do not require metabolic activation to induce CNS injury include lead, arsenic, ethylene oxide, carbon disulfide, and organophosphate insecticides.

The close interrelationship between enzymes of phase I and phase II facilitates the detoxification and excretion process. Disruption of the activity of any key enzymes in this process can increase the effect of toxic exposure from either the parent compound or its metabolites. For example, an individual with increased activity of the phase I enzyme CYP-2E1 along with decreased activity of the phase II enzyme glutathione-S-transferase could be at greater risk for oxidant injury than an individual who only carries the gene encoding for the inactive form of glutathione-S-transferase.

Toxic injury from endogenous free radicals may play a role in dementia. Oxidative insults in the frontal cortex and hippocampus from Alzheimer dementia patients are dependent on the apoE genotype (59). Individuals with impaired antioxidant defense, such as carriers of the inactive form of glutathione-S-transferase theta 1 (*GSTT1*) or polymorphisms in the glutathione S-transferase omega-1 (*GSTO1*) gene, are more likely to develop dementia, suggesting that the exposure to neurotoxicants metabolized to free radicals is a significant risk factor in the pathogenesis of dementia (60,61).

Environmental Toxins and Metabolic Dementia in the Developing Brain

The prenatal period of neurodevelopment is the most sensitive to the effects of toxins; its study encompasses the field of teratology. Neurodevelopmental processes that are adversely affected by environmental toxins include prenatal migration of neurons to the cortex, prenatal and postnatal formation of synapses in the cortex, and postnatal myelination processes. Determining the timing of prenatal and postnatal neurotoxic exposure and its neurodevelopmental consequences remains an important diagnostic issue for clinicians as well as a public health policy issue for governments.

Model Disorder: Prenatal and Postnatal Methylmercury Toxicity

The combination of studies in experimental animals and in major human poisoning episodes in Japan and in Iraq has firmly established methylmercury as a severe neurotoxic agent. The effects of methylmercury are particularly toxic to the developing fetus, when exposure at higher levels can lead to significant cerebral malformation (62,63). Postnatal low dose methylmercury toxicity causes subtle and diffuse cognitive disturbances that are clinically indistinguishable from non-specific learning disabilities.

Mercury occurs in nature in three forms, and each form has its own profile of toxicity. *Metallic elemental mercury* is used in liquid form in thermometers and other instruments, dental amalgam, fluorescent light bulbs, and disc batteries. Waste disposal of these objects has led to a striking increase in environmental mercury contamination, estimated to be two to five times greater than preindustrial levels. Excessive ingestion or inhalation of mercury vapor primarily affects the CNS. Classical mercury poisoning is characterized by a triad of signs, namely tremor, erethism, and gingivitis. Mercurial erethism is also characterized by memory loss, behavioral changes with excitability, loss of appetite, red palms, and insomnia.

Inorganic mercury salts were once used in numerous consumer products but are now banned in the United States. These compounds are predominantly nephrotoxic.

Organic mercury compounds (methylmercury, ethylmercury, and phenyl-mercury) are most toxic to the CNS, although the extent of toxicity is dependent on the type of compound, route of exposure, dose, and age of the person at exposure (64). Exposure to organic mercury typically occurs by ingestion. Infants are exposed to methylmercury through consumption of human milk. Children and pregnant women who consume excessive amounts of either freshwater or ocean fish can have a significant exposure to organic mercury. Methylmercury is demethylated to mercury in the nervous system, where it maintains a long half-life (62). Signs of toxicity progress from paresthesias and ataxia to tremor and weakness, hearing impairment and dementia to spasticity and coma.

Methylmercury is toxic to the developing cerebral and cerebellar cortex. In sufficient dosage, it leads to focal necrosis of neuronal and glial tissue (63). In the Minamata Bay disaster and the Iraq seed grain epidemic, mothers were either asymptomatic or had transient paresthesias, but their infants developed a range of cognitive deficits, blindness, deafness, and seizures (65). Prospective studies conducted in the Faroe Islands and Seychelles assessed mercury concentrations in the hair of pregnant women who consume various fish diets and the neuro-developmental outcomes in their children. The Faroe Islands study suggested that low level prenatal exposure is associated with subtle neurodevelopmental disorders, in which memory, attention, and language scores were inversely associated with higher methylmercury exposures in children up to seven years of age (66). Adverse effects on development or IQ were not found in the Seychelles study at up to 66 months of age, although exposures were in the same range as the Faroe Islands study (67).

Prior to autumn 1999, thimerosal was used as a preservative for most diphtheria and tetanus toxoids and acellular pertussis vaccines, as well as some *Hemophilus influenzae* type B, influenza, meningococcal, pneumococcal, hepatitis B, and rabies vaccines. Thimerosol contains upto 50% mercury and is metabolized to ethylmercury and thiosalicylate. Because of the concern that cumulative doses of up to 187 μg mercury by six months of age are considered to be potentially toxic, all new vaccines in the recommended childhood immunization schedule do not contain thimerosal as a preservative (68).

Dental amalgam, which is a composite metal used to fill teeth, contains about 50% elemental mercury. Although mercury exposure from dental amalgams has prompted concern about its association with numerous inexplicable neurological disorders, an expert panel for the National Institutes of Health concluded that current evidence indicates dental amalgams do not cause a health risk and should not be replaced on the basis of concerns of mercury exposure (69).

Environmental Toxins and Metabolic Dementia in the Developed Brain

Environmental or occupational exposure to solvents, lead, and other chemicals can exert direct neurotoxic effects on the brain and can promote systemic diseases. Both acute high-level exposures and chronic low-level exposures can negatively affect cognition. Young children are at a greater risk than adolescents and adults. However, current data on childhood exposures and activities are insufficient to adequately assess exposures to most environmental contaminants. As a result, regulators use a series of default assumptions and exposure factors when conducting exposure assessments (70).

Model Disorder: Low-Level Lead Exposure in Young Children and Secondary Toxic Dementia

Landmark studies by Needleman et al. (71) demonstrated an inverse effect between blood lead concentrations in 3-year-old children and later measures of IQ, which was estimated as a decline of three IQ points for every 10 μg/ 100 mL blood lead over 10 μg/100 mL. Clinical studies further suggest that such neurotoxic secondary childhood dementia can occur after low levels of lead exposure. Lead appears to affect three interrelated steps in synaptic neurotransmission: through interruption of presynaptic neurotransmitter release from nerve terminals, through blockade of excitatory amino acid receptors and through alteration of protein kinases downstream from synaptic receptors (72). These clinical observations, combined with evidence of impaired neuronal circuitry directly involved in learning and memory, support the notion of an age-dependent selective vulnerability to the toxic effects of lead (73,74).

Children less than two years of age are most susceptible to lead exposure; its effects result not only in a permanent drop of IQ, but also an increase in attentional deficits and behavioral disorders. Chelation therapy with succimer (dimercaptosuccinic acid) transiently lowers average blood lead concentrations, but results in no benefit in cognitive, behavioral, and neuromotor endpoints (75–77). Primary prevention and preventing additional increases in blood lead levels among children whose blood lead levels are high remain the most effective means of managing lead poisoning.

Environmental Toxins and Metabolic Dementia in the Aging Brain

Although there is some epidemiological evidence that certain metals increase the risk of various neurodegenerative diseases, it is unlikely that metals are the sole cause for any of them. Toxic lead, mercury, manganese, or copper exposure have been linked to amyotrophic lateral sclerosis and Parkinson disease (73). Past occupational exposure to organic solvents and agricultural chemicals may be associated with onset of dementia (78).

Aluminum Toxicity and Secondary Dementia in the Aging Brain

Aluminum is a highly potent neurotoxin. High-aluminum exposure, usually resulting from kidney dialysis at home with well water containing high-aluminum concentrations, has resulted in dementia similar to Alzheimer dementia (79). Affected dialysis patients developed osteomalacia, anemia, progressive myoclonus, speech dysfluency, and irreversible dementia. Efforts to eliminate dialysis dementia succeeded after dialysis methods were modified to use water with low aluminum concentration (80).

However, in non-dialysis patients, recent evidence generally argues against aluminum as a possible risk factor for dementia (81). Neuropathological studies have found no difference in aluminum content between Alzheimer dementia and control brains (82). Except for one case-control study in Ontario (83), most epidemiological studies that compared exposure to drinking water with high versus low aluminum concentration found negligible increased risk for Alzheimer dementia in high-aluminum geographic regions (84,85).

THYROID DISORDERS

Thyroid disorders must be considered in the differential diagnosis of any patient with altered mental status, depression, or hallucinations. A gradually progressive dementia may result from hypothyroidism secondary to inadequate synthesis of thyroxine (T4) and tri-iodothyronine (T3) (primary hypothyroidism), inadequate pituitary secretion of thyroid-stimulating hormone (secondary hypothyroidism), and insufficient production of thyrotropin-releasing hormone by the hypothalamus (tertiary hypothyroidism).

Primary hypothyroidism is the most common form; its causes include chronic autoimmune thyroiditis, surgical or radioiodine thyroid gland ablation, iodine deficiency, iodine excess, congenital anomalies, and drugs that impair hormone biosynthesis, such as amiodarone, lithium, sulfonamides, interleukins, propylthiouracil, and methimazole (86). The key laboratory finding in primary hypothyroidism is an elevated serum thyrotropin (TSH) concentration, which gradually increases after lack of inhibitory feedback from the thyroid gland to the hypothalamus and anterior pituitary. A rare cause of elevated TSH is a syndrome of generalized thyroid hormone resistance (87).

Secondary and tertiary hypothyroidism can result from thyrotropin-producing pituitary tumors, granulomatous disease, surgery, hemorrhage, infarction, and irradiation. In secondary hypothyroidism, TSH and T4 concentrations are both low. In tertiary hypothyroidism, the pituitary still produces TSH, despite the absence of hypothalamic stimulation, but usually T4 concentrations are low, and TSH concentrations stay within the high-normal range. A thyroid-releasing hormone stimulation test may help distinguish between secondary and tertiary hypothyroidism. Patients with secondary hypothyroidism frequently have low levels of other pituitary hormones (87). Focused MRI studies can rule out mass lesions, hemorrhage, infarction, and other diseases and can distinguish hypothalamic disorders from pituitary disorders.

Hypothyroidism can affect the CNS and the peripheral nervous system at multiple levels, resulting in a spectrum of neurological signs and symptoms. The direct effects of thyroid hormones include stimulation of oxygen consumption, increased carbohydrate absorption, and mobilization of mucopolysaccharides and lipids in metabolically active tissues. In the brain, circulating levels of T4 are the main source of T3, which is the more active metabolite. Significant interaction of thyroid hormone with catecholamines in the reticular activating system act to regulate electrolytes and blood flow (88). Brain T3 receptors are expressed in a developmentally specific pattern with strict, age-dependent requirements (89). Concentrations of both T4 and T3 are tightly regulated within narrow ranges; small alterations in thyroid hormone concentrations may lead to significant changes in mental status.

Treatment of hypothyroidism is well established. Successful primary prevention of endemic hypothyroidism is attained after dietary iodine supplementation, mostly through iodized salt. Only myxedema coma necessitates parenteral levothyroxine. Other forms of hypothyroidism are treated with oral levothyroxine by starting a single low daily dose of thyroxine and then gradually increasing the dosage over months until a euthyroid state is achieved. Hyperthyroidism can be treated by antithyroid medication, by definitive therapy using radioactive iodine therapy, or by surgical thyroid ablation therapy. A surgical biopsy is indicated if there is suspicion of thyroid cancer.

Thyroid Disorders and Metabolic Dementia in the Developing Brain

In congenital hypothyroidism, secondary cognitive deficiency can result from iodine deficiency or from defects in thyroid hormone biosynthesis (90,91). The incidence of congenital hypothyroidism has decreased conspicuously because of newborn screening, early recognition, and thyroxine replacement therapy. However, long-term outcome studies in adolescents with congenital hypothyroidism reveal persistent memory, attention, and visuospatial skill deficits, all of which correlate with severity of early hypothyroidism (92). These clinical findings demonstrate the critical role of thyroid hormone in cognitive development.

Model Disorder: Iodine Deficiency in Infancy and Childhood

Primary iodine deficiency can lead to a severe diffuse developmental encephalopathy, which was termed "cretinism" in the early nineteenth century. Iodine deficiency constitutes the world's most prevalent single cause of preventable metabolic dementia (90). According to the WHO, iodine deficiency affects over 740 million people, or about 13% of the world's population. It is still a public health concern in parts of Africa and Asia where water and food lack iodine or where the consumption of iodized salt is inadequate (93).

As would be expected with any deficiency disorder, there is a wide range of severity in the clinical features within affected populations. Serious iodine deficiency during pregnancy results in miscarriage, stillbirth, and congenital malformations. In postnatal endemic iodine deficiency, the main neurological findings are cognitive impairment, hearing loss, and spasticity. Historically, cretinism was recognized as a severe form of mental retardation. However, a milder iodine deficiency encephalopathy currently affects an estimated 50 million children worldwide and produces an average loss of 15 IQ points (94). In addition, hearing impairment and deafness are common features of iodine deficiency. Auditory brainstem-evoked potential studies show impaired cochlear responses at all sound frequencies. Motor disorders are characterized by marked spasticity of proximal arm, leg, and trunk muscles with relative preservation of function in the hands and feet.

Model Disorder: Iodine Excess During Pregnancy

Because the fetal thyroid is particularly susceptible to iodine-induced goiter, iodine should not be given in large doses during pregnancy, and pregnant women should not receive radioactive iodine.

Thyroid Disorders and Metabolic Dementia in the Developed Brain

In older children and adults, even mild hypothyroidism can be associated with altered mental status, typically characterized as short-term memory loss, inattention, apathy, lethargy, depression, or behavioral changes. The systemic manifestations of hypothyroidism in older children and adults include cold intolerance, fatigue, constipation, menorrhagia, reduced appetite, weight gain, dry skin, alopecia, and deepening of the voice.

Model Disorder: Encephalopathy Associated with Autoimmune Thyroid Disease

The most common cause of acquired hypothyroidism in adolescents and adults is Hashimoto thyroiditis. This condition probably stems from an autoimmune disorder and is characterized by chronic lymphocyticinfiltration of the thyroid gland and high serum titers of anti-thyroid antibodies. Most children and young adults remain euthyroid or hypothyroid, but thyrotoxicosis can occur (95,96).

Encephalopathy associated with autoimmune thyroid disease is a neurological syndrome comprised of mental confusion, depression, tremor, myoclonus, or hallucinations in association with high anti-thyroid antibody titers. Other terms for this disorder include Hashimoto encephalopathy (97) and steroid responsive encephalopathy associated with Hashimoto thyroiditis (SREHT), which, as its name implies, markedly improves following corticosteroid treatment (98).

SREHT can have either an insidious onset with progressive worsening of cognition, fatigue, and psychosis or a more rapid onset with stroke-like episodes, focal neurological deficits and seizures. Young women are most often affected, and symptoms may be exacerbated during menses (99). Common laboratory findings include elevated CSF protein without pleocytosis and focal or diffuse EEG slowing. Variable MRI findings include normal images, generalized atrophy, and focal white matter abnormalities, which may be reversible (98,100–102). There is only limited evidence that pathological changes in the brain are directly caused by thyroid antibodies, which may represent an epiphenomenon relating to other autoimmune disorders (96). The true prevalence of autoimmune thyroid disease and its clinical recognition is unknown (103,104).

Thyroid Disorders and Metabolic Dementia in the Aging Brain

Although hypothyroidism is always considered as one of the potentially reversible causes of secondary dementia in the elderly, there is a lack of consensus about its prevalence, its exact diagnostic criteria, and its scale of recovery after thyroid hormone replacement (105). On one side of the clinical spectrum of mild chronic hypothyroidism, subtle cognitive dysfunction without serious additional medical problems may persist for many years. Conversely, it is argued that unrecognized and untreated dementia from hypothyroidism is rare, especially in the absence of additional systemic manifestations. Complete recovery, even with appropriate thyroid replacement therapy, may not be attained until after a year of treatment (106,107).

Model Disorder: Subclinical Hypothyroidism in the Elderly

Hypothyroidism appears to be relatively common after the age of 60, affecting approximately 5–7% of persons (105,108,109). The most common co-existing findings of hypothyroidism are depression, mental slowness, and social withdrawal. However, thyroid disease may be overlooked when mildly elevated serum TSH and "low normal" thyroxine concentrations are associated with minimal cognitive slowing in the elderly (106,109–111). Thus, it is often uncertain whether elderly hypothyroid patients have a greater degree of cognitive impairment than is recognized during routine medical examinations.

In older, physically impaired women who were followed through The Women's Health and Aging Study (112), thyroxine concentrations within the low normal range were associated with a greater risk of cognitive decline over a 3-year period (111). In a study of patients with hypothyroidism without the diagnosis of dementia, the majority of hypothyroid subjects had lower mental status test scores, lower word fluency, worse visuospatial abilities, and poorer learning than euthyroid controls (105,113).

In the elderly, hypothyroidism frequently presents with the development of cardiac disease or thyroid myopathy. Physical examination of the thyroid gland is normal to palpation in the majority of elderly patients. Hypothyroidism can present with non-specific constitutional and neuropsychiatric complaints, or with hypercholesterolemia, hyponatremia, hyperprolactinemia, or hyperhomo-cysteinemia. Although these manifestations are neither specific nor sensitive, the diagnosis is confirmed or excluded by measurements of serum thyrotropin and free thyroxine. An increased metabolic rate can precipitate adrenocortical insufficiency, so patients with secondary or tertiary hypothyroidism must be evaluated for adrenal insufficiency. If adrenal insufficiency is present, hydrocortisone replacement must be initiated before starting thyroxine.

Myxedema

Severe untreated hypothyroidism can lead to heart failure and coma with high rates of mortality (114). "Myxedema madness," a term first described in 1949, is associated with a severe psychotic illness and marked hypothyroidism. This condition is now rare because of sensitive thyroid screening tests and thyroxine therapy (115). Myxedema includes the clinical findings of doughy induration of skin, depressed consciousness, hypothermia, hypoventilation, cardiomegaly, bradycardia, adynamic ileus, and seizures. It occurs most commonly in elderly women during the winter.

Hyperthyroidism

Low TSH and high-thyroxine concentrations are also associated with dementia, especially in the elderly. Thyrotoxicosis may present as apathy, memory impairment, confusion, or other behavioral changes. Chronic over-replacement with levothyroxine (iatrogenic thyrotoxicosis) may cause cardiac hypertrophy and atrial fibrillation, and can lead to osteoporosis (116).

In summary, hypothyroidism is a treatable medical disorder and, if managed correctly, no adverse long-term consequences are likely. Thyroxine replacement therapy is highly effective and safe, but suboptimal dosing is common in clinical practice, in part because of patient non-compliance, drug interactions, and pregnancy. Improvement in both cerebral hypoperfusion and cognitive deficits are possible after correction of hypothyroidism (117).

AMINO ACID METABOLISM DISORDERS

Most amino acids act as a supply of brain nutrients or precursors to neurotransmitters. Circulating amino acids cross the blood–brain barrier depending upon many factors, including the dietary content of amino acids and other nutrients, the actual plasma amino acid concentrations, the inherent regulation of protein synthesis, individual enzyme kinetics, and blood–brain barrier transport mechanisms.

Amino Acid Metabolism Disorders and Metabolic Dementia in the Developing Brain

Model Disorder: Maternal Hyperphenylalaninemia

An example of a secondary dementia from an amino acid injury to the developing brain is maternal phenylketonuria (PKU) or secondary hyperphenylalanemia. Genetically unaffected offspring of mothers with the autosomal recessive disorder PKU will acquire this encephalopathy from prenatal exposure to high tissue concentrations of phenylalanine (Phe). Poorer long-term outcome of offspring in maternal PKU is inversely correlated with dietary discontinuation and with higher blood Phe concentrations. The condition is preventable if mothers with PKU adhere to the recommended PKU diet before conception and throughout pregnancy.

Infants exposed to hyperphenylalaninemia may have a range of mild to severe birth defects, especially involving brain and heart development. The major clinical signs of this disorder are mental retardation (92–94%), microcephaly (73–100%), intrauterine growth retardation (40%), and congenital heart disease (15%). Less common signs of hyperphenylalaninemia embryopathy include seizure disorders, autistic-like behaviors, mild craniofacial dysmorphic features, and postnatal growth retardation (118).

For persons with classic PKU, early discontinuation of a Phe-restricted diet is associated with lower intellectual ability and achievement test scores as well as increased rates of behavioral problems and abnormal MRI findings (119). In addition, individuals with PKU who discontinue the restricted diet report more health problems, such as eczema, asthma, mental disorders, headache, and hyperactivity.

Although the exact mechanism of the toxic effect of Phe is uncertain, recent studies show that exposure of human or rat astroglial cells to Phe results in decreased cell proliferation and cell cycle arrest. Phe and its metabolites are not directly cytotoxic to neurons but Phe metabolites may have an adverse effect on glial cells (120).

In addition to the maternal history and physical findings of hyperphenylalaninemia embryopathy, a number of medical and genetic tests can be used to assess the diagnosis of secondary hyperphenylalanemia. Maternal concentrations of Phe can be monitored throughout pregnancy. The current recommended Phe concentrations during pregnancy (60–250 μmol/L or 1–4 mg/dL) are at least as strict as the currently recommended levels of PKU treatment during early childhood. This dietary adherence requires a strong commitment by the woman, her family, and her caregivers. It is expected that approximately half of all infants surviving toxic in-utero exposure to high maternal concentrations of Phe are otherwise unaffected heterozygous carriers of the disorder. As with all infants, however, the Guthrie test can be used at birth to detect the unlikely chance of a homozygous state and the diagnosis of PKU.

Amino Acid Metabolism Disorders and Metabolic Dementia in the Developed Brain

Model Disorder: Severe Hyperhomocysteinemia

Homocysteine is a sulfur amino acid whose metabolism is closely interrelated with the methionine and folate cycles. The metabolism of homocysteine depends on several B vitamins, including folate, B_{12} (cobalamin), B_6 (pyridoxine), and B_2 (riboflavin). Homocysteine is formed from methionine via the numerous adenosylmethionine-dependent methyl transfer reactions. The reactions of importance to brain metabolism include the enzyme GAMT, which catalyzes the formation of creatine. An imbalance between homocysteine formation and removal will lead to changes in plasma homocysteine concentrations. Homocysteine assays are not straightforward, but measurements of plasma total homocysteine generally use chromatographic or enzyme and immunoassay methods (121).

Signs of severe hyperhomocystinemia include unexplained secondary dementia, neuropsychiatric disorders, thromboembolism, megaloblastic anemia, osteoporosis, Marfan-like appearance, and lens dislocation with progressive myopia. Urinary excretion of large amounts of homocysteine (homocystin*uria*) combined with markedly increased plasma homocysteine concentrations (severe homocystein*emia*) above 100-times normal values is usually secondary to cystathionine beta-synthase (CBS) deficiency. This rare autosomal recessive disorder, which has a variable worldwide prevalence between 1:100,000 and 1:300,000 births, is known to have pyridoxine-responsive and pyridoxine-non-responsive clinical variants. Premature vascular disease, thromboembolic events, and a progressive encephalopathy are common. Certain functional genetic variants, such as the 844ins68 allele, are associated with lower IQ, possibly because of vasculopathy or higher risk for thromboembolic events. Other genetic etiologies of severe hyperhomocystinemia include homozygous deficiency of 5,10-methylenetetrahydrofolate reductase and severe disorders of cobalamin utilization.

Amino Acid Metabolism Disorders and Metabolic Dementia in the Aging Brain

Determinants of plasma homocysteine concentration include other genetic, physiologic, and lifestyle factors, such as diet (e.g., B-vitamin consumption), drugs (e.g., nicotine, caffeine, methotrexate), and certain diseases (e.g., obesity, hypertension, renal disease) (122–127). Milder, chronic forms of hyperhomocysteinemia result from impaired homocysteine re-methylation attributable to enzyme defects in methionine synthase, methylenetetrahydrofolate reductase (MTHFR), or factors involved in the transport or metabolism of cobalamin (128). In addition, mildly increased plasma total homocysteine is a relatively sensitive marker of folate and cobalamin deficiency and an independent risk factor for cardiovascular disease (122,126,129–131).

Age, gender, and renal function all influence plasma homocysteine values. Total plasma homocysteine concentrations increase throughout life and nearly double between childhood and old age. Males and persons with renal impairment have elevated homocysteine concentrations. Homozygosity for the MTHFR C677>T polymorphism is the most common genetic determinant of mild hyperhomocysteinemia (128). Population studies suggest that the MTHFR T677T genotype produces a slightly higher homocysteine concentration than the C677C variant, but that the levels are influenced by both folate and riboflavin (130,132,133).

Low folate or cobalamin stores or renal impairment account for the majority of cases of increased homocysteinemia (122,124). In the elderly who consume a folic acid-fortified diet, renal impairment and cobalamin deficiency are the major determinants of hyperhomocysteinemia (125). In North America, after introduction of folic acid fortification of the diet, folate and MTHFR C677>T polymorphisms are less likely to cause elevation in plasma total homocysteine (134).

Model Disorder: Mild Hyperhomocysteinemia in the Elderly

Elevated plasma homocysteine is also linked to neuropathologically confirmed cases of AD in the absence of any vascular neuropathology (135). In large longitudinal population-based studies, mildly elevated plasma homocysteine, especially concentrations ≥ 15 μM, is associated with a significant risk factor for cognitive decline in healthy elderly people. The association between mild hyperhomocysteinemia and cognitive deficits is independent of other established vascular risk factors, such as hypertension, diabetes, hypercholesterolemia, or apolipoprotein E polymorphism and is observed in various domains of cognitive functions (136,137). Other studies in healthy elderly persons show a clear correlation between mild hyperhomocysteinemia and cognitive dysfunction, even in the absence of folate or B12 deficiency (135,138–140). These findings are present across ethnic and sociodemographic lines (141).

Beyond adequate dietary sources, supplements of folate, cobalamin, and pyridoxine are probably effective in lowering plasma homocysteine concentrations; however, the extent to which vitamin supplementation reduces the risks of cerebrovascular disease and dementia in aging populations deserves further study.

B$_{12}$ COBALAMIN DEFICIENCY

Vitamin B$_{12}$ (cobalamin) deficiency is the most frequently identified laboratory abnormality in patients with memory impairment, confusion, and behavioral changes. However, cobalamin deficiency can have highly variable presentations, insidious onset, and age-dependent manifestations (142). A few common observations about clinical diagnosis deserve initial consideration.

First, cognitive impairment secondary to cobalamin deficiency is common but is rarely the sole manifestation of a reversible metabolic deficit (143,144). The presentation of the disorder is usually gradual, in part because normal body stores of cobalamin are adequate to prevent acute clinical manifestations of deficiency after temporary dietary restriction or malabsorption by any mechanism.

Second, the most common signs of cobalamin deficiency are hematological and gastrointestinal. Cobalamin is essential for the normal maturation of erythrocytes, and hypersegmentation may be a sensitive marker for cobalamin deficiency, even in the absence of anemia or macrocytosis. However, megaloblastic ("pernicious") anemia may produce neurological manifestations in the absence of hematological abnormalities in up to one-third of all established cases of cobalamin deficiency (145). Glossitis and diarrhea are common gastrointestinal symptoms.

Third, the most common cerebral manifestations of cobalamin deficiency are memory impairment, depression, irritability, confusion, or delirium (146). Although subacute cognitive impairment associated with subtle white matter changes in MRI may resolve after cobalamin replacement, long-standing dementia in patients with cobalamin deficiency is poorly responsive to treatment (144,147).

Fourth, the most common neurological finding in cobalamin deficiency is myeloneuropathy. The initial complaints are usually paresthesia in the feet or hands followed by ataxia and weakness. The most common finding on neurological examination is decreased vibratory sensation, but up to one-fifth of patients with cobalamin deficiency will have a normal examination. In the advanced stages of subacute combined degeneration of the posterior and lateral columns of the spinal cord, patients will have marked loss of sensation, diffuse muscle weakness, hyper-reflexia, spasticity, incontinence, and orthostatic hypotension in addition to dementia.

The biological basis and causes of cobalamin deficiency: Cobalamin is a cobalt-containing corrin compound with a chemical structure similar to porphyrin. It is available in animal foods, such as meat, dairy products, and yeast in the diet. Cobalamin has two biologically active forms:

1. Methylcobalamin, a cofactor in the transfer of a methyl-group from N^5-methyltetrahydrafolate to homocysteine in the biosynthesis of methionine. Abnormalities in this metabolism lead to elevated concentrations of plasma and tissue homocysteine.
2. Adenosylcobalamin, a cofactor necessary for the conversion of methylmalonyl-coenzyme A (CoA) to succinyl-CoA. Deficiencies in this metabolism lead to elevated concentrations of urine and serum methymalonic acid. Deficits in this metabolism affect synthesis of neural lipids, phospholipids, and fatty acids.

Pernicious anemia from a functional cobalamin deficiency most often results from abnormal gastrointestinal absorption. Bioactive cobalamin is extracted from the diet through a sequential process. After gastric digestion, cobalamin is first bound to a protein in the duodenum and later bound to "intrinsic factor," a protein produced by gastric parietal cells. The cobalamin-intrinsic factor complex transverses through the distal ileum where it is absorbed into the enteral cell and is then bound to the transporter protein transcobalamin II.

Making the accurate diagnosis of cobalamin deficiency is not always straightforward, and there are no gold standard tests for diagnosis (147,148). Megaloblastic changes develop late in the disease process, and dementia symptoms may begin without hematologic findings (146,147,149). The diagnosis of cobalamin deficiency in dementia usually starts with direct measurement of the serum vitamin B_{12} concentration (3). Commonly used assays of serum cobalamin may not be adequately sensitive to discover all patients with cobalamine deficiencies. Patients with early deficits in cobalamin metabolism can have low normal serum vitamin B_{12} concentrations, and there is no definite correlation between the level of deficiency and the severity of neurological impairment (150).

After the initial serum B_{12} screening, subsequent tests may aid in the assessment of cobalamin status:

- Testing for elevation of plasma homocysteine, and plasma or urine methylmalonic acid (MMA) concentrations is a more sensitive method to identify cobalamin-deficient patients than measurements of the cobalamin itself. MMA cannot be metabolized without cobalamin and is probably the best reflection of cobalamin tissue supply. Although an increased MMA concentration is reasonably specific for cobalamin deficiency, false positive values are often noted in patients with renal insufficiency. Normalization of elevated MMA concentrations after parenteral vitamin B_{12} replacement may represent a valid functional assessment of cobalamin metabolism (129,151–153).
- The homocysteine concentration in plasma is a supportive but less specific test than MMA. Elevations in homocysteine are present in CBS and MTHFR deficiency (see section on "Amino Acid Metabolism Disorders"), as well as in renal insufficiency and folate deficiency (129).
- If plasma MMA or homocysteine concentrations are elevated, then serum intrinsic factor antibodies, antiparietal cell antibodies, and gastrin should be measured. If serum intrinsic factor antibodies are elevated in this context, then the diagnosis of pernicious anemia is confirmed, and a Schilling test is not necessary. If antiparietal cell or intrinsic factor antibodies are present, treatment with 1000 µg vitamin B_{12} should be given intramuscularly each day for five days, followed by 500 to 1000 µg monthly as an intramuscular injection.
- The serum gastrin level is often elevated in pernicious anemia and is a marker for achlorhydria, a cause of food-cobalamin malabsorption.

- Oral replacement is an alternative for those patients who cannot tolerate intramuscular injections, or for whom injections are impractical. Because 1% of all ingested cobalamin may be absorbed by passive diffusion, cobalamin requirements can be satisfied with oral therapy, even in patients with pernicious anemia (154).
- Serum folate concentration should be measured in patients suspected of cobalamin deficiency. Folic acid deficiency is aggravated by deficiencies of vitamins C and B_{12} as well as iron deficiencies. Isolated folate deficiency can produce megaloblastic anemia, but neurological abnormalities are uncommon.
- In patients with low serum vitamin B_{12} concentration, elevated plasma MMA and homocysteine, and normal antiparietal cell antibodies, a Schilling test should be performed to assess the ability to absorb oral radioactive-labeled vitamin B_{12} given with a concomitant parenteral dose of cyanocobalamin. Absorption of less than 7% of the radioactive-labeled vitamin B_{12} indicates malabsorption. In a modified test, labeled vitamin B_{12} is administered in food, which may provide a more realistic determination of absorptive capacity.

Electrodiagnostic studies may show signs of functional cobalamin deficiency even in patients without neurological symptoms. Nerve conduction studies typically demonstrate mixed decreases in conduction velocity and in amplitude of motor sensory potentials.

Pathologic examination of brain, spinal cord, and peripheral nerve from patients with cobalamin deficiency demonstrates diffuse demyelination and neuronal degeneration at multiple levels of the nervous system. Thus, it is postulated that demyelination plays a major role in the pathogenesis of cobalamin deficiency. The most likely biochemical mechanism for demyelination is explained by the depletion of S-adenosylmethionine (SAM) through impairment of vitamin B_{12}-dependent methionine synthase. Markedly reduced concentrations of SAM, which is a major methyl donor in the brain, may alter gene expression, biosynthesis of phospholipids, and the metabolism of hormones and neurotransmitters. Other possible mechanisms include a cycle of age-related cerebral oxidative stress changes that impair methionine synthase activity, leading to an increase in intermediate forms (analogs) of vitamin B_{12} [cob(46)alamin] and further induced hyperhomocystinemia (155).

Vitamin B_{12} Deficiency Leading to Secondary Dementia in the Developing Brain

Model Disorder: Infant Cobalamin Deficiency

Neurological signs of infant cobalamin deficiency range from mild (apathy with visual inattention) to moderate (hypotonia with lethargy) to severe (coma with marked anemia) (156–159). Hypotonia is probably the most frequent sign of vitamin B_{12} deficiency in infancy and may be accompanied by peripheral sensory motor neuropathy (156–158,160–162). Non-specific involuntary movements are reported before and after replacement therapy (158,159). Both generalized and localized skin hyperpigmentation is often a characteristic feature of infant cobalamin deficiency. MRI findings in infants with vitamin B_{12} deficiency typically show a symmetric T2-weighted increased signal in frontal and parietal white matter in addition to diffuse cerebral atrophy.

Newborns frequently have low cobalamin (163). Age-independent causes include maternal pernicious anemia, malnourishment, or inadequate intake from an unfortified maternal vegan diet. Congenital disorders also have been described with transcobalamin-II deficiency, R-binder protein deficiency, and other less well-specified abnormalities in cobalamin metabolism.

Vitamin B_{12} Deficiency Leading to Secondary Dementia in the Developed Brain

In contrast to the pronounced findings in infantile cobalamin deficiency, adolescents and adults may show only mild neuropsychiatric signs (164,165). Possible causes of cobalamin deficiency in younger adults include: (i) the "blind loop syndrome" caused by fish tapeworm infestation (*diphyllobothrium latum*) or other causes of competition for intraluminal cobalamin; (ii) gastrectomy, leading to deficient intrinsic factor production; (iii) pancreatic insufficiency leading to the failure of digestion of the cobalamin-R-binder complex and the subsequent failure of binding of cobalamin to intrinsic factor; (iv) disorders of the distal ileum, such as tropical sprue, Crohn disease, or surgical resection, leading to deficient absorption of the cobalamin-intrinsic factor complex; and (v) inhalation of nitrous oxide leading to irreversible oxidization of the cobalt in cobalamin to the 3+ state, inhibition of the activity of vitamin B_{12}-dependent methionine synthetase, and subsequent methionine deficiency.

In addition to their role in dementia, chronic, low-normal cobalamin and folate concentrations are related to other conditions, such as neural tube defects, cardiovascular disease, cancer, and pregnancy complications (166,167). Consequently, the ultimate goal of cobalamin deficiency screening is for early diagnosis in a presymptomatic state.

Model Disorder: Unsupplemented, Strict Vegetarian Diets

In a study of adolescents who had no hematological abnormalities, the cognitive performance of the cobalamin-deficient group who consumed a vegan diet with marginal vitamin B_{12} status was found to be lower than the control group (164). However, as a result of the large quantity of vitamin B_{12} in animal products and the availability of vitamin B_{12} supplements, insufficient dietary intake of cobalamin is now uncommon even in strict vegetarians.

Vitamin B$_{12}$ Deficiency Leading to Secondary Dementia in the Elderly

Model Disorder: Pernicious Anemia

Cobalamin deficiency is most often observed in the elderly, and its prevalence may be as high as 10–15% in persons over 70 years of age. The Kungsholmen Project, a large community-based population study, revealed that low serum concentrations of cobalamin or folate were associated with a higher incidence of dementia (168). The most common cause in this population was pernicious anemia attributable to malabsorption secondary to lack of intrinsic factor, gastric atrophy, or ileal disease. In addition, laboratory evidence of an autoimmune process is often found. Antiparietal cell antibodies are present in up to 90% of the elderly patients; however, a high false positive rate is also reported. Intrinsic factor antibodies are found in approximately 60% of the patients and the finding is highly specific for the disorder.

OTHER VITAMIN DEFICIENCIES

The consequences of other isolated vitamin deficiencies have been well known for decades. However, the exact biological mechanisms of vitamin deficiency-related dementia under ordinary dietary conditions are less clear, especially in relation to the aging process. Furthermore, it is difficult to measure the effects of suboptimal vitamin status on human cognition and behavior and to separate these effects from the wide-ranging signs of complete malnutrition. Nonetheless, vitamins of the B-complex are vital for optimal neuronal metabolism, and both vitamins E and C appear to be potent antioxidants in the brain.

Vitamin deficiency states may also result from the adverse effects of medications and alcohol (see Chapter 12 and section on Alcohol-Related Dementia in this chapter). Alcohol is related to nutritional deficiency states through displacement of food in the diet, the relative excess of carbohydrate calories, and malabsorption of vitamins.

Effects of Folate Deficiencies in the Developing Brain

Through decades of concerted interdisciplinary effort worldwide, evidence has emerged that mammalian development is critically dependent upon a cluster of folic acid-dependent processes, and that perturbation of these by nutritional deficiency or by metabolic defect can induce various serious developmental disorders, including neural tube defects (NTD). This evidence was dramatically confirmed through the successful intervention with folic acid supplementation in human populations at high risk for NTD (169,170).

Extensive clinical studies of NTD have demonstrated a high frequency of abnormal folic acid assimilation and methyl group metabolism during the mother's pregnancy. Two enzymes that are potentially involved at this level are methyl-tetrahydrofolate homocysteine-methionine methyltransferase and

MTHFR. A thermolabile isoform of MTHFR is associated with risk for NTD in humans (171) and also certain forms of cardiovascular disease (172). The clinically observed metabolic perturbations related to these enzyme variants are resolved by dietary supplementation of folic acid, pyridoxine and cobalamine. Part of the protective effect of folic acid may reflect tissue-specific expression and temporal patterns of gene expression, established through gene imprinting, gene silencing, and gene activation (173).

Model Disorder—The Effect of Folic Acid on Cognition and Dementia

Folic acid is a major B-vitamin in the family of folate compounds. Folic acid deficiency results from a depletion in folic acid reserves due to increased demands during pregnancy, decreased dietary intake, decreased absorption due to gastrointestinal disturbances, or the action of certain drugs (including many antiepileptic drugs). In later life, folate deficiency may produce a characteristic form of anemia (megaloblastic or "pernicious" anemia). Degrees of folate inadequacy not severe enough to produce anemia have been associated with high plasma homocysteine concentrations (see the section on Amino Acid Metabolism Disorders in this chapter). Such mild folate insufficiency can arise because of inadequate folate in the diet, inefficient absorption, or irregular utilization of folate due to genetic variations, such as the common polymorphisms in MTHFR.

Uncertainties remain about whether vitamin deficiency states adversely affect learning ability and behavior. In a double-blind, placebo-controlled study of vitamin and mineral supplements in school-age children, a significant increase in non-verbal intelligence was demonstrated in a multivitamin-supplemented study group (174). However, folic acid deficiency can be exacerbated by deficiencies in iron, and vitamins C and B_{12}. Although folate deficiency produces megaloblastic anemia, isolated CNS disorders are usually not reported. Learning disabilities and behavioral disorders can occur in hyperhomocystinemia states and hematological disorders common to both folic acid and B_{12} metabolism. Isolated deficiency of folate does not effect cerebral glucose utilization, whereas glucose metabolism is suppressed in B_{12} deficiency. Folic acid plus vitamin B_{12} is effective in reducing the serum homocysteine concentrations; however, there are no apparent beneficial effects of folic acid supplementation on measures of cognition or mood in otherwise healthy elderly persons (175). Altogether, the exact roles of B_{12} and folate as significant causes or potential treatments for dementia are still uncertain.

Other B-Vitamin Deficiencies and Metabolic Dementia in the Developed Brain

Model Disorder—Thiamine (Vitamin B_1) Deficiency

Vitamin B_1 (thiamine) acts as an essential coenzyme and plays a role in ion transport. Thiamine deficiency leads to a reduction in the neurotransmitters, glutamate and aspartate, possibly due to decreased entry of pyruvate into the tricarboxylic cycle. Thiamine plays an important role in Wernicke-Korsakoff syndrome (see section on "Alcohol-Related Dementia" in this chapter). This encephalopathy occurs most commonly in chronic alcoholics who rely on alcohol for nutrition and maintain an excess of carbohydrates in the diet relative to thiamine. The initial stages of thiamine deficiency are usually reversible through injection of large doses of thiamine. Typical organic brain syndromes in alcoholics, including early signs of dementia, should be considered as variants of the Wernicke-Korsakoff syndrome. Careful attention should be paid to the nutritional status in all persons who abuse alcohol (176).

Thiamine deficiency also can occur in any condition with poor intake of vitamins, such as anorexia nervosa, gastric plication, hyperemesis gravidarum, and prolonged fasting. Elevation of the red blood cell transketolase activity is the most reliable assay of thiamine deficiency. The assay is most sensitive when performed before and after a thiamine pyrophosphate challenge. Abnormal T2 signal in the periaqueductal gray matter in brain MRI is an additional indicator of possible thiamine deficiency. Measurements of serum thiamine concentrations are unreliable because of low sensitivity and specificity.

The cholinergic system and Alzheimer disease have been implicated in the pathophysiology of thiamine deficiency because acetylcholine synthesis and synaptic transmission are secondarily decreased. Similar relationships between beriberi amnesia, Wernicke encephalopathy, and senile dementia have been postulated. However, there is currently no evidence that thiamine is a useful treatment for the symptoms of primary dementia (177).

Other Vitamin Deficiencies and Metabolic Dementia in the Aging Brain

Deficiencies in various micronutrients and other vitamin deficiencies could contribute to age-associated cognitive impairment and dementia. As discussed in the "Amino Acids Metabolism Disorders" section of this chapter, high blood levels of homocysteine have been linked to cerebrovascular disease and dementia. There are questions about whether additional dietary supplements of folic acid could improve homocysteine metabolism and affect cognitive function or long-term outcome of persons at risk for metabolic vascular disease. Vitamin B_{12} deficiency produces an anemia identical to that of folate deficiency, but also causes irreversible CNS impairment. Folic acid will correct the anemia of vitamin B_{12} deficiency; however, there is a risk that folic acid given to persons who have undiagnosed vitamin B_{12} deficiency may lead to progressive neurological impairment. For this reason, clinical trials of folic acid supplements should either involve simultaneous administration of vitamin B_{12} or a thorough assessment for concurrent B_{12} deficiency.

There is longstanding interest in vitamin B_6 in the elderly because of studies suggesting the possibility of B_6 deficiency in aging populations (178). Vitamin B_6

consists of three chemically distinct compounds: pyridoxal, pyridoxamine, and pyridoxine. Vitamin B_6 is also an essential cofactor for homocysteine re-methylation, and deficiency is associated with increase in blood homocysteine levels. Vitamin B_6 deficiency is associated with neurological dysfunction in the elderly, including cognitive impairment, seizures, migraine, chronic pain, and depression.

Model Disorder—The Effect of Vitamin B_6 (Pyridoxine) on Cognition

Despite the plausible benefits of vitamin B_6 supplementation in reducing the risk of developing cognitive impairment by older healthy people, or of improving cognitive functioning of people with cognitive decline and dementia, no statistically significant differences have been found in double-blind, randomized, placebo-controlled trials (179). Trials in elderly persons found evidence that vitamin B_6 supplements improve biochemical indices of vitamin B_6 metabolism, but these short-term trials showed no benefits from vitamin B_6 in improving symptoms of depression, fatigue, and or cognitive dysfunction.

Model Disorder—Niacin Deficiency and Dementia (Pellagra)

Niacin (vitamin B_3) is comprised of nicotinic acid and nicotinamide. These compounds are precursors for the coenzymes nicotinamide adenine dinucleotide (NAD) and nicotinamide adenine dinucleotide phosphate (NADP), which function in numerous oxidation–reduction reactions. The causes of niacin deficiency include corn as an exclusive staple in the diet, excessive alcohol consumption, and drugs, such as 6-mercaptopurine and isonicotinic acid hydrazide. The classic signs of niacin deficiency, or pellagra, are characterized by dementia, dermatitis, and diarrhea. The dermatitis begins as a sunlight sensitive erythema, which resembles sunburn in its initial stages but with absent or delayed tanning (180). The initial neurological manifestations are apathy, memory impairment, and cognitive slowing followed by confusion or other thought disorders. Symptoms of pellagra are usually reversible after treatment with niacinamide.

LIPID DISORDERS AND SECONDARY DEMENTIAS

A multitude of dementias are related to the sequelae of lipid metabolism disorders. The dyslipidemias and premature atherogenesis are well-established risk factors for vascular dementia. The cerebral lipidoses are a diverse group of metabolic disorders involving abnormal synthesis, storage, or degradation of brain lipids. The growing field of lipidomics refers to the large-scale study of lipid quantity and function.

In blood, there are four major subtypes of lipoproteins, which vary in size, density, protein, and fat content. Chylomicrons and very low-density lipoproteins (VLDL) are the least dense lipoproteins and consist mainly of a triglyceride-rich core. Low-density lipoprotein (LDL) and high-density lipoprotein (HDL) are the smallest and most dense lipoproteins, each of which has a core comprised mostly of cholesterol. Accordingly, these neutral lipids are able to circulate in aqueous environments packaged as lipoproteins, complexes composed of a shell of proteins, phospholipids, and free cholesterol surrounding the distinctive triglyceride or cholesterol-ester core.

In the brain, lipids act as structural components of the hydrophobic "tail-to-tail" bilayers in mitochondrial, plasma (cell), and myelin membranes, and as signal transducers across cell membranes. Cholesterol accounts for 20–25% of the lipid molecules in the plasma membrane of most cells, whereas various phospholipids, sphingomyelin, and glycolipids make up the remainder. The concentration of unesterified cholesterol in the membrane is tightly regulated and plays an important role in the permeability characteristics of the membrane as well as the function of both the transporters and signaling proteins. The brain contains high concentrations of other isoprenoid substances, such as the dolichols, very long (up to C_{100}) branched-chain alcohols, squalene, the carotenoids, and retinoic acid. In addition, the brain contains numerous fatty acids with variable long carbon chains and hydroxy groups, which are prevalent in the cerebrosides and other complex molecules. It also contains relatively large concentrations of arachidonic acid, a 20-carbon fatty acid with four double bonds. Lipids, such as steroid hormones, eicosanoids, inositides, and phosphatidylcholine coupled to proteins, act as biomessengers.

Sphingolipids are a group of unique lipids comprised of the long chain hydrocarbon amino alcohol sphingosine. Fatty acids of varying chain length are linked covalently at the amino group to form ceramides. Specific sphingolipids are then formed by the addition of phosphorylcholine (to form sphingomyelin) or specific sugars to the terminal alcohol group forming the respective sphingolipids. For example, the addition of sulfate or sialic acid (*N*-acetylneuraminic acid) yields either a sulfatide or one of the various gangliosides, respectively. Sphingomyelins and ceramides are important constituents of specialized signaling domains known as lipid rafts (181).

The lipoprotein complexes are stabilized by surface proteins known as apoproteins. The apoproteins function as ligands for lipoprotein receptors, act as membrane stabilizers, serve as cofactors in the activation of enzymes that modify the lipoproteins, and are required for synthesis, secretion, and degradation of certain lipoproteins. Apolipoprotein E (ApoE) is a component of several classes of lipoproteins, including chylomicron remnants, VLDL, and a subset of HDL that regulate plasma lipid transport and clearance. ApoE is the most abundant apoprotein in the CSF and is produced in the brain where it serves paracrine-like functions. Astrocytes and microglia are the primary producers of ApoE.

A common variant of the ApoE gene, the epsilon 4 (E4) allele, is a strong determinant of higher risk for several neurological diseases, including Alzheimer dementia, and is associated with poor outcome after stroke, traumatic brain injury, cerebral hemorrhage, and possibly HIV-associated dementia. (182–186). ApoE is postulated to act as an acute phase inflammatory protein or as a chaperone in the formation of cleaved pathogenic proteins, such as ß-amyloid. Additional potential mechanisms by which ApoE may effect disease include the variable effects of *ApoE* alleles on neurite outgrowth, ApoE-mediated effects on free cholesterol efflux from macrophages, and the regulation of oxidative/nitrosative stress in neural cells leading to an increased risk of vascular disease (187). Routine use of *ApoE* genotyping as predictive testing or in patients with suspected dementia is not recommended at this time (3).

Lipid Disorders and Metabolic Dementia in the Developing Brain

Most growth and differentiation of the human CNS occurs in the first year after birth. During perinatal and early postnatal development, when the plasma cholesterol concentrations are gradually rising, there are maximally high rates of tissue synthesis in the brain and spinal cord with assembly of plasma membranes and compact myelin by oligodendrocytes. Unesterified cholesterol is an essential structural component of the plasma membrane and is a major architectural component of compact myelin (188). The concentrations of sterols circulating in lipoproteins vary markedly during the periods of development when brain size, degree of myelination, and cholesterol content are rapidly changing. The average concentration of cholesterol in the brain increases from 6 mg/g at birth to 23 mg/g in the young adult. The breast-fed human newborn ingests 18 mg cholesterol/day/kg body weight while endogenous synthesis is about 25 mg/day/kg. When infants decrease intake of high cholesterol breast milk, endogenous sterol synthesis increases (189,190). There is no evidence for the net transfer of sterol from the blood into the brain or spinal cord, strongly suggesting that cholesterol required for brain growth comes exclusively from de novo synthesis.

Multiple non-cholesterol lipid disorders result in early onset, severe progressive encephalopathy in infancy or childhood. Milder phenotypes of such disorders may present in adolescence or adulthood with signs of dementia. Examples of lipidoses include metachromatic leukodystrophy (arylsulfatase A or saposin B deficiency), adrenoleukodystrophy (*ABCD1* gene mutation with elevated very long-chain fatty acids), Fabry disease (sphingomyelinase deficiency), Krabbe disease (galactocerebroside beta-galactosidase deficiency), GM1 gangliosidosis (beta galactosidase deficiency), and GM2 gangliosidosis (Tay-Sachs disease, hexosaminidase A deficiency).

Overlying the lipidoses are a group of conditions known as lysosomal storage disorders, which now represent more than 45 distinct genetic diseases. All of these disorders result in an accumulation of substrates that are normally degraded within lysosomes, either because of a deficiency of a particular lysosomal protein or from non-lysosomal proteins that are involved in lysosomal biogenesis. The particular substrates stored and the sites of storage vary with disease type, but most have CNS involvement and result in various degrees of dementia. The nature of the substrate is used to group the lysosomal storage disorders into broad categories, including mucopolysaccharidosis (MPS), lipidoses, glycogenoses, and oligosaccharidoses. These categories show many clinical similarities within groups as well as significant similarities between groups. Non-neurological features of these disorders include coarse hair and facies, organomegaly, and bone abnormalities. During the modern era of molecular genetics and the discovery of many of the lysosomal storage disorder genes, it became clearer that the range of disease severity can often be ascribed to the nature of the mutation within a given gene. In addition, it is evident that other genetic factors and environmental factors may play a role in disease progression of an individual.

Many of the lipidoses and lysosomal storage disorders are potentially treatable. Bone marrow transplantation may be clinically efficacious in metachromatic leukodystrophy and Krabbe disease if the transplant takes place before significant brain injury occurs. Enzyme replacement therapy for Fabry disease and MPS I has become available, and clinical trials of this type of therapy for MPS II, MPS VI, and Pompe disease (a glycogen-storage disease caused by a deficiency of alpha-glucosidase) are in progress (191). Enzyme replacement therapy is generally limited to those disorders that do not develop CNS disease. Enzyme enhancement therapy also offers the possibility of treating neurodegenerative lysosomal disorders since these small therapeutic molecules may cross the blood–brain barrier. The effectiveness of these therapies still relies on early diagnosis before the onset of irreversible pathology. In addition, early bone marrow transplant therapy takes advantage of the naturally immature immune system in infancy to maximize the chance of successful engraftment. When the procedure is applied early, bone marrow and umbilical cord blood stem cell transplantation have been reported to benefit a number of disorders that develop CNS pathology at a later stage (192).

Model Disorder—Niemann-Pick Type C

Niemann-Pick disease type C (NPC; categorically distinct from types A and B) is a complex lysosomal lipidosis that can present with dementia in infants, children, or adults. In early life, the wide range of manifestations includes severe liver disease in the newborn and non-specific hypotonia and developmental delay in older infants. A typical presentation occurs in middle to late childhood with gradual onset ataxia, vertical supranuclear gaze palsy, dystonia, and dementia. A progressive encephalopathy in the later stages of the disease includes seizures and severe dysphagia. Dementia and psychiatric disorders are more likely to present in adult-onset NPC.

Niemann-Pick disease type C can result from mutations in either the *NPC1* gene or the *NPC2* gene (193,194). Although the exact function of the NPC proteins have not yet been established, errors result in abnormal intracellular transport of LDL-derived exogenous cholesterol and accumulation of non-esterified cholesterol in lysosomes (193). These errors further disrupt cholesterol transfer to the plasma membrane and the regulatory role in cell sterol metabolism (195).

In practice, the diagnosis of NPC is frequently overlooked because of the lack of organomegaly or other signs of storage disease and the lack of abnormal blood screening tests for the metabolic disturbances. Brain MRI may be normal until later stages of the disease, at which time cerebral and cerebellar atrophy and increased T2 signal in periatrial white matter are noted. The diagnosis of NPC is confirmed by biochemical testing that demonstrates absent or very low intracellular cholesterol esterification and positive filipin staining in cultured fibroblasts. Filipin staining appears as a punctate fluorescence pattern around the nucleus consistent with the accumulation of unesterified cholesterol. The large majority of patients with NPC have NPC1, but molecular genetic sequencing of both the *NPC1* and *NPC2* genes is clinically available (196).

Lipid Disorders and Metabolic Dementia in the Developed Brain

Many clinical studies of neurological aspects of human immunodeficiency virus (HIV) and the acquired immunodeficiency syndrome (AIDS) have focused on the prevalence of HIV-related dementia and risk of dyslipidemias secondary to antiretroviral therapy. Significant interactions between antiretroviral regimens and individual susceptibility genes associated with HIV-related dementia suggest pathological mechanisms relevant to secondary dementias in general.

Model Disorder—HIV-Associated Dementia in Young Adults

In HIV-associated dementia, higher brain and CSF concentrations of sphingomyelin, ceramide, cholesterol, and the lipid peroxidation product 4-hydroxynonenal have been measured in autopsied patients with the ApoE E4/4 and E3/4 genotypes than in patients with ApoE E3/3. This altered lipid metabolism is also present when compared with HIV/AIDS patients without dementia and uninfected control patients (197). In addition, altered lipid metabolism leads to changes in ceramide levels that correlate with increased neurotoxicity caused by certain viral proteins. Sphingomyelin, ceramide, and cholesterol also are increased in the brains and CSF of patients with HIV-associated dementia (186).

Lipid Disorders and Metabolic Dementia in the Aging Brain

There is no certain evidence that the concentration of cholesterol in the plasma directly influences cholesterol metabolism in the CNS. However, there is preliminary evidence that cholesterol-lowering treatments, such as inhibitors of 3-hydroxy-3-methylglutaryl coenzyme A (HMG-CoA) reductase inhibitors (statins), may directly decrease the incidence of dementia. Retrospective clinical studies suggest a decreased prevalence of dementia in patient groups who used statins to treat hypercholesterolemia, compared with patients with untreated hyperlipidemia or groups who used other lipid-lowering drugs (fibrates, cholestyramine, or nicotinic acid) (198,199). HMG-CoA reductase inhibitors cross the blood–brain barrier and appear to reduce de novo cholesterol synthesis in the CNS, possibly slowing cholesterol movement through the astrocyte/neuron hydroxycholesterol pathway and affecting the rate of processing of amyloid precursor protein (188,200).

Model Disorder—Cholestanol Lipidosis (Cerebrotendinous Xanthomatosis)

Cholestanol lipidosis (cerebrotendinous xanthomatosis) is a rare secondary dementia that results from mutation in the sterol 27-hydroxylase gene (*CYP27A1*), deficient cholesterol 27-hydroxylase activity, and excess conversion of cholesterol to cholestanol (dihydrocholesterol) (201). Clinical manifestations may begin in adolescence and consist of cataracts and xanthomas over extensor tendons (especially Achilles tendons), with slowly progressive spasticity, cerebellar ataxia, and subsequent dementia. Hallucinations, delusions, or other psychiatric disturbances often occur in the early stages of the disease. Survival into the 50s or 60s, with marked dementia and deterioration in overall neurological function, is common. MR imaging in advanced stages demonstrates diffuse white matter hypodensity, as well as cerebral and cerebellar atrophy, presumably reflecting sterol infiltration with demyelination (202). Xanthomas containing cholesterol and cholestanol are present over tendons and within brain white matter, particularly in the cerebellum. Atherosclerotic deposits lead to cardiovascular failure or myocardial infarction in most patients. Metabolic testing demonstrates normal serum cholesterol, elevated cholestanol and bile acid intermediates in serum, CSF, and red cells, and decreased cholesterol 27-hydroxylase activity in cultured skin fibroblasts. Treatment with chenodeoxycholic acid or cholic acid can reduce plasma cholestanol levels by reducing cholesterol synthesis through feedback inhibition of the rate-limiting reaction, hydroxymethylglutaryl CoA reductase. These treatments stabilize or improve neurologic manifestation. Hydroxymethylglutaryl CoA reductase inhibitors, such as lovastatin, also reduce cholestanol (203).

IRON METABOLISM AND SECONDARY DEMENTIA

Iron-deficiency anemia is the most common nutritional disorder in the world, affecting all age groups. Two billion people, or approximately one-third of the world population, are anemic due to iron deficiency. Roughly 90% of individuals affected by iron deficiency live in developing countries.

The biological basis of the cognitive and neurobehavioral disorders observed in iron-deficient persons is not completely understood, but possible mechanisms include changes in neurotransmitter metabolism, disturbances in myelin formation, and alterations in brain energy metabolism (204,205). The CNS has highly regulated, age-dependent mechanisms for iron acquisition (transferrin receptor), mobilization (transferrin and ceruloplamin), and cell-specific iron storage (H and L isoforms of ferritin). MRI can track iron distribution in the brain during development (206). The basal ganglia, deep cerebellar nuclei, and substantia nigra are particularly rich in iron, although substantia nigra iron does not fully evolve until puberty. The total concentration of iron is highest in the brain at birth, decreases during early postnatal life, and then begins to increase coincident with the onset of myelination. Early iron deficiency in experimental animals results in altered behavior and neurotransmitter disorders, including altered postsynaptic responses to serotonin and dopamine, and these disorders are irreversible if uncorrected (207).

Iron Deficiency and Secondary Dementia in the Developing Brain

Model Disorder—Iron-Deficiency Anemia in Infancy and Subsequent Cognitive Impairment

Iron-deficiency anemia in infancy is consistently associated with cognitive and motor developmental disorders if untreated (208). Through extrapolation of animal data, iron-deficiency anemia in early life causes irreversible adverse effects on cognitive performance and altered behavioral and neural development. These pathological effects may result from chemical changes in neurotransmitters, dysmyelination, or dysmorphology of neuronal networks (204,205). In a double-blind clinical trial with iron-supplementation in Thai school children, an association was shown between iron status and IQ (209). Low consumption of foods rich in bioavailable iron, such as red meat, and high consumption of foods rich in inhibitors of iron absorption, such as phytate, certain dietary fibers, and calcium, cause iron deficiency and subsequent cognitive disability (210). However, it is not certain whether iron deficiency is the dominant cause of these neurodevelopmental disorders or whether they are primarily due to other factors, such as different types of malnutrition, environmental factors, such as lead poisoning, or social deprivation. The most persuasive studies in favor of long-term effects of iron deficiency in infancy are those by Lozoff et al., who followed a group of Costa Rican children, originally described in 1987, for over 10 years (211,212). They found that severe chronic iron deficiency in infancy has long-term negative neurodevelopmental and behavioral effects on children, even after remedial iron treatment. Similar prospective, randomized trials in Chilean infants demonstrate that otherwise healthy full-term infants who are iron-deficient are less likely to interact socially and are slower to process information than their peers who have sufficient iron intake (213). Despite some uncertainty about whether long-term cognitive defects are the sole result of iron deficiency in infancy or to other factors, these results provide a strong argument to prevent iron deficiency with adequate food fortification strategies or for screening programs to identify affected infants and provide supplemental iron therapy.

Iron Deficiency and Secondary Dementia in the Developed Brain

Model Disorder—Iron Deficiency Anemia in Older Children and Adolescents

Although most research in iron deficiency has focused on early development as the "critical period," it is not certain that such a period has been exactly defined or is limited to infants less than two years of age. Children who are deficient in iron often show poor behavioral development, and iron supplementation therapy is usually beneficial (209). Randomized, supplementation trials in adolescents who were iron-deficient, but not anemic, revealed alterations in cognitive functioning that could be attributed to iron depletion but not to anemia (214). When specific tests of attention were performed, iron-deficient anemic adolescents performed worse than iron-sufficient teens. Although there was no significant difference between treatment groups on measures of attention, the iron metabolism status of the iron-supplementation group improved significantly, as did their performance on tests of verbal learning and memory.

Iron Deficiency and Metabolic Dementia in the Aging Brain

Recent studies in adults with iron deficiency in renal disease, restless leg syndrome, and simple postpartum iron deficiency all suggest that neural functioning and behavioral consequences to brain iron deficits are not limited to infants and children. Aging is often associated with a dysregulation of immune function, and iron deficiency in older adults may further impair their immune systems and render them more vulnerable to infections (215).

Model Disorder—Hereditary Aceruloplasminemia and Secondary Dementia

Aceruloplasminemia is a rare autosomal recessive disorder of iron homeostasis due to loss-of-function mutations in the ceruloplasmin gene. Characteristic findings in the disorder include dementia, dystonia, dysarthria, diabetes, peripheral retinal degeneration, and signs of hepatic iron overload (216). MRI reveals iron deposition in the CNS and shows decreased T2-weighted signal in the striatum, thalamus, dentate nucleus, and substantia nigra. Laboratory diagnosis is made by the elevation of serum ferritin, low serum copper, and undetectable serum ceruloplasmin. Mutations in the ceruloplasmin gene on chromosome 3q23-25 can be identified by PCR amplification and gene sequencing. Histopathology shows excess iron deposition in hepatocytes, reticuloendothelial cells of the liver, spleen, and pancreatic beta cells, as well as in the basal ganglia and astrocytes. Aceruloplasminemia demonstrates the essential role of ceruloplasmin as an iron-transport molecule and as an endogenous antioxidant. Ceruloplasmin, a multi-copper ferroxidase, affects the distribution of tissue iron and has antioxidant properties through the oxidation of ferrous iron to ferric iron. The disorder is associated with increased CSF iron concentration, elevated superoxide dismutase, increased products of lipid peroxidation, and accumulation of very long-chain fatty acids in erythrocytes (217). These indices of abnormal antioxidant status, along with the apparent improvement in patients after desferrioxamine therapy, support a major role for iron in the oxidant pathogenesis of aceruloplasminemia (218).

CARBOHYDRATE METABOLISM DISORDERS IN DEMENTIA

Brain glucose concentration has an important effect on cognitive brain functions, such as memory, executive functions, attention, and learning ability. Overall, cognitive function is superior after a balanced meal when compared with water only. Dietary carbohydrates, such as potatoes, enhance cognition in subjects with poor memory and impaired pancreatic beta cell function independently of plasma glucose (219). In addition to glucose, optimal brain function requires a balance of nutrients and cofactors that are directly involved in conversion of glucose into energy, including thiamin, riboflavin, niacin, pyridoxine, pantothenic acid, magnesium, manganese, iron, phosphates, and lipoic acid.

Animal studies suggest that a chronic high-fat, carbohydrate-poor diet hinders cognitive function (220). The connection between such high-fat diets and impaired brain function may be either diabetes or obesity, since both of these conditions are linked to decline in cognitive functions, such as long-term memory. High-fat diets may decrease brain function by promoting insulin resistance.

Impairment in glucose regulation, resulting in either hypoglycemia or hyperglycemia, can alter cell-to-cell communication, cerebral blood flow, and oxygen uptake. Early biochemical studies of Alzheimer dementia noted deficiencies in key enzymes of glucose utilization and energy metabolism, most consistently α-ketoglutarate dehydrogenase and pyruvate dehydrogenase (221). In some patients with genetic predisposition for dementia, a reduction in glucose utilization has been reported before the onset of clinical symptoms (222,223). Reduced glucose transporter activity has been noted in the vasculature of dementia patients, but it is uncertain whether decreased glucose uptake is secondary to lower metabolic demand in response to cellular pathology or reflects a primary inability of the vasculature to facilitate glucose uptake (224). The amyloid ß (Aß) protein, a histopathologic hallmark of Alzheimer dementia, interacts with the insulin receptor, functioning as a competitive inhibitor of insulin binding as well as a glucose transporter protein (225–227). These findings suggest a role of metabolic contribution of glucose utilization pathways in the pathophysiology of dementia.

Carbohydrate Metabolism Disorders and Metabolic Dementia in the Developing Brain

The numerous inherited disorders of carbohydrate metabolism include galactosemia, galactokinase deficiency, and the glycogen storage diseases. Although most of these disorders do not directly involve the CNS, hypoglycemia is a common primary clinical manifestation that has both acute and chronic effects on mental status. Many carbohydrate metabolism disorders can be treated effectively to prevent adverse sequelae.

Model Disorders—Glycogen-Related Diseases and Early Dementia

The glycogen storage diseases are a group of hereditary disorders caused by a lack of specific enzymes that involve glycogen synthesis or breakdown. In most of these disorders, excessive liver glycogen deposition leads to palpable hepatomegaly. Prominent CNS involvement is associated with glycogen storage disease type IV (Andersen disease) and type VIII. Muscle findings are predominant in type II (Pompe disease), type V (McArdle disease), and type VII (Tarui disease). Pompe disease is also classified among the lysosomal storage diseases. Glycogen storage diseases that do not involve the CNS or muscle directly, such as glycogenosis type I (von Gierke disease), are associated with hypoglycemia and hepatic glycogen storage and may present with acute or chronic hypoglycemia.

Dysregulation of glycogen synthase kinase-3 (GSK3) is linked to several common disorders, including insulin resistance, diabetes, and dementia. Increases in GSK3 activity have been associated with neuronal death, paired helical filament tau formation and neurite retraction, as well as a decline in cognitive performance. Current research is focused on potential selective inhibitors capable of diminishing the deleterious impact of GSK3 dysregulation (228,229).

Carbohydrate Metabolism Disorders and Metabolic Dementia in the Developed Brain

A common metabolic disorder associated with chronic cognitive dysfunction is diabetes mellitus. Diabetes is characterized by hyperglycemia due to either deficiency of insulin, resistance to insulin, or both (230). Specifically, diabetes is defined by the American Diabetes Association as: diabetes is reproducible fasting blood glucose concentrations exceeding 126 mg/dL (7 mM) and/or two-hour peak glucose concentrations of at least 200 mg/dL (11.1 mM) after an oral glucose tolerance test (OGTT) (1.75 gm/kg upto 75 gm) in the absence of symptoms or as a random glucose level exceeding 200 mg/dL in the presence of symptoms, such as polyuria, polydipsia, and weight loss suggesting underlying insulin insufficiency (231).

Type 1 and type 2 diabetes are linked to distinctive patterns of cognitive impairment. It is less certain whether these differences in clinical patterns are due to etiology, the variable ages of onset, the effect of insulin in the brain, the effects of inadequately rigorous treatments for each diabetes type, the role of obesity, or other environmental factors.

Model Disorder—Type 1 Diabetes Mellitus

Type 1 diabetes is caused by an absolute shortage in the production of insulin due to the destruction of pancreatic β cells (230). This type of diabetes, which was previously referred to as insulin-dependent diabetes mellitus, is not as common as type 2 diabetes; only 5–10% of the patients with diabetes have type 1 diabetes.

Younger individuals with type 1 diabetes often show mild performance deficits in a wide range of neuropsychological tests compared with non-diabetic controls (232,233). Chronic type 1 diabetes may develop into a more severe syndrome of cerebral dysfunction known as diabetic encephalopathy, which is a heterogeneous disorder characterized by cognitive impairment, neuroanatomical changes, neuropsychological dysfunction, and behavioral disorders (234,235). No consensus on strict clinical diagnostic criteria of diabetic encephalopathy is available.

Persons with type I diabetes may experience fluctuating levels of cognitive function related to abnormal blood glucose concentrations throughout the day. Even with strict diurnal injections or subcutaneously implanted pumps, exogenous insulin therapies cannot fully compensate for the tightly regulated insulin secretions of a normally functioning pancreas. Nevertheless, careful control of systemic glucose concentrations through diet and insulin administration is the best therapeutic action known to prevent diabetic encephalopathy.

Carbohydrate Metabolism Disorders and Metabolic Dementia in the Aging Brain

Diabetes mellitus is a common metabolic disorder in the elderly, affecting about 20% of persons older than 65 years. Diabetes is associated with many adverse health effects, including neuropathy, retinopathy, minimal cognitive impairment, and increased risk of dementia (236). Diabetes almost doubled the risk of dementia in a large prospective study in the Netherlands (237). In another large prospective study in Israel, diabetes in mid-life was associated with a threefold higher rate of dementia (238). Diabetic subjects taking medication (either oral hypoglycemic or insulin therapy) had similar rates of dementia compared with diabetic subjects not taking medication.

Model Disorder—Type 2 Diabetes Mellitus

Type 2 diabetes, the most common form of diabetes, is characterized by resistance to insulin or an inadequate compensation in the secretion of insulin. Numerous studies demonstrate greater risk for persons with type 2 diabetes to develop impaired cognitive performance, minimal cognitive impairment, or dementia (239,240).

The biological basis underlying the relationship between dementia and diabetes is not well established, but some mechanisms have been proposed. Insulin-degrading enzyme in neurons and microglia degrades Abeta, the principal component of beta-amyloid, which is one of the neuropathologic hallmarks of Alzheimer dementia (241). Diabetes may reduce the availability of this enzyme, thus decreasing degradation of Abeta. Advanced glycation end products (AGE) result from naturally occurring reactions between glucose and protein or lipid amino groups. These compounds are elevated in diabetes and are found in plaques and tangles in the early stages of Alzheimer dementia. The AGE receptor, which is overexpressed in the brain in Alzheimer dementia, is activated by beta-amyloid, which may lead to increased oxidative stress and subsequent cell injury (242,243).

DRUG ADVERSE EFFECTS (SEE ALSO CHAPTER 11: DRUG-INDUCED CONGNITIVE IMPAIRMENT)

Exposure to numerous therapeutic and illicit drugs may induce acute or chronic neurotoxic effects on cognitive function. However, because only a limited portion of the drugs currently in use have been thoroughly studied for neurotoxicity, many drug risks cannot be completely estimated based on available information. Individuals under evaluation for cognitive impairment or possible dementia should be scrutinized for the potential adverse metabolic effects of drug toxicity.

Drug Adverse Effects in the Developing Brain

Teratology is the study of the effects that drugs, medications, chemicals, and other exposures may have on the fetus. Neurological birth defects (prenatal onset encephalopathy) attributable to drug therapy represent about 1% of congenital defects of known etiology. Teratology Information Services (TIS) are comprehensive, multidisciplinary resources for medical consultation on prenatal exposures. TIS interpret information regarding known and potential reproductive risks into risk assessments that are communicated to healthcare providers and individuals of reproductive age. The Organization of Teratology Information Services (OTIS) provides regional telephone consultation for professionals and internet resources (http://www.otispregnancy.org).

Model Disorder—Teratogenic Effects of Drugs on Brain Development

Over 20 current prescription drugs (e.g., isotretinoin) with proven teratogenic effects are in use in the United States. Due to insufficient human exposure, testing or reporting, newer pharmaceutical drugs may have teratogenic effects that are not yet recognized and it can be assumed that yet unidentified adverse effects of both therapeutic and illicit drugs are impending (244).

Overall, the most prominent developmental neurotoxic effects of drugs are mental retardation syndromes and non-specific learning disabilities. However, the neurotoxic effects of any drug exposure depend on the dosage, the mechanism of drug action, and the period of exposure during brain development. It often is not possible to predict the periods when the fetus is most vulnerable to the induction of cognitive disorders. Critical periods of exposure during development and recognizable patterns of malformation are illustrated by the animal models of teratogenicity for isotretinoin, phenytoin, and methamphetamine (245).

Drug Adverse Effects in the Developed Brain

Illicit drug use should be considered in the differential diagnosis during the evaluation of early-onset dementia. Urine toxicology screens can reveal the presence of a multitude of drug metabolites in persons whose impaired cognitive performance is a consequence of drug abuse.

Model Disorder—Chronic Marijuana Abuse

Marijuana (d-9-tetrahydrocannabis or THC) is the most widely used illicit drug in the United States, especially by teenagers and young adults. According to surveys, approximately one-third of Americans aged 12–17 years and two-thirds of those aged 18–25 years of age had used marijuana, 40% of the latter group more than 100 times. One-quarter of U.S. high school students reported using marijuana within the previous month (246). One marijuana cigarette typically delivers approximately 2.5–5 mg of THC, but the drug effects depend on its dose and purity. Marijuana produces jitteriness, anxiety, or fear followed by a relaxed, dreamy ("stoned") euphoria with subjective sensations of altered body proportion and slowing of time (247–249).

It has been difficult to collect epidemiological data on whether exposure to cannabis in humans affects the risk of developing dementia. However, higher doses of marijuana are associated with acute and subacute memory loss and impaired problem solving (249–252). Although the euphoria sensation typically resolves within a few hours of use, impaired performance on cognitive tasks can last for more than 24 hours (253). Marijuana-related cognitive dysfunction consists of difficulty in digit repetition, serial subtraction, concept formation, reading comprehension, and coherent speaking (250,254–258). Balance and hand steadiness are usually impaired, compromising complex motor tasks, such as driving (259–262).

At very high doses, marijuana can cause confusion, disorientation, markedly impaired memory, anxiety, and psychotic depression or excitement. Flashbacks, hallucinations, and other feelings associated with the original marijuana use are reported weeks to months after its use (263–265). Abstinence symptoms in humans who have used marijuana for several weeks can include emotional lability, anxiety, restlessness, insomnia, anorexia, tremor, hyperreflexia, and sweating (266,267). Chronic cannabis use is often associated with personality change and an "antimotivational syndrome" consisting of diminished drive and ambition, apathy and flat effect, decreased attentiveness, and impaired recent memory (268–272). Improvement of symptoms is reported after discontinuing the drug.

Positron emission tomography (PET) studies in chronic marijuana users show decreased glucose metabolism in the cerebellum at baseline and increased glucose metabolism in the orbitofrontal cortex, prefrontal cortex, and basal ganglia after administration of d-9-THC (273). Other PET studies showed reduced regional cerebral blood flow (rCBF) in temporal lobe auditory regions, in visual cortex, and in brain regions that may be part of an attentional network (parietal lobe, frontal lobe, and thalamus) (274). These rCBF decreases may be the neural basis of perceptual and cognitive alterations that occur with acute marijuana intoxication.

Other clinical studies found impaired psychomotor, poor visual-motor performance, and impaired memory in cannabis users (275), as well as decreased work output among cannabis smokers compared with controls (276,277). Studies in heavy and light marijuana users on the first day of abstinence demonstrate that heavy users perform less well on tests of attention and executive function; however, whether this results from residual drug action, withdrawal, or specific neurotoxic effects is uncertain (278). Overall, the published research suggests that chronic marijuana abuse causes significant cognitive and behavioral changes in humans.

Drug Adverse Effect in the Aging Brain

See Chapter 11: Drug-induced Congnitive Impairment.

ENERGY METABOLISM DISORDERS

Metabolism is the process of chemical actions that transform food into smaller molecules and energy. Brain energy requirements must be met continuously for optimal function. The organ-specific basal metabolic rate of the brain (230 kcal/kg/day) is approximately nine times higher than the average basal metabolic rate (25 kcal/kg/day) for the whole body. The high level of brain energy expenditure is associated with the maintenance of ion pumping channels across axonal membranes and the continual synthesis of neurotransmitters. The human brain has evolved the capability to supply itself with the high concentrations of substrate and oxygen required to fuel this expenditure, a task made more difficult by the inability of the brain to store significant energy reserves or switch to glycogen when glucose concentrations are low.

In evolution, an "expensive-tissue hypothesis" suggests that the development of the neocortex in humans came at the expense of the splanchnic organs (liver and gastro-intestinal tract), which are as metabolically expensive as brains (250 kcal/kg/day) (279,280). Primitive humans with gradually enlarging brains became more efficient hunter-gatherers, gained greater access to more nutritious foods, conserved energy by greatly reducing the size of the intestine, and then shifted the basal energy expenditure to support the brain. Gut size is highly correlated with diet, and relatively small guts are compatible only with high-quality, easy-to-digest food. The assimilation of greater amounts of highly nutritious foods into the diet, including animal products, was essential in the evolution of the large human brain.

Disorders of energy metabolism, exemplified by mitochondrial electron transport chain (ETC) disorders, most commonly present with diverse neuromuscular symptoms; however, other features such as dementia or hearing loss may co-exist. The two primary substrates for energy production in mitochondria are carbohydrates and fatty acids. Carbohydrate metabolism is initiated in the cytosol, where glycolysis generates pyruvate from glucose. Pyruvate subsequently is metabolized in mitochondria to form acetyl-CoA, which enters the Krebs cycle. Fatty acids undergo beta-oxidation to produce acetyl-CoA, which also enters the Krebs cycle. Oxidation of these products of carbohydrate and fatty acid metabolism in the Krebs cycle provides electrons to the mitochondrial ETC, a complex system of cytochromes, non-heme iron proteins and quinones that ultimately produces adenosine triphosphate (ATP) by oxidative phosphorylation.

Energy Metabolism Disorders and Metabolic Dementia in the Developing Brain

Early brain energy failure and secondary dementia may result from genetically determined metabolic disorders, such as various hypoglycemic syndromes, hypoketonemic syndromes associated with fatty acid oxidation defects, glycolytic enzymopathies, and mitochondrial defects.

Model Disorder—Glucose Transporter (GLUT) Deficiency Syndromes and Secondary Dementia

Glucose transporter deficiency syndromes are illustrative of the energy-failure states that lead to a secondary dementia (281). Glucose transporter 1 deficiency (De Vivo) syndrome was the first of these disorders to be described. The typical clinical presentation is an infant with epileptic encephalopathy, acquired microcephaly, apnea, and oscillatory eye movements reminiscent of opsoclonus. Characteristic EEG changes appear in late infancy as 2.5- to 4-Hz spike-wave discharges. However, the laboratory hallmark of glucose transporter protein syndromes is markedly reduced CSF glucose (hypoglycorrhachia) with normal blood glucose. CSF lactate levels are reduced, reflecting the reduced CSF glucose.

Glucose transporter protein syndromes result from a deficiency of glucose transporter proteins secondary to a mutation in one of the GLUT genes. These transporter proteins are necessary for glucose transport in erythrocytes, placenta, and brain microvessels constituting the blood–brain barrier. Glucose transporter proteins are multifunctional, as indicated by the demonstration that vitamin C is also transported by these mechanisms, suggesting that the disorder is not related to glucose deficiency alone (282). Early recognition of the glucose transporter deficiency lessens long-term sequelae because the available treatment with a ketogenic diet is very effective. Thioctic acid (lipoic acid) also may be of benefit, whereas barbiturates and methylxanthines are glucose transporter 1 inhibitors and should be avoided.

Energy Metabolism Disorders and Metabolic Dementia in the Developed Brain

Energy metabolism disorders can be separated into primary and secondary disorders and classified according to clinical, biochemical, and genetic criteria.

There is no single identifying feature of these disorders, but tissues with high energy demand and substrate utilization, such as brain and muscle, are predominantly affected. Most patients will have a range of clinical problems, varying ages of onset, and a fluctuating clinical course. The mitochondriopathies serve as the best model of energy metabolism disorders.

Model Disorders—Biologically Defined Mitochondrial Disorders

Dementia secondary to a mitochondriopathy is related to deficient ATP production in the brain. This group of disorders has marked clinical heterogeneity due to variable rates of heteroplasmy with varying thresholds of biochemical expression depending upon the mutation and the tissue involved. Modulating effects of nuclear and other mitochondrial genes may contribute to the protean nature of these disorders. Numerous typical mitochondrial syndromes have been identified, but they frequently overlap and many individual patients appear to have clinically unique phenotypes.

Biochemical classification of mitochondrial disorders distinguishes defects of intramitochondrial protein transport, defects of substrate utilization, defects of the Krebs cycle, defects of the ETC, and defects in oxidative phosphorylation. Genetic classification of mitochondrial disorders distinguishes causative DNA mutations that are either nuclear (nDNA) or mitochondrial (mtDNA) affecting either ETC or non-ETC mitochondrial proteins. The large majority of mitochondiopathies are caused by nDNA mutations, although very few specific mutations have been identified so far. Less than 5% of these disorders are due to mtDNA mutations. MtDNA-derived mitochondrial disorders may be due to germline (hereditary) or somatic (acquired) mutations. Individuals with a high degree of abnormal mtDNA heteroplasmy (high mutant to wild-type DNA ratios) will typically have more severe manifestations.

There is no standard diagnostic approach to the mitochondrial disorders; however, the relative overall diagnostic certainty can be graded according to clinical, metabolic, imaging, histopathological, biochemical, and genetic features (283). Although a known pathogenic mutation in a symptomatic individual is regarded as diagnostic, there is a considerable lack of consensus about the minimal inclusion criteria for a mitochondriopathy. Suspicion for a mitochondrial disorder as a cause of dementia should increase with a familial history of maternally inherited, poorly defined disorders of brain, muscles, or gut. Blood, CSF, histopathological, biochemical, and DNA studies may be initiated in a stepwise fashion combined with longitudinal examinations by a physician familiar with mitochondrial disorders. Treatments of the mitochondriopathies depend upon the individual disorder.

Energy Metabolism Disorders and Metabolic Dementia in the Aging Brain

Mitochondrial alterations and oxidative damage have been linked to the aging process and secondary dementia. MtDNA mutation analysis shows a marked increase in point mutations in mitochondrial brain DNA associated with an increase in age. The majority of the recognized mutations lead to an amino acid change that has a substantial effect on the function of the proteins involved, such as decreases in the activities of cytochrome b, ATP synthase, or other enzymes.

The mechanisms responsible for these age-related changes may be secondary to chronic oxidative and molecular injuries and a lack of neutralization of reactive oxygen species (ROS). Analysis of DNA injury and gene regulation in aging human brains demonstrates a number of overexpressed or underexpressed genes when compared with younger controls. Among the less functional genes with aging are those encoding for mitochondrial proteins as well as for molecules involved in synaptic regulation, vesicular transport, and synaptic plasticity. Genes involved in DNA repair and protection against ROS-mediated damage are overexpressed in older individuals. The ROS theory of aging assigns these mediators a critical role of compromising cell homeostasis and survival of the individual as a whole.

Model Disorder—Mitochondrial Oxidative Deficiency in the Elderly

Numerous studies have linked dementia-associated biochemical changes to oxidative stress and cell injury. Some of these changes include disruptions in metal ion homeostasis, mitochondrial injury, reduced cellular glucose metabolism, decreased intracellular pH, and inflammation. The causes and effects of these oxidative stress-related injuries are not certain. Increases in the concentrations of A-peptides, the main protein components of the cerebral amyloid deposits of Alzheimer dementia, have been demonstrated to occur in inherited early-onset forms of dementia and in association with certain environmental and genetic risk factors. A-peptides have been shown to exhibit superoxide dismutase activity that increases hydrogen peroxide and may be responsible for the neurotoxicity exhibited by this peptide in vitro (284,285).

Antioxidant therapies may be effective in preventing or counteracting some of the injuries caused by free radicals and oxidative stress. Several experimental studies indicate that increasing dietary intake of fruits and vegetables high in antioxidant activity may be an important component of a healthy living strategy designed to maximize neuronal and cognitive functioning into old age (286). Preliminary controlled trials in patients with the clinical diagnosis of dementia suggested a modest delay in cognitive loss after acetyl-L-carnitine supplementation (2–3 g/day for 6–12 months) (287–289). Another study suggested that some patients under age 65 with early-onset dementia experienced a more rapid cognitive decline that could be diminished by acetyl-L-carnitine supplements (290). However, a subsequent, larger multi-center, randomized controlled trial involving 431 patients diagnosed with Alzheimer dementia found no benefit of acetyl-L-carnitine (3 g/day for 12 months) in delaying cognitive decline (291). A multi-center, randomized controlled trial conducted in 229 subjects with early-onset Alzheimer dementia between 45 and 65 years of age also failed to demonstrate a benefit from acetyl-L-carnitine (3 g/day for 12 months) in most measures of cognitive decline with the exception of slightly decreased declines in attention compared with placebo (292).

MICRONUTRIENT AND TRACE ELEMENT DEFICIENCY STATES

The human body contains at least 60 elements and minerals including many that perform essential functions as integral components of metalloenzymes or as activating cofactors for other enzymes. Trace elements are those minerals present in pictogram-to-microgram quantity per gram of tissue and constitute less than 0.01% of total body weight. The 13 trace elements believed to be nutritionally important, in order of importance, are iron, zinc, copper, iodine, fluoride, selenium, manganese, chromium, cobalt, molybdenum, nickel, silicon, and vanadium. Trace elements are said to be essential if their deficiency consistently results in impairment of function. Conversely, excesses in minerals may arise through changes in intrinsic control mechanisms or by consumption in extra quantity. Deficiency states and toxic quantities of diverse elements have the potential to produce non-specific clinical syndromes including secondary dementia. Dietary reference intakes (DRIs) have been established by the Food and Nutrition Board of the Institute of Medicine for zinc, copper, iodine, selenium, manganese, chromium, and molybdenum (293).

Micronutrient Deficiency and Metabolic Dementia in the Developing Brain

Many health consequences are associated with micronutrient deficiency in the developing brain, including premature birth, low birth weight, and a higher rate of infections and death (294). However, research examining the effects of micronutrient deficiencies on early cognitive development suffers from the same methodological problems inherent to research on the effects of malnutrition. Micronutrient deficiencies most often occur in the context of poverty, frequently with confounding physical and social stressors that may interfere with health and optimal development. Furthermore, if children are deficient in multiple micronutrients, it may be difficult to interpret the effects of individual micronutrient deficits or the meaning of dietary supplementation trials.

Model Disorder—Chloride Deficiency in Infancy and Cognitive Disorders

A selective form of micronutrient malnutrition, often induced by use of a chloride-deficient infant formula, appears to generate a permanent residual syndrome of cognitive, language, visuomotor, and attentional deficits (295–297). Chloride is an essential element, but its concentrations in the body are much higher than those of trace elements. Humans contain up to 100 g of chloride, or about

0.15% of total weight. Chloride is found mainly in the extracellular fluids and is an integral part of the digestive juice hydrochloric acid. Chloride ion is also essential for maintaining osmotic pressure and acid–base balance.

Clinical signs of a chloride-deficient diet in infancy include hypochloremic alkalosis, deceleration of head growth, linear growth, and body weight, and subsequent cognitive deficits. Compared to growth parameters in generally malnourished control infants, chloride-deficient diet infants have more severe deceleration of head growth and more frequent and more severe cognitive deficits.

Model Disorder—Zinc Deficiency and the Developing Brain

The brain has the highest zinc content of all organs and its highest concentrations are in the cortex, certain forebrain regions, hippocampus, and amygdale (298). Zinc is an essential cofactor for many enzymes, structural proteins, and transcription factors. Zinc has unique vesicular localization in presynaptic terminals where it probably plays a modulatory role in synaptic transmission, but the physiological significance of this phenomenon is poorly understood (299). It is suggested that excessive synaptic $Zn(2+)$ release may lead to accumulation in postsynaptic neurons and selective neuronal loss associated with certain acute degenerative disorders including dementia.

Clinical evidence links zinc deficiency with various systemic signs as well as impairment of cognitive function (300). Zinc deficiency is common in both developing and developed countries. Several studies on zinc-deficient children and adults have shown beneficial effects of zinc repletion on growth, health, and neuropsychologic function (301). Zinc deficiency is particularly relevant to brain development because of its fundamental roles in cell division and maturation (302,303). In trials among nutritionally deprived infants and toddlers, zinc supplementation has been associated with vigorous play activity among Indian infants (304), functional activity among Guatemalan toddlers (305), motor development among Canadian infants born at <1500 g (306), motor quality among Chilean infants (307), and co-operative behavior during testing among Brazilian infants (308). In elderly populations, borderline zinc concentrations have been associated with deteriorating immune function, especially when associated with diabetes mellitus or alcohol abuse. Zinc supplementation may protect against the deteriorating vision associated with age-related macular degeneration (309).

Micronutrient Deficiency and Metabolic Dementia in the Developing and Developed Brain

Worldwide, at least half of all otherwise healthy children in regions of poverty have sub-clinical or biochemical deficiencies of vitamins A, C, B_2, B_6, and folate, trace elements, such as iodine and zinc, and other essential elements, such as iron (310). Such sub-clinical deficiencies of micronutrients are commonly referred to as "hidden hunger" and may contribute to sub-optimal growth and cognitive development during infancy and childhood. Children with a deficiency of micronutrients are more vulnerable to developing recurrent severe infections, further aggravating a cycle of undernutrition and infections. In areas of poverty, it may not be possible to meet 100% of the recommended dietary allowance (RDA) requirements of micronutrients from dietary sources alone. Most preschool children in these areas need supplements to optimize their genetic potential for physical growth and mental development (311).

Model Disorder—Selenium Deficiency and Secondary Myxedematous Dementia

Although selenium is an essential trace element with multiple functions in metabolism, it plays its most prominent role as a selenoprotein in the antioxidant enzyme glutathione peroxidase, which acts to protect lipids in polyunsaturated membranes from hydrogen peroxide (H_2O_2) and oxidative degradation (312). Animal models suggest that dietary selenium restriction does not directly cause spontaneous neurological defects, but sensitizes the brain to increased damage after experimental challenge with neurotoxins (313). Under dietary restriction, brain selenium is only slightly reduced, as is cellular glutathione peroxidase activity. In glutathione peroxidase knockout mice, no spontaneous neurological deficits are observed, but these mice are more vulnerable to brain ischemia and neurotoxins. In selenoprotein P-deficient mice, brain selenium is strongly reduced as are the activities of the selenoenzymes (313). Thus, these models suggest that adequate brain selenium concentrations are essential to guarantee normal selenoprotein expression, which is necessary to counteract the neurotoxicity of metals, such as mercury, cadmium, lead and vanadium, and the oxidative injury associated with cancer, aging, Parkinson's disease, and dementia (314).

Dietary sources of selenium from grain reflect the soil in which the grain was grown and human consumption varies markedly between different parts of the world. Although selenium deficiency is not usually reported in healthy populations in North America, severe selenium deficiency occurs in central African populations where myxedematous cretinism is endemic. This secondary dementia associated with the combination of selenium and iodine deficiency, as well as thiocyanate overload, is thought to be the consequence of excess H_2O_2 accumulation within thyroid cells, subsequent cell death, thyroid fibrosis, and myxedema dementia (315). In areas of China where severe endemic selenium deficiency occurs without iodine deficiency, an isolated cardiomyopathy (Keshan disease) is reported without higher incidence of thyroid disease or dementia. Relative selenium deficiency and low intake have been linked to adverse mood states (312). Although the underlying biological mechanisms are unclear, responses to supplementation are found with doses greater than those needed to produce maximal activity of the selenoprotein glutathione peroxidase.

Micronutrient Disorders in the Aging Brain

Approximately two-thirds of American adults do not eat the recommended five portions of fruits and vegetables per day (285). Lower dietary consumption of fruits and vegetables is associated with higher cancer rates for most types of cancer when compared with groups of higher consumption. Common micronutrient deficiencies may cause DNA alterations by the same mechanisms as radiation and many toxins. Similarly, the aging of the brain appears to be closely related to the oxidants produced by mitochondria as by-products of normal metabolism.

Model Disorder—Magnesium Deficiency and Cognitive Dysfunction

Magnesium has an essential function in cellular physiology and is involved in the activation of about 300 enzymes including numerous enzymes catalyzing energy-producing and energy-consuming reactions. Magnesium is an extracellular cell membrane stabilizer and a non-competitive N-methyl-D-aspartate (NMDA) channel antagonist.

A large part of the elderly population may have an inadequate magnesium intake and may be prone to chronic latent magnesium deficiency compounded by a deficiency of other vitamins and minerals. Magnesium deficiencies are frequently observed in alcoholics and diabetic patients, in whom a combination of factors contributes to its pathogenesis. Signs of magnesium deficiency are decreased cognition, fatigue, lethargy, and depression. Systemically administered magnesium sulfate can block NMDA receptors in the brain and afford neuronal protection in cerebral ischemia and seizures (316). Ionized magnesium acts as a sedative and CNS depressant, which is the basis for its efficacy in reduction of seizures in women with eclampsia and severe pre-eclampsia (317).

ENDOCRINE DISORDERS AND SECONDARY DEMENTIA

Besides thyroid disorders (See the section "Thyroid Disorders" in this chapter), other key endocrinopathies relating to secondary dementia include parathyroid, pituitary, and adrenal disorders (318,319). In addition, small quantities of steroids, termed neurosteroids, are synthesized de novo in brain tissue (320).

Endocrine Disorders and Metabolic Dementia in the Developing Brain

Brain hormones and neuroregulators play important roles in control of appetite and body weight. Neuropeptide Y is a major regulator of food consumption and energy homeostasis. Opioid peptides can promote rewards of eating. Corticotropin-releasing factor can affect stress-induced eating, and leptin controls energy homeostasis and feeding behavior; however, the link between dysregulation in these signaling pathways, the development of type 2 diabetes, and its risk for dementia remains speculative.

Model Disorder—Persistent Hyperinsulinemic Hypoglycemia of Infancy

Deficient insulin release causes hyperglycemia and diabetes, whereas excessive insulin can lead to significant hypoglycemia-related metabolic disorders. Persistent hyperinsulinemic hypoglycemia of infancy, previously termed nesidioblastosis, is a disorder characterized by dysregulated insulin secretion that can lead to secondary CNS injury, dementia, and seizures. Known causes for the disorder include aberrant regulation of ATP-sensitive potassium channels, defective carbohydrate glycosylation, or abnormal glucokinase and glutamate dehydrogenase activities (321).

Endocrine Disorders and Metabolic Dementia in the Developed Brain

Ionized calcium plays essential roles in learning and memory but it is also involved in neuronal survival and death (322). Endocrine dysregulation of neuronal calcium/phosphate homeostasis by glucocorticoids, vitamin D, or parathyroid hormone could have pathogenetic implications in the development of dementia.

Model Disorder—Primary Hyperparathyroidism

Increasing calcium availability has been shown to ameliorate age-related deficits in neurotransmission, but hypercalcemia is a manifestation of several systemic disorders. CNS symptoms of hypercalcemia include impaired short-term memory, depression, confusion, somnolence, or stupor. Primary hyperparathyroidism is diagnosed by elevated serum calcium and parathyroid hormone concentrations, and decreased serum phosphate (318). Primary hyperparathyroidism is most commonly diagnosed in elderly women, but the disorder can present with signs of cognitive impairment, affective disorders, nervousness, and personality or behavioral changes in younger persons. Parathyroidectomy is the effective treatment when a parathyroid adenoma is present.

Model Disorder—Hypoparathyroidism

Chronic hypocalcemia due to hypoparathyroidism is another disorder that may produce dementia without other obvious systemic manifestations. The presumed pathological mechanism in the disorder is the hypocalcemia rather than the underlying hypoparathyroidism, but rare cases of dementia due to hypoparathyroidism without hypocalcemia have been effectively reversed with 1,25-dihydroxy-cholecalciferol therapy (323).

Endocrine Disorders and Metabolic Dementia in the Aging Brain

In men, neural androgen depletion appears to be a natural consequence of aging. Lower brain testosterone concentrations have been reported as a possible risk factor for mild neurological changes and dementia (324). However, studies of the correlation between serum concentrations of testosterone and dementia have lead to contradictory results. Benefits of testosterone replacement therapy in male hypogonadism, with or without dementia, is uncertain (325).

In women, lack of estrogen after menopause was considered to be a possible risk factor for dementia. This hypothesis led to several epidemiological studies proposing that postmenopausal estrogen replacement protects from cognitive decline (326,327).

Model Disorder—Hormone Replacement Therapy (HRT) and Cognitive Performance in Elderly Women

Despite supportive evidence from animal, basic science, and observational studies, current clinical evidence does not support a role for HRT in the prevention or treatment of dementia. However, a number of questions about the biologic effects of HRT in the brain remain unresolved, including the potential benefits of HRT given in forms other than conjugated equine estrogens (CEE), with alternative schedules of administration and various timings of therapy initiation.

Data from the Women's Health Initiative Memory Study show that HRT did not lower the risk of dementia in women over the age of 64, contradicting previous studies that suggested HRT could protect against age-related memory loss in postmenopausal women (328,329). These studies of women aged 65–79 years show that regimens of CEE or CEE plus medroxyprogesterone acetate (MPA) *increase* the risk of global cognitive dysfunction or of dementia with mild cognitive impairment, respectively, when given to women after menopause. Higher rates of stroke and hypertension also were reported in elderly women taking HRT.

These studies do not answer the questions about the relative risk of dementia if HRT is taken for symptomatic relief of symptoms during menopause. Animal research suggests that estrogen preserves cognitive abilities through effects on cholinergic neurons in the basal forebrain that project into the hippocampal formation and cerebral cortex (330). However, pooling human data for estrogen alone and estrogen plus progestin, use of hormone therapy to prevent dementia or cognitive decline in women aged 65 years or older is not recommended.

NEUROTRANSMITTER DISORDERS

Neuronal synaptic function is facilitated through action potentials and a multitude of molecules acting as neurotransmitters and neuromodulators. Early stages of dementia may begin with diminished neurotransmission of acetylcholine, glutamate, norepinephrine, serotonin, and dopamine, or with abnormalities in second messengers and protein kinases.

Neurotransmitter Disorders and Dementia in the Developing Brain

Neurotransmitters have diverse tasks in the developing brain ranging from early developmental functions in morphogenesis to later functions in neurite outgrowth, target selection, and synapse formation. The growth cones of developing neurons are known to release transmitters and to respond to transmitters released from other neurons. Depletion of transmitters during embryonic development results in developmental deficits of the brain, which suggests that neurotransmitters may play critical roles as neurotrophic factors.

Model Disorder—Creatine Deficiency Syndromes

Creatine (methylguanido-acetic acid) is an intermediate molecule synthesized mainly in the liver and the pancreas by the action of arginine:glycine amidinotransferase (AGAT) and GAMT. Creatine reaches muscle and brain via an active transmembrane creatine transport system (CRTR). Along with creatine kinase and ATP/ADP, creatine is utilized in a high-energy-phosphate buffering system that utilizes the release of a phosphate molecule from its structure. Disorders in creatine metabolism are distinguished according to the metabolic pathway of creatine and disorders of creatine synthesis including AGAT and GAMT deficiency and disorders of cellular creatine transport (CRTR deficiency).

GAMT deficiency is an early childhood-acquired dementia. Clinical manifestations include severe language deficits, hyperkinesis, dystonia, and seizures (331). The biochemical hallmark of creatine deficiency syndromes is the striking cerebral creatine deficiency in MRS. Further discrimination of the causes of creatine deficiency can be accomplished by measurement of blood guanidinoacetate concentration, which is increased in GAMT deficiency, decreased in AGAT deficiency, and normal in CRTR deficiency. GAMT and AGAT deficiency are treatable by oral creatine supplementation (7).

Neurotransmitter Disorders and Dementia in the Developed Brain

Model Disorder—Serotonin and Catecholamine Deficiency

Neurotransmitter systems involving serotonin and dopamine are most directly related to the regulation of emotion, mood, and memory (also see Chapter 12, Cognitive Impairment in Depression). In studies of Alzheimer dementia, variants of serotonin promoter, transporter, and receptor genes have been linked to neuropsychiatric symptoms including agitation, aggression, depression, and psychosis (332).

Metabolic disorders may interrupt the eventual synthesis of the monoaminergic neurotransmitters. Tetrahydrobiopterin (BH4) is the cofactor in the hydroxylation of phenylalanine, tyrosine, and tryptophan, which are the amino acids involved in the synthesis of dopamine, norepinephrine, and serotonin, respectively. Decreased CSF biopterin concentrations in patients with dementia suggest that a CNS biopterin deficiency may play an important role in the pathogenesis of the disorder (333,334). In addition, BH4 is an essential cofactor in all nitric oxide synthase (NOS) isoforms (335). These enzymes utilize molecular oxygen for nitric oxide (NO) synthesis, which is elevated in Alzheimer dementia, suggesting an important role for NO in the neurodegenerative process (336,337).

Neurotransmitter Disorders and Dementia in the Aging Brain

Model Disorder—Acetylcholine Metabolism in Dementia

Cholinergic neurotransmitter deficiency is a distinguishing feature of Alzheimer dementia. Prior to neuronal loss and the formation of plaques and neurofibrillary tangles, a decrease in both nicotinic and muscarinic acetylcholine receptors occurs (338). Such decreases in acetylcholine receptors may explain the effects of anti-cholinergic drugs in precipitating confusion and transient memory deficits in the elderly (see Chapter 11: Drug-Induced Cognitive Impairment). Cholinergic therapy by stimulation of nicotinic or muscarinic acetylcholine receptors may exert a neuroprotective effect, leading to the reduction of amyloid and the slowing of the disease process. Nicotine is known to act on presynaptic nicotinic acetylcholine receptors and epidemiological studies suggest that smoking may lower the incidence of dementia (339).

Cholinesterase inhibitors, such as donepezil, act to reduce breakdown of acetylcholine. Additionally, galantamine acts as a positive allosteric modulator of brain nicotinic acetylcholine receptors and appears to render receptors in the presynaptic nerve terminals more sensitive to available acetylcholine, whereas memantine shows moderate affinity CNS glutamate receptor antagonist properties. This class of drugs provides small benefits in cognitive abilities for persons with Alzheimer dementia based on measures of global function. However, recent non-industry-sponsored studies did not show significant improvements in ratings of disability, dependency, behavioral and psychological symptoms, caregiver psychopathology, or delay in institutionalization, subsequently raising the question whether cholinesterase inhibitors are truly cost-effective (340). Large, prospective, placebo-controlled dementia studies using rational combinations of cholinesterase inhibitors with statins, antioxidants, non-steroidal anti-inflammatory agents, or other non-pharmacological treatments are yet to be performed.

TRACE ELEMENT DISORDERS

In contrast to environmentally induced trace element toxicity or deficiency states, genetic disorders of trace element synthesis, regulation, and degradation can also cause recognizable cerebral disorders.

Trace Metal Disorders and Dementia in the Developing Brain

Model Disorder—Molybdenum Cofactor Deficiency

Current understanding of the essentiality of molybdenum in humans is based on the study of rare genetic disorders involving the synthesis of molybdenum cofactor. This molybdenum-containing cofactor is necessary to the function of three enzymes: sulfite oxidase, xanthine dehydrogenase, and aldehyde oxidase. Neurological manifestations usually occur in infancy or early childhood and include seizures, dislocated lenses, and severe cognitive stagnation or decline.

Mutations causing molybdenum cofactor deficiency have been traced to several sites in the genes *MOCS1A*, *MOCS1B*, *MOCS2*, and the gephyrin gene (*GEPH*) (341). The most straightforward screening test for molybdenum cofactor deficiency is a strip test for excess urinary sulfite in a fresh urine sample. It is uncertain whether the pathological mechanisms of molybdenum deficiency are the result of accumulation of toxic sulfite metabolites, inadequate sulfate production, or the depletion of cysteine, cystine, other thiols, or thiol-dependent proteins through reaction with the excess sulfite (342,343).

Dietary molybdenum deficiency has been described only as acquired molybdenum deficiency in Crohn disease or after receiving long-term total parenteral nutrition (TPN) without molybdenum supplementation. The protein intolerance and acquired encephalopathy associated with molybdenum deficiency is reversible with molybdenum supplementation (160 mcg/day).

Trace Metal Disorders and Dementia in the Developed Brain

Copper is a metallic cofactor of dopamine-beta-carboxylase. Although it is present in the brain in reasonably high concentrations, it is affected by nutritional status, particularly during development. Copper metabolism is altered in numerous disorders with distinct neurologic and behavioral sequelae.

Model Disorder—WD and Secondary Dementia in Young Adults

Wilson disease (WD) is a rare autosomal recessive disorder characterized by inadequate excretion of absorbed dietary copper via bile, resulting in accumulation of toxic quantities of copper in liver, brain, and other organs. Although the most common presentation of WD is hepatic dysfunction, in about one-third of patients, cerebral dysfunction is initially present with signs of dementia, psychosis, or a distinctive involuntary "wing-beating" tremor. Other neurological manifestations include irritability, depression, disinhibition, dysarthria, dystonia, gait abnormalities, and muscular rigidity (344,345). Wilson disease should be suspected in adolescents and adults under age 40 with these neurological findings combined with unexplained signs of liver disease, such as elevated serum transaminase concentrations. A ceruloplasmin test screening for a decreased serum concentration is helpful; however, false negatives and false positives can occur in numerous systemic disorders. Other supportive diagnostic tests include elevated 24-hour urine copper, the presence of a Kaiser-Fleischer ring in the cornea by a slit-lamp examination, and findings of bilateral T2-weighted MRI hyperintensity in the lentiform nuclei and thalamus with corresponding bilateral hypointensity of the globus pallidus. An elevated hepatic copper concentration exceeding 250 mcg/g of dry weight is the most definitive test available for the diagnosis of WD.

Reduced concentration of plasma ceruloplasmin is a key diagnostic biochemical marker of Menkes (kinky hair) syndrome and WD (hepatolenticular degeneration) (346). Both of these conditions involve genes that encode P-type copper-transporting ATPases (347). The gene for WD encodes 7.5-kb mRNA for a protein synthesized in hepatocytes as a single chain polypeptide that is localized to the trans-Golgi network. Over 240 heterogeneous mutations have been found in WD patients, consisting of a small number of frequent mutations in the related patients and large numbers of rare mutations in unrelated patients (345,348). A database of WD mutations can be found at http://www. uofa-medical-genetics.org/wilson/index.php. Putative molecular mechanisms include gene mutations resulting in abnormal Wilson protein structure with rapid degradation or abnormal intracellular trafficking and defective chaperone interactions with the Wilson protein.

Considerable controversy remains in the current treatment approach to WD. Depending on the stages of the disease at the time of diagnosis, the exact protocols of penicillamine, trientene, and tetrathiomolybdate in the initial treatment of symptomatic WD, and the role of zinc monotherapy for maintenance treatment in asymptomatic WD remain to be optimized (345). It is currently not certain whether neurological manifestations alone are an indication for liver transplantation in WD.

Trace Metal Disorders and Dementia in the Aging Brain

Model Disorder—Chronic Trace Element Accumulation and Depletion in the Elderly

In a study of patients with Alzheimer dementia without clinical signs of malnutrition, decreased CSF zinc concentrations were lower than in controls (349). In the same patients, CSF and serum levels of iron, copper, and manganese, and serum concentrations of zinc did not differ significantly between dementia and control groups, suggesting that low CSF zinc concentrations were related to the dementia rather than nutritional deficits.

IMMUNE RESPONSE DISORDERS

Systemic and local inflammatory responses are associated with cerebrovascular disease and may be associated with primary and secondary dementias (350,351). Patients with vascular disease who have low levels of acute-phase reactants, such as C-reactive protein (CRP), after statin therapy have better clinical outcomes than those with higher CRP, regardless of the resultant level of LDL cholesterol (352). In patients with Alzheimer dementia, CRP is present in neuritic plaques and neurofibrillary tangles and proinflammatory cytokines are present in high concentrations in serum (353,354). Such findings are the basis for the hypothesis that inflammatory mechanisms are a precursor to some dementias (355).

Immune Response Disorders Leading to Pseudodementia in the Developing Brain

Model Disorder—Pediatric AIDS–Dementia Complex
(See Also Chapter 2: HIV-1-Associated Dementia.)

According to the WHO, approximately 2.2 million children under the age of 15 years are infected with HIV/AIDS. Neurodevelopmental sequelae of HIV/AIDS infection in children are most common when infants are infected during the perinatal period (356). Neurologic disorders include cognitive impairments, impaired brain growth, and motor dyspraxias. Despite the trend of increasing rates of infection, advances in therapies have led to survival past five years of age in two out of three infected children. Increased survival has lead to greater recognition of secondary cognitive disabilities and an increasing array of adverse metabolic effects, including insulin resistance and glucose intolerance, dyslipidemia, changes in body fat distribution, lactic acidemia, and osteopenia (357). The mechanisms underlying metabolic abnormalities and their relationship to specific antiretroviral therapies and long-term risks for developing dementia remain unclear.

Immune Response Disorders Leading to Pseudodementia in the Developed Brain

Model Disorder—Celiac Disease and Other Inflammatory
Gastrointestinal Diseases and Secondary Dementia

Celiac disease is a multisystem autoimmune disorder associated with dementia and numerous other neurological disorders, including cerebellar ataxia, epilepsy, myoclonic ataxia, and chronic neuropathies, mainly in middle-aged adults (358,359). There are limited data linking celiac disease with milder neurological disorders in children, but recent studies have explored the possible associations with headache, learning disorders, attention-deficit/hyperactivity disorder (ADHD), and tic disorders (360). In celiac disease associated with neurological disorders, evidence for a beneficial clinical response to a gluten-free diet is inconsistent in most studies. CNS symptoms of celiac disease generally show a poor response to gluten restriction, while peripheral symptoms are more likely to respond to elimination of gluten from the diet. The underlying pathological mechanisms of the neurological conditions associated with celiac disease are not completely certain, but are thought to be more likely related to immunological-inflammatory processes rather than to intestinal malabsorption and secondary vitamin deficiencies (361,362).

Model Disorders—Whipple Disease

Whipple's disease is caused by the gram-positive bacillus Tropheryma whipplei. Patients with a CNS manifestation of Whipple's disease may develop a variety of symptoms, including dementia, supranuclear gaze palsy, movement disorders, hypothalamic dysfunction, and myorhythmia. The CNS-infection is diagnosed by amplification of DNA in the CSF by PCR. Long-term antibiotic treatment is required, and relapses may occur after withdrawal of antimicrobial therapy. Crohn disease and ulcerative colitis are often complicated by polyneuropathy and cerebrovascular disease (363).

Immune Response Disorders and Dementia in the Aging Brain

Model Disorder—Hyponatremia and Memory Loss in VGKC Antibody-Associated Limbic Encephalitis—A Treatable Metabolic Disorder with Pseudodementia

Various clinical syndromes have been classified as limbic encephalitis. Consideration of the diagnosis is often based on the subacute development of disorientation, agitation, and short-term memory loss. Behavioral changes are common and include irritability, physical violence, apathy, and lethargy. Language function is preserved and the main findings on examination are usually impaired memory and attention. Patients may present with mild hyponatremia (serum sodium, 120–131 mEq/L) (364,365). In voltage-gated potassium channel (VGKC) antibody-associated limbic encephalitis, VGKC antibodies are elevated and a sustained clinical response to immunosuppression with clinical improvement of symptoms typically is noted (366). VGKC antibodies are also associated with neuromyotonia and Morvan's syndrome, in which cholinergic symptoms, such as excess secretions, sweating, lacrimation, and salivation are common.

In VGKC antibody-associated limbic encephalitis, symptoms and morbidity are often only vaguely correlated with the magnitude and duration of hyponatremia. However, a faster rate of acute metabolic changes can lead to overwhelming neurological disturbances. A rapid decline in serum sodium correlates with the usual relationship between a net increase in brain water and the loss of brain electrolytes. As the condition progresses, focal neurological signs develop including hemiparesis, aphasia, tremor, ataxia, nystagmus, pupillary asymmetry, and long-tract signs. Myelinolysis is more likely to occur after the treatment of chronic rather than acute hyponatremia, and is more likely with a rapid rate of correction. The exact pathogenesis of myelinolysis has not been determined. Optimal management of hyponatremic patients involves weighing the risk for illness and death from untreated hyponatremia against the risk for myelinolysis due to correction of hyponatremia. Experiments in animals and clinical experience suggest that correction of chronic hyponatremia should be kept at a rate less than 10 mmol/L in any 24-hour period.

ALCOHOL-RELATED DEMENTIA

Approximately 2–10% of persons who drink alcohol show signs of chronic or excessive alcohol consumption. Estimates of the exact frequency of alcohol abuse vary between cultures, social groups, age groups, and geographic regions. Alcohol-related dementia has been defined as a clinical diagnosis of dementia after more than 60 days from the last exposure to alcohol, combined with a history of excessive alcohol consumption for more than five years (367). However, alcohol-related dementia can be viewed as a syndrome with a range of clinical signs and biological effects depending on genetic risk factors, concurrent nutrition, dosage, and age of exposure. In practice, controversies surrounding the diagnosis of alcohol-related dementia include questions of cognitive impairment related to ongoing intoxication, principal effects of vitamin and nutrient deficiencies, effects of chronic liver disease, and possible occult head injuries. Arguably, alcoholism alone is not the exclusive cause of dementia in most cases (368).

Alcohol-Related Dementia in the Developing Brain

Model Disorder—Fetal Alcohol Spectrum Disorders

Prenatal alcohol exposure can influence embryological and fetal development, resulting in a range of functional deficits and structural malformations described as fetal alcohol spectrum disorders (369). Classic fetal alcohol syndrome (FAS) is a relatively severe syndrome in infants born to mothers who abuse alcohol during pregnancy (370). Physical signs of FAS include short stature, characteristic dysmorphic facial features with narrow palpebral fissures, a long flat philtrum, thin upper lip, flat mid-face, and relative microcephaly. Neurological findings consist of significant cognitive impairment, receptive and expressive language disorders, hyperactivity, hypotonia, and motor dyspraxia (371,372). Life-long CNS sequelae of milder prenatal alcohol teratogenicity include learning disabilities, attention deficits, and other similar behavioral disorders.

Alcohol-Related Dementia in the Developed Brain

The effects of chronic alcohol abuse on cognition in adolescents and adults begin with mild clinical signs, such as loss of recent memory, delayed response times, and deterioration of abstract reasoning skills (373). Other disorders associated with alcohol-related dementia include hyponatremia, liver disease, Marchiafava-Bignami disease, cerebellar degeneration, head trauma, cerebrovascular disease, and hypertension (374).

Model Disorder—Metabolic Changes from Thiamine Deficiency Leading to Wernicke-Korsakoff Syndrome

Korsakoff syndrome and Wernicke encephalopathy are clinical and neuropathological conditions secondary to vitamin deficiency in dementia (see the section on

Other Vitamin Deficiencies in this chapter) (374,375). Wernicke-Korsakoff syndrome results primarily from thiamine and niacin deficiency. The initial clinical features of Wernicke encephalopathy are lethargy, apathy, disorientation, memory impairment, inattention, and sleepiness. If fundamental thiamine and other nutritional deficiencies are not corrected, the encephalopathy is progressive. Physical findings in advanced stages of the disorder include abducens palsies, nystagmus, and ataxia (376,377). Kofsakoff syndrome is characterized by retrograde amnesia (an inability to recall events), anterograde amnesia (an inability to learn new information), denial of memory dysfunction, confabulation, and occasional psychosis. Characteristic neuropathological findings are neuronal loss, neuroglial proliferation, dendritic simplification, reduction in synaptic complexity, loss of the medial thalamus and Purkinje cell dendritic structure, and atrophy of the mamillary bodies (378).

Alcoholic disorders tend not to appear in dementia pathology series other than as Wernicke-Korsakoff syndrome. In addition, only a minority of pathologically diagnosed Wernicke encephalopathy cases are clinically recognized, suggesting that thiamine-deficiency-related dementia may be more common than currently reported (376,379).

Alcohol Abuse and Metabolic Dementia in the Aging Brain

Excessive alcohol use as a cause of dementia in the elderly may overlap with the wide spectrum of age-related dementias. There is considerable debate about whether alcohol-related dementia is under-diagnosed in the geriatric population, or whether there is even sufficient evidence to justify a distinct clinical category besides Wernicke-Korsakoff syndrome. However, some geriatric studies suggest that between 6% and 24% of all elderly persons chronically consume excessive alcohol (380–383). The risk of alcohol consumption increases significantly in certain groups, such as those with social isolation or divorced status (383). A lifetime history of heavy drinking is associated with a fourfold increase in dementia diagnoses (367). Alcohol-related dementia patients may be up to 10 years younger than non-alcohol-related dementia patients. Although there are no validated instruments for alcoholism screening in cognitively impaired elderly patients, clinical evaluation should attempt to accurately estimate a past and present alcohol consumption history including a search for alcoholic beverages at home visits (381).

Model Disorder—Alcoholism Masquerading as Dementia in the Elderly

Despite the high prevalence of alcohol use in the elderly population, the risks of alcohol-related disorders are often under-recognized. Determinants of alcohol use and abuse may include "self treatment" of major depression, social isolation, and reduced mobility. In addition to cognitive impairment, the consequences of excessive alcohol use include risks of hip fracture from falls, liver disease, peripheral neuropathy, insomnia, late-onset seizure disorders, poor nutrition, incontinence, diarrhea, myopathy, inadequate self-care, and adverse effects from medication due to altered metabolism.

SYSTEMIC ILLNESS

Many metabolic disorders related to primary systemic illnesses lead to secondary dementia. Clinical manifestations of these metabolic disorders may be associated with dysfunction of the liver, kidney, eye, bone, blood, muscle, gastrointestinal tract or integument. Examples of these associations are listed in Table 2. Clinicians should keep in mind the relative infrequency of these disorders, their mode of inheritance, key metabolic markers, and the possibility of milder phenotypes with atypical features.

Systemic Illness and Metabolic Dementia in the Developing Brain

Improvements in medical technology and greater knowledge of the human genome are resulting in significant changes in the diagnosis, classification, and treatments of inherited metabolic disorders that can lead to secondary dementia in infants and children. Hundreds of known "inborn errors" of metabolism will be recognized earlier or treated differently because of these changes. Although most physicians rarely encounter these individual metabolic disorders in daily practice, their collective incidence is at least one in 1,500 persons (384).

Model Disorder—Other Inborn Errors of Metabolism Causing Cognitive Loss in Infancy and Early Childhood

Current approaches to inborn errors of metabolism (IEM) revolve around: (i) laboratory screening of certain disorders in asymptomatic newborns, (ii) prompt physician recognition of unscreened disorders in symptomatic individuals, (iii) follow-up and verification of abnormal laboratory results, and (iv) rapid implementation of appropriate therapies. The increasing application of new technologies such as electrospray ionization-tandem mass spectrometry (MS/MS, Fig. 2) to newborn screening allows earlier identification of a larger number of IEM with clear cost benefits. Table 2 lists those IEM typically detected, and also those usually not detected by MS/MS. However, there are ongoing changes in screening laboratories and technology, with large variations in screening policy between geographic regions.

Many of the inborn errors of metabolism, including urea cycle defects, organic acidemias, and certain disorders of amino acid metabolism, often present in infants with symptoms of acute or chronic metabolic encephalopathy. Characteristic symptoms include lethargy, poor feeding, apnea or tachypnea, and recurrent vomiting. Individuals at all ages may have metabolic disorders that present with systemic findings, such as hepatic, renal or cardiac syndromes, dysmorphic syndromes, ocular findings, or significant orthopedic abnormalities.

A "pattern recognition" approach helps guide the physician toward a differential diagnosis and targeted molecular testing (Table 3). These clinical indications for advanced laboratory studies are the standard of practice in modern children's hospitals.

Hypoglycemia is a common manifestation of a number of inborn errors of metabolism, including glycogen storage diseases and defects in gluconeogenesis. Fatty acid oxidation defects, galactosemia, hereditary tyrosinemia, and neonatal hemochromatosis may have a variable clinical presentation including a sub-acute encephalopathy with hepatic dysfunction or cardiomyopathy. Certain lysosomal storage disorders may come to attention because of organomegaly or coarse facial features. Recognizable facial patterns and clearly dysmorphic features may lead to the diagnosis of other metabolic disorders, such as Smith-Lemli-Opitz syndrome (cholesterol synthesis defect) or Zellweger syndrome (peroxisome biogenesis deficiency). Metabolic acidosis or hyperammonemia are observed in many small-molecule disorders, but there are notable exceptions including non-ketotic hyperglycinemia and molybdenum cofactor deficiency.

Early diagnosis and treatment of certain inherited inborn errors of metabolism may allow the reduction of many secondary metabolic dementias of childhood. Traditional therapies for metabolic diseases include dietary therapy, such as protein restriction, avoidance of fasting, or cofactor supplements. Evolving therapies for IEM may now include organ transplantation, enzyme replacement, pharmacologic intervention, or other strategies. Efforts to provide treatment through somatic gene therapy are still in early stages but there is hope that this approach will provide additional therapeutic possibilities. Even when no effective therapy exists or an infant dies from a metabolic disorder, an accurate diagnosis is still imperative for family clarification, reassurance, genetic counseling, and potential prenatal screening.

Systemic Illness and Metabolic Dementia in the Developed Brain

Model Disorder—Uremia and Metabolic Effects of Renal Insufficiency

Renal insufficiency and failure result in systemic retention of toxic nitrogenous compounds; it is usually diagnosed without difficulty by the characteristic clinical signs and laboratory markers of uremia. Uremic encephalopathy is a complication of uremia that leads to dementia-like cognitive changes, such as confusion, memory loss, inattentiveness, delayed motor responses, and fatigue. Dialysis treats uremic encephalopathy through clearance of small- to moderate-sized molecules from blood and usually results in resolution of the CNS disturbances. Dialysis encephalopathy secondary to intoxication of aluminium was a common occurrence prior to 1980 and the strict use of purified water in dialysis (see the subsection on Environmental Toxins and Metabolic Dementia in the Aging Brain in this chapter). Seizures occur in approximately one-third of patients with uremia from acute renal failure. Patients with chronic uremia and signs of dialysis-associated dementias should be thoroughly evaluated for metabolic and toxic encephalopathies, heavy metal or trace element intoxication, hypertension, and structural neurological lesions, such as cerebrovascular disease. Moderate renal impairment, reflected by chronic elevations of serum creatinine, is associated with an increased risk of carotid atherosclerosis, stroke, and an excess risk of incident dementia among individuals in good to excellent health (385).

Systemic Illness and Metabolic Dementia in the Aging Brain

Model Disorder—Chronic Hypoxemia, Sleep Apnea, and Effects of Cardiopulmonary Failure

Disturbances in nighttime sleep are common in patients with advanced age, obstructive apnea, and dementia. Chronic obstructive pulmonary disease (COPD) can lead to cognitive impairment and hypoxemia secondary to poor cerebral perfusion. Brain perfusion single-photon emission computed tomography (SPECT) studies in patients with COPD demonstrate anterior cerebral hypoperfusion with hypoxemia that correlates with diminished performance in neuropsychological tests of frontal lobe function, such as verbal attainment, attention, and deductive thinking (386). The findings in COPD are in contrast to those in patients with Alzheimer dementia, who show signs of hypoperfusion in brain associative areas and more severely affected cognitive performance tests. Thus, COPD and mild hypoxemia usually can be distinguished from dementia-based clinical patterns of neuropsychological test results and response to oxygen therapy (387).

SUMMARY

Errors of metabolism can lead to defects in the structure or function of essential proteins in metabolic pathways. Innumerable metabolic changes have the potential to cause secondary dementia. As knowledge of the genesis and nature of dementia increases, new opportunities arise to investigate disease expression. Studies in dementia must continue to correlate markers of risk with specific environmental, physical, and psychological profiles.

Dementia is typically a chronic condition that is present long before the diagnosis is made. The major challenge in the diagnosis of any patient with minimal cerebral dysfunction or dementia is early recognition of treatable disorders before dementia develops. No single biomarker or metabolic assay will detect all forms of dementia. The best diagnostic approach is organized, systematic, and individualized based on clinical clues. The metabolic diagnostic evaluation usually includes a combination of general screening and focused testing. Early treatment of metabolic risk factors, such as cobalamin deficiency, hypothyroidism, hyperhomocysteinemia, hypercholesterolemia, insulin resistance, and diabetes should delay the onset of microangiopathy and cerebral atrophy in the majority of individuals.

Thus, as in most neurological disorders, the prognosis for secondary metabolic dementia still hinges on an accurate and timely diagnosis. Ruling out the presence of a medically treatable disorder provides reassurance to family members and allows the palliative care plan to focus care on minimizing the disability of dementia while maintaining respectable quality of life for the patient as well as the family.

ABBREVIATIONS

AAMR	American Association on Mental Retardation
Abeta	amyloid beta peptide
AChE	acetylcholine esterase
ADHD	attention-deficit/hyperactivity disorder
AGAT	arginine:glycine amidinotransferase
AGE	advanced glycogen end products
ApoE	apolipoprotein E
AST	aspartate aminotransferase
ATP	adenosine triphosphate
CBF	cerebral blood flow
CBS	cystathionine beta-synthase
CEE	conjugated equine estrogens
COPD	chronic obstructive pulmonary disease
CNS	central nervous system
CRTR	creatine transport
CRP	C-reactive protein
CSF	cerebrospinal fluid
CT	computed tomography
DNA	deoxyribonucleic acid
FAS	fetal alcohol syndrome
EEG	electroencephalogram
GSK	glycogen synthase kinase
GLUT	glucose transporter
GABA	gamma-aminobutyric acid
GAMT	guanidino acetate methyltranferase
ETC	electron transport chain
HDL	high-density lipoproteins
IQ	intelligence quotient
LCL	low density lipoproteins
HIV/AIDS	human immunodeficiency virus/acquired immunodeficiency syndrome
HRT	hormone replacement therapy
MMA	methylmalonic acid

MPS	mucopolysaccharidosis
MRA	magnetic resonance angiography
MRI	magnetic resonance imaging
MS/MS	electrospray ionization-tandem mass spectrometry
MTHFR	methylenetetrahydrofolate reductase
NAD/NADP	nicotinamide adenine dinucleotide/phosphate
NMDA	N-methyl-D-aspartate
NO/NOS	nitric oxide/synthase
NPC	Niemann-Pick type C
NTD	neural tube defects
PET	positron emission tomography
Phe	phenylalanine
PKU	phenylketonuria
RDA	recommended dietary allowance
ROS	reactive oxygen species
SAM	S-adenosylmethionine
SPECT	single photon emission computed tomography
SREHT	steroid responsive encephalopathy associated with Hashimoto thyroiditis
SSADH	succinic semialdehyde dehydrogenase
T3	tri-iodothyronine
T4	thyroxine
THC	tetrahydrocannabis
TIS	Teratology Information Services
TPN	total parenteral nutrition
TSH	thyrotropin
VGKC	voltage-gated potassium channel
VLCL	very low-density lipoproteins
WD	Wilson disease
WHO	World Health Organization

REFERENCES

1. American Psychiatric Association. Diagnostic and Statistical Manual of Mental Disorders Fourth Edition, Text Revision [DSM-IV-TR]. Washington, DC, 2000.
2. World Health Organization. International Classification of Diseases: 10th Revision [ICD-10]. Commission on Professional and Hospital Activities, 2004.
3. Knopman DS, DeKosky ST, Cummings JL, Chui H, Corey-Bloom J, Relkin N, et al. Practice parameter: diagnosis of dementia (an evidence-based review). Report of the Quality Standards Subcommittee of the American Academy of Neurology. Neurology 2001; 56:1143–1153.
4. Clarfield AM. The reversible dementias: do they reverse? Ann Intern Med 1988; 109:476–486.

5. Novotny E, Ashwal S, Shevell M. Proton magnetic resonance spectroscopy: an emerging technology in pediatric neurology research. Pediatr Res 1998; 44(1): 1–10.

6. Herminghaus S, Frolich L, Gorriz C, Pilatus U, Dierks T, Wittsack HJ, et al. Brain metabolism in Alzheimer disease and vascular dementia assessed by in vivo proton magnetic resonance spectroscopy. Psychiatry Res Neuroimag 2003; 123:183–190.

7. Stockler S, Hanefeld F, Frahm J. Creatine replacement therapy in guanidinoacetate methyltransferase deficiency, a novel inborn error of metabolism. Lancet 1996; 348(9030):789–790.

8. Gropman A. Vigabatrin and newer interventions in succinic semialdehyde dehydrogenase deficiency. Ann Neurol 2003; 54(suppl 6):S66–S72.

9. Hyland K. The lumbar puncture for diagnosis of pediatric neurotransmitter diseases. Ann Neurol 2003; 54(suppl 6):S13–S17.

10. Knight SJ, Regan R, Nicod A, Horsley SW, Kearney L, Homfray T, et al. Subtle chromosomal rearrangements in children with unexplained mental retardation. Lancet 1999; 354:1676–1681.

11. Rooms L, Reyniers E, van Luijk R, Scheers S, Wauters J, Ceulemans B, et al. Subtelomeric deletions detected in patients with idiopathic mental retardation using multiplex ligation-dependent probe amplification (MLPA). Hum Mutat 2004; 23:17–21.

12. Kriek M, White SJ, Bouma MC, Dauwerse HG, Hansson KB, Nijhuis JV, et al. Genomic imbalances in mental retardation. J Med Genet 2004; 41:249–255.

13. Yao Y, Zhukareva V, Sung S, Clark CM, Rokach J, Lee VM, et al. Enhanced brain levels of 8,12-iso-iPF2alpha-VI differentiate AD from frontotemporal dementia. Neurology 2003; 61:475–478.

14. Fam SS, Morrow JD. The isoprostanes: unique products of arachidonic acid oxidation—a review. Curr Med Chem 2003; 10:1723–1740.

15. Irizarry MC, Hyman BT. Brain isoprostanes: a marker of lipid peroxidation and oxidative stress in AD. Neurology 2003; 61:436–437.

16. Prasad A, Kaye EM, Alroy J. Electron microscopic examination of skin biopsy as a cost-effective tool in the diagnosis of lysosomal storage diseases. J Child Neurol 1996; 11(4):301–308.

17. Salthouse TA, Berish DE, Miles JD. The role of cognitive stimulation on the relations between age and cognitive functioning. Psychol Aging 2002; 17: 548–557.

18. Coffey CE, Lucke JF, Saxton JA, Ratcliff G, Unitas LJ, Billig B, et al. Sex differences in brain aging: a quantitative magnetic resonance imaging study. Arch Neurol 1998; 55:169–179.

19. Resnick SM, Goldszal AF, Davatzikos C, Golski S, Kraut MA, Metter EJ, et al. One-year age changes in MRI brain volumes in older adults. Cereb Cortex 2000; 10:464–472.

20. Hazlett EA, Buchsbaum MS, Mohs RC, Spiegel-Cohen J, Wei TC, Azueta R, et al. Age-related shift in brain region activity during successful memory performance. Neurobiol Aging 1998; 19:437–445.

21. Della-Maggiore V, Sekuler AB, Grady CL, Bennett PJ, Sekuler R, McIntosh AR. Corticolimbic interactions associated with performance on a short-term memory task are modified by age. J Neurosci 2000; 20:8410–8416.

22. Liu J, Raine A, Venables PH, Dalais C, Mednick SA. Malnutrition at age 3 years and lower cognitive ability at age 11 years: independence from psychosocial adversity. Arch Pediatr Adolesc Med 2003; 157:593–600.
23. Wauben IP, Wainwright PE. The influence of neonatal nutrition on behavioral development: a critical appraisal. Nutr Rev 1999; 57:35–44.
24. Cockburn F. Role of infant dietary long-chain polyunsaturated fatty acids, liposoluble vitamins, cholesterol and lecithin on psychomotor development. Acta Paediatr 2003; 92:19–33.
25. Morgane PJ, Mokier DJ, Galler JR. Effects of prenatal protein malnutrition on the hippocampal formation. Neurosci Biobehav Rev 2002; 26:471–483.
26. Galler JR, Ramsey FC, Forde V, Salt P, Archer E. Long-term effects of early kwashiorkor compared with marasmus. II. Intellectual performance. J Pediatr Gastroenterol Nutr 1987; 6:847–854.
27. Chase HP, Martin HP. Undernutrition and child development. N Engl J Med 1970; 282:933–939.
28. Brandt I. Head circumference and brain development. Growth retardation during intrauterine malnutrition and catch-up growth mechanisms. Klin Wochenschr 1981; 59:995–1007.
29. Oyedeji GA, Olamijulo SK, Osinaike AI, Esimai VC, Odunusi EO, Aladekomo TA. Head circumference of rural Nigerian children – the effect of malnutrition on brain growth. Cent Afr J Med 1997; 43:264–268.
30. Pollitt E. Poverty and child development: Relevance of research in developing countries to the United States. Child Dev 1994; 65:283–295.
31. Hoffman DR, Birch EE, Castaneda YS, Fawcett SL, Wheaton DH, Birch DG, et al. Visual function in breast-fed term infants weaned to formula with or without long-chain polyunsaturates at 4 to 6 months: a randomized clinical trial. J Pediatr 2003; 142:669–677.
32. Rey J. Breastfeeding and cognitive development. Acta Paediatr 2003; 92(suppl 442): 11–18.
33. Jain A, Concato J, Leventhal JM. How good is the evidence linking breastfeeding and intelligence? Pediatrics 2002; 109:1044–1053.
34. Gordon N. Nutrition and cognitive function. Brain Dev 1997; 19(3):165–170.
35. Zeisel SH. Choline: an essential nutrient for humans. Nutrition 2000; 16: 669–671.
36. Li Q, Guo-Ross S, Lewis DV, Turner D, White AM, Wilson WA, et al. Dietary prenatal choline supplementation alters postnatal hippocampal structure and function. J Neurophysiol 2004; 91:1545–1555.
37. Frongillo EA, de Onis M, Hanson KM. Socioeconomic and demographic factors are associated with worldwide patterns of stunting and wasting of children. J Nutr 1997; 127:2302–2309.
38. Grant J. The State of the World's Children. Oxford: Oxford University Press, 1991.
39. Brown JL, Pollitt E. Malnutrition, poverty and intellectual development. Sci Am 1996; 274(2):38–43.
40. Grantham-McGregor SM, Powell C, Walker S, Chang S, Fletcher P. The long-term follow-up of severely malnourished children who participated in an intervention program. Child Dev 1994; 65:428–439.
41. Barrett DE. Nutrition and school behavior. In: Yogman MW, ed. Theory and Research in Behavioral Pediatrics. New York: Plenum, 1986:147.

42. Boddy J, Skuse D, Andrews B. The developmental sequelae of nonorganic failure to thrive. J Child Psychol Psychiatry 2000; 41:1003–1014.

43. Galler JR, Ramsey FC, Morley DS, Archer E, Salt P. The long-term effects of early kwashiorkor compared with marasmus. IV. Performance on the national high school entrance examination. Pediatr Res 1990; 28:235–239.

44. Kleinman RE, Hall S, Green H, Korzec-Ramirez D, Patton K, Pagano ME, et al. Diet, breakfast, and academic performance in children. Ann Nutr Metab 2002; 46(suppl 1):24–30.

45. Grantham-McGregor SM, Scafeld W, Powell C. Development of severely malnourished children who received psychosocial stimulation: Six-year follow-up. Pediatrics 1987; 79:247–254.

46. Abalan F, Manciet G, Dartigues JF, Decamps A, Zapata E, Saumtally B, et al. Nutrition and SDAT. Biol Psychiatry 1992; 31(1):103–105.

47. Idoate MA, Martinez AJ, Bueno J, Abu-Elmagd K, Reyes J. The neuropathology of intestinal failure and small bowel transplantation. Acta Neuropathol (Berl) 1999; 97(5):502–508.

48. White LR, Petrovitch H, Ross GW, Masaki K, Hardman J, Nelson J, et al. Brain aging and midlife tofu consumption. J Am Coll Nutr 2000; 19(2):242–255.

49. Whalley LJ, Fox HC, Lemmon HA, Duthie SJ, Collins AR, Peace H, et al. Dietary supplement use in old age: associations with childhood IQ, current cognition and health. Int J Geriatr Psychiatry 2003; 18:769–776.

50. McDaniel MA, Maier SF, Einstein GO. "Brain-specific" nutrients: a memory cure? Nutrition 2003; 19:957–975.

51. Sano M, Ernesto C, Thomas RG, Klauber MR, Schafer K, Grundman M, et al. A controlled trial of selegiline, alpha-tocopherol, or both as treatment for Alzheimer's disease. The Alzheimer's Disease Cooperative Study. N Engl J Med 1997; 336:1216–1222.

52. Luchsinger JA, Tang MX, Shea S, Mayeux R. Antioxidant vitamin intake and risk of Alzheimer disease. Arch Neurol 2003; 60:203–208.

53. Morris MC, Evans DA, Bienias JL, Tangney CC, Bennett DA, Aggarwal N, et al. Dietary intake of antioxidant nutrients and the risk of incident Alzheimer disease in a biracial community study. JAMA 2002; 287:3230–3237.

54. Miller ERr, Pastor-Barriuso R, Dalal D, Riemersma RA, Appel LJ, Guallar E. Meta-analysis: high-dosage vitamin E supplementation may increase all-cause mortality. Ann Intern Med 2004; (November 10):Epub.

55. Coyle JT, Price DL, DeLong MR. Alzheimer's disease: a disorder of cortical cholinergic innervation. Science 1983; 219·1184 1190.

56. Higgins JP, Flioker L. Lecthin for dementia and cognitive impairment: Cochrane Database Syst Rev 2003.

57. Fioravanti M, Yanagi M. Cytidinediphosphocholine (CDP choline) for cognitive and behavioural disturbances associated with chronic cerebral disorders in the elderly. Cochrane Database Syst Rev 2000; 4:CD000269.

58. Cohen RA, Browndyke JN, Moser DJ, Paul RH, Gordon N, Sweet L. Long-term citicoline (cytidine diphosphate choline) use in patients with vascular dementia: neuroimaging and neuropsychological outcomes. Cerebrovasc Dis 2003; 16:199–204.

59. Ramassamy C, Averill D, Beffert U, Bastianetto S, Theroux L, Lussier-Cacan S, et al. Oxidative damage and protection by antioxidants in the frontal cortex of Alzheimer's disease is related to the apolipoprotein E genotype. Free Radic Biol Med 1999; 27:544–553.

60. Stroombergen MC, Waring RH. Determination of glutathione S-transferase mu and theta polymorphisms in neurological disease. Hum Exp Toxicol 1999; 18:141–145.
61. Kölsch H, Linnebank M, Lütjohann D, Jessen F, Wüllner U, Harbrecht U et al. Polymorphisms in glutathione S-transferase omega-1 and AD, vascular dementia, and stroke. Neurology 2004; 63(12):2255–2260.
62. National Research Council CotTEoM. Toxicology effects of methylmercury. Washington, DC: National Academy Press, 2000.
63. Choi BH, Lapham LW, Amin-Zaki L, Saleem T. Abnormal neuronal migration, deranged cerebral cortical organization, and diffuse white matter astrocytosis of human fetal brain: a major effect of methylmercury poisoning in utero. J Neuropathol Exp Neurol 1978; 37:719–733.
64. Goldman LR, Shannon MW, Health CoE. American Academy of Pediatrics: Technical Report: Mercury in the Environment: Implications for Pediatricians. Pediatrics 2001; 108:197–205.
65. Amin-Zaki L, Majeed MA, Elhassani SB, Clarkson TW, Greenwood MR, Doherty RA. Prenatal methylmercury poisoning. Clinical observations over five years. Am J Dis Child 1979; 133:172–177.
66. Grandjean P, Weihe P, White RF. Cognitive deficit in 7-year-old children with prenatal exposure to methylmercury. Neurotoxicol Teratol 1997; 19:417–428.
67. Davidson PW, Myers GJ, Cox C. Effects of prenatal and postnatal methylmercury exposure from fish consumption on neurodevelopment: outcomes at 66 months of age in the Seychelles Child Development Study. JAMA 1998; 280:701–707.
68. Centers for Disease Control and Prevention, American Academy of Family Physicians, American Academy of Pediatrics, Advisory Committee on Immunization Practices, Public Health Service. Summary of the joint statement on thimerosal in vaccines. MMWR Morb Mortal Wkly Rep 2000; 49:622–631.
69. US Public Health Service, Committee to Coordinate Environmental Health and Related Programs, Subcommittee on Risk Management. Dental Amalgam: A Scientific Review and Recommended Public Health Service Strategy for Research, Education, and Regulation. Washington, DC, US Public Health Service, 1993.
70. Cohen Hubal EA, Sheldon LS, Burke JM, McCurdy TR, Berry MR, Rigas ML, et al. Children's exposure assessment: a review of factors influencing children's exposure, and the data available to characterize and assess that exposure. Environmental Health Perspectives 2000; 108:475–486.
71. Needleman HL, Schell A, Bellinger D, Leviton A, Alred EN. The long-term effects of exposure to low doses of lead in childhood. N Engl J Med 1990; 322: 83–88.
72. Bressler JP, Goldstein GW. Mechanisms of lead neurotoxicity. Biochem Pharmacol 1991; 41:479–484.
73. Alkondon M, Costa ACS, Radhakrishnan V, Aronstam RS, Albuquerque EX. Selective blockade of NMDA-activated channel currents may be implicated in learning deficits caused by lead. FEBS Lett 1990; 261:124–130.
74. Alfano DP, Petit TL. Neonatal lead exposure alters the dendritic development of hippocampal dentate granule cells. Exp Neurol 1982; 75:275–288.
75. Rogan WJ, Dietrich KN, Ware JH, Dockery DW, Salganik M, Radcliffe J, et al. The effect of chelation therapy with succimer on neuropsychological development in children exposed to lead. N Engl J Med 2001; 344:1421–1426.

76. Liu X, Dietrich KN, Radcliffe J, Ragan NB, Rhoads GG, et al. Do children with falling blood lead levels have improved cognition? Pediatrics 2002; 110:787–791.
77. Dietrich KN, Ware JH, Salganik M, Radcliffe J, Rogan W, Rhoads G, et al. Effect of chelation therapy on the neuropsychological and behavioral development of lead-exposed children after school entry. Pediatrics 2004; 114:19–26.
78. Kukull WA, Larson EB, Bowen JD, McCormick WC, Teri L, Pfanschmidt ML, et al. Solvent exposure as a risk factor for Alzheimer's disease: a case-control study. Am J Epidemiol 1995; 141:1059–1071.
79. Arieff AI, Cooper JD, Armstrong D, Lazarowitz VC. Dementia, renal failure, and brain aluminum. Ann Intern Med 1979; 90:741–747.
80. Alfrey AC. Dialysis encephalopathy. Clin Nephrol 1985; 24(suppl 1):S15–S19.
81. Munoz DG. Is exposure to aluminum a risk factor for the development of Alzheimer disease? No. Arch Neurol 1998; 55:737–739.
82. Bjertness E, Candy JM, Torvik A, Ince P, McArthur F, Taylor GA, et al. Content of brain aluminum is not elevated in Alzheimer disease. Alzheimer Dis Assoc Disord 1996; 10:171–174.
83. McLachlan DR, Bergeron C, Smith JE, Boomer D, Rifat SL. Risk for neuropathologically confirmed Alzheimer's disease and residual aluminum in municipal drinking water employing weighted residential histories. Neurology 1996; 46:401–405.
84. Salib E, Hillier V. A case-control study of Alzheimer's disease and aluminium occupation. Br J Psychiatry 1996; 168:244–249.
85. Martyn CN, Barker DJ, Osmond C, Harris EC, Edwardson JA, Lacey RF. Geographical relation between Alzheimer's disease and aluminum in drinking water. Lancet 1989; 1(8629):59–62.
86. Kaplan MM. Clinical perspectives in the diagnosis of thyroid disease. Clin Chem 1999; 45(8 Pt 2):1377–1383.
87. Peery WH, Meek JC. Interpretation of thyroid function tests: an update. Compr Ther 1998; 24(11–12):567–573.
88. Loosen PT. Effects of thyroid hormones on central nervous system in aging. Psychoneuroendocrinology 1992; 17(4):355–374.
89. Bernal J, Guadano-Ferraz A, Morte B. Perspectives in the study of thyroid hormone action on brain development and function. Thyroid 2003; 13:1005–1012.
90. Delange F. The role of iodine in brain development. Proc Nutr Soc 2000; 59(1): 75–79.
91. Calaciura F, Mendorla G, Distefano M, Castorina S, Fazio T, Motta RM, et al. Childhood IQ measurements in infants with transient congenital hypothyroidism. Clin Endocrinol (Oxf) 1995; 43:473–477.
92. Rovet JF. Congenital hypothyroidism: long-term outcome. Thyroid 1999; 9(7): 741–748.
93. Sankar R, Pulger T, Rai B, Gomathi S, Gyatso TR, Pandav CS. Epidemiology of endemic cretinism in Sikkim, India. Indian J Pediatr 1998; 65(2):303–309.
94. Bleichrodt N, Born MP. A metaanalysis of research on iodine and its relationship to cognitive development. In: Stanbury JB e, ed. The Damaged Brain of Iodine Deficiency. New York: Cognizant Communication, 1994:195–200.
95. Canton A, de Fabregas O, Tintore M, Mesa J, Codina A, Simo R. Encephalopathy associated to autoimmune thyroid disease: a more appropriate term for an underestimated condition? J Neurol Sci 2000; 176:65–69.

96. Chong JY, Rowland LP, Utiger RD. Hashimoto encephalopathy: syndrome or myth? Arch Neurol 2003; 60(2):164–171.

97. Shaw PJ, Walls TJ, Newman PK, Cleland PG, Cartlidge NE. Hashimoto's encephalopathy: a steroid-responsive disorder associated with high anti-thyroid antibody titers—report of 5 cases. Neurology 1991; 41(2 Pt 1):228–233.

98. Mahmud FH, Lteif AN, Renaud DL, Reed AM, Brands CK. Steroid-responsive encephalopathy associated with Hashimoto's thyroiditis in an adolescent with chronic hallucinations and depression: case report and review. Pediatrics 2003; 112: 686–690.

99. Sellal F, Berton C, Andriantseheno M, Clerc C. Hashimoto's encephalopathy: exacerbations associated with menstrual cycle. Neurology 2002; 59(10):1633–1635.

100. Vasconcellos E, Pina-Garza JE, Fakhoury T, Fenichel GM. Pediatric manifestations of Hashimoto's encephalopathy. Pediatr Neurol 1999; 20(5):394–398.

101. McCabe DJ, Burke T, Connolly S, Hutchinson M. Amnesic syndrome with bilateral mesial temporal lobe involvement in Hashimoto's encephalopathy. Neurology 2000; 54:737–739.

102. Bohnen NILJ, Parnell KJ, Harper CM. Reversible MRI findings in a patient with Hashimoto's encephalopathy. Neurology 1997; 49:246–247.

103. v Maydell B, Kopp M, v Komorowski G, Joe A, Juengling FD, Korinthenberg R. Hashimoto encephalopathy – is it underdiagnosed in pediatric patients? Neuropediatrics 2002; 33(2):86–89.

104. Sawka AM, Fatourechi V, Boeve BF, Mokri B. Rarity of encephalopathy associated with autoimmune thyroiditis: a case series from Mayo Clinic from 1950 to 1996. Thyroid 2002; 12:393–398.

105. Robuschi G, Safran M, Braverman LE, Gnudi A, Roti E. Hypothyroidism in the elderly. Endocr Rev 1987; 8(2):142–153.

106. Clarnette RM, Patterson CJ. Hypothyroidism: does treatment cure dementia? J Geriatr Psychiatry Neurol 1994; 7(1):23–27.

107. Haupt M, Kurz A. Reversibility of dementia in hypothyroidism. Z Gesamte Inn Med 1993; 48(12):609–613.

108. Ganguli M, Burmeister LA, Seaberg EC, Belle S, DeKosky ST. Association between dementia and elevated TSH: a community-based study. Biol Psychiatry 1996; 40:714–725.

109. Shetty KR, Duthie EH, Jr. Thyroid disease and associated illness in the elderly. Clin Geriatr Med 1995; 11(2):311–325.

110. Dugbartey AT. Neurocognitive aspects of hypothyroidism. Arch Intern Med 1998; 158(13):1413–1418.

111. Volpato S, Guralnik JM, Fried LP, Remaley AT, Cappola AR, Launer LJ. Serum thyroxine level and cognitive decline in euthyroid older women. Neurology 2002; 58(7):1055–1061.

112. Kasper JD, Shapiro S, Guralnik JM, Bandeen-Roche KJ, Fried LP. Designing a community study of moderately to severely disabled older women: the Women's Health and Aging Study. Ann Epidemiol 1999; 9(8):498–507.

113. Osterweil D, Syndulko K, Cohen SN, Pettler-Jennings PD, Hershman JM, Cummings JL, et al. Cognitive function in non-demented older adults with hypothyroidism. J Am Geriatr Soc 1992; 40(4):325–335.

114. Jordan RM. Myxedema coma. Pathophysiology, therapy, and factors affecting prognosis. Med Clin North Am 1995; 79(1):185–194.

115. Swanson JW, Kelly JJ, Jr., McConahey WM. Neurologic aspects of thyroid dysfunction. Mayo Clin Proc 1981; 56(8):504–512.

116. Roberts CG, Ladenson PW. Hypothyroidism. Lancet 2004; 363(9411):793–803.

117. Kinuya S, Michigishi T, Tonami N, Aburano T, Tsuji S, Hashimoto T. Reversible cerebral hypoperfusion observed with Tc-99m HMPAO SPECT in reversible dementia caused by hypothyroidism. Clin Nucl Med 1999; 24(9): 666–668.

118. Waisbren SE, Chang P, Levy HL, Shifrin H, Allred E, Azen C, et al. Neonatal neurological assessment of offspring in maternal phenylketonuria. J Inherit Metab Dis 1998; 21(1):39–48.

119. Koch R, Burton B, Hoganson G, Peterson R, Rhead W, Rouse B, et al. Phenylketonuria in adulthood: a collaborative study. J Inherit Metab Dis 2002; 25(5): 333–346.

120. Oberdoerster J, Guizzetti M, Costa LG. Effect of phenylalanine and its metabolites on the proliferation and viability of neuronal and astroglial cells: possible relevance in maternal phenylketonuria. J Pharmacol Exp Ther 2000; 295(1): 295–301.

121. Powers HJ, Moat SJ. Developments in the measurement of plasma total homocysteine. Curr Opin Clin Nutr Metab Care 2000; 3:391–397.

122. Jacques PF, Bostom AG, Wilson PW, Rich S, Rosenberg IH, Selhub J. Determinants of plasma total homocysteine concentration in the Framingham Offspring cohort. Am J Clin Nutr 2001; 73:613–621.

123. Lievers KJ, Kluijtmans LA, Blom HJ. Genetics of hyperhomocysteinaemia in cardiovascular disease. Ann Clin Biochem 2003; 40:46–59.

124. Selhub J, Jacques P, Wilson P, Rush D, Rosenberg I. Vitamin status and intake as primary determinants of homocysteinemia in an elderly population. JAMA 1993; 270:2693–2698.

125. Johnson MA, Hawthorne NA, Brackett WR, Fischer JG, Gunter EW, Allen RH. Hyperhomocysteinemia and vitamin B-12 deficiency in elderly using Title IIIc nutrition services. Am J Clin Nutr 2003; 77:211–220.

126. Desouza C, Keebler M, McNamara DB, Fonseca V. Drugs affecting homocysteine metabolism: impact on cardiovascular risk. Drugs 2002; 62:605–616.

127. Francis ME, Eggers PW, Hostetter TH, Briggs JP. Association between serum homocysteine and markers of impaired kidney function in adults in the United States. Kidney Int 2004; 66:303–312.

128. Harmon DL, Woodside JV, Yarnell JW, McMaster D, Young IS, McCrum EE. The common 'thermolabile' variant of methylene tetrahydrofolate reductase is a major determinant of mild hyperhomocysteinaemia. QJM 1996; 89:571–577.

129. Savage DG, Lindenbaum J, Stabler SP, Allen RH. Sensitivity of serum methylmalonic acid and total homocysteine determinations for diagnosing cobalamin and folate deficiencies. Am J Med 1994; 96:239–246.

130. Hustad S, Ueland PM, Vollset SE, Zhang Y, Bjorke-Monsen AL, Schneede J. Riboflavin as a determinant of plasma total homocysteine: effect modification by the methylenetetrahydrofolate reductase C677T polymorphism. Clin Chem 2000; 46:1065–1071.

131. Rosenblatt DS, Whitehead VM. Cobalamin and folate deficiency: acquired and hereditary disorders in children. Semin Hematol 1999; 36:19–34.

132. Klerk M, Verhoef P, Clarke R, Blom HJ, Kok FJ, Schouten EG. MTHFR 677CT polymorphism and risk of coronary heart disease: a meta-analysis. JAMA 2002; 288:2023–2031.

133. Ueland PM, Hustad S, Schneede J, Refsum H, Vollset SE. Biological and clinical implications of the MTHFR C677T polymorphism. Trends Pharmacol Sci 2001; 22:195–201.

134. Selhub J, Jacques PF, Bostom AG, Wilson PW, Rosenberg IH. Relationship between plasma homocysteine and vitamin status in the Framingham study population. Impact of folic acid fortification. Public Health Rev 2000; 28:117–145.

135. Clarke R, Smith AD, Jobst KA, Refsum H, Sutton L, Ueland PM. Folate, vitamin B12, and serum total homocysteine levels in confirmed Alzheimer disease. Arch Neurol 1998; 55(11):1449–1455.

136. Seshadri S, Beiser A, Selhub J, Jacques PF, Rosenberg IH, D'Agostino RB, et al. Plasma homocysteine as a risk factor for dementia and Alzheimer's disease. N Engl J Med 2002; 346:476–483.

137. Dufouil C, Alperovitch A, Ducros V, Tzourio C. Homocysteine, white matter hyperintensities, and cognition in healthy elderly people. Ann Neurol 2003; 53: 214–221.

138. Joosten E, Lesaffre E, Riezler R, Ghekiere V, Dereymaeker L, Pelemans W, et al. Is metabolic evidence for vitamin B-12 and folate deficiency more frequent in elderly patients with Alzheimer's disease? J Gerontol A Biol Sci Med Sci 1997; 52(2): M76–M79.

139. Lehmann M, Gottfries CG, Regland B. Identification of cognitive impairment in the elderly: homocysteine is an early marker. Dement Geriatr Cogn Disord 1999; 10(1):12–20.

140. McCaddon A, Davies G, Hudson P, Tandy S, Cattell H. Total serum homocysteine in senile dementia of Alzheimer type. Int J Geriatr Psychiatry 1998; 13(4):235–239.

141. Wright CB, Lee HS, Paik MC, Stabler SP, Allen RH, Sacco RL. Total homocysteine and cognition in a tri-ethnic cohort: the Northern Manhattan Study. Neurology 2004; 63:254–260.

142. Green R, Kinsella LJ. Current concepts in the diagnosis of cobalamin deficiency. Neurology 1995; 45:1435–1440.

143. Healton EB, Savage DG, Brust JC, Garrett TJ, Lindenbaum J. Neurologic aspects of cobalamin deficiency. Medicine (Baltimore) 1991; 70(4):229–245.

144. Ovsiew F. Seeking reversibility and treatability in dementia. Sem Clin Neuropsych 2003; 8:3–11.

145. Lindenbaum J, Healton EB, Savage DG, Brust JC, Garrett TJ, Podell ER, et al. Neuropsychiatric disorders caused by cobalamin deficiency in the absence of anemia or macrocytosis. N Engl J Med 1988; 318(26):1720–1728.

146. Lindenbaum J, Healton EB, Savage DG, Brust JC, Garrett TJ, Podell ER, et al. Neuropsychiatric disorders caused by cobalamin deficiency in the absence of anemia or macrocytosis. 1988. Nutrition 1995; 11(2):181; discussion 180, 182.

147. Carmel R. Cobalamin deficiency. In: Carmel R, Jacobsen D, eds. Homocysteine in Health and Disease. Cambridge, UK: Cambridge University Press, 2001:289–305.

148. Klee GG. Cobalamin and folate evaluation; measurement of methylmalonic acid and homocysteine vs vitamin B12 and folate. Clin Chem 2000; 46:1277–1283.

149. Herbert V. Staging vitamin B-12 (cobalamin) status in vegetarians. Am J Clin Nutr 1994; 59(suppl 5):1213S–1222S.

150. Snow CF. Laboratory diagnosis of vitamin B12 and folate deficiency: a guide for the primary care physician. Arch Intern Med 1999; 159(12):1289–1298.

151. Hvas AM, Ellegaard J, Nexo E. Increased plasma methylmalonic acid level does not predict clinical manifestations of vitamin B12 deficiency. Arch Intern Med 2001; 161(12):1534–1541.

152. Hvas AM, Juul S, Nexo E, Ellegaard J. Vitamin B-12 treatment has limited effect on health-related quality of life among individuals with elevated plasma methylmalonic acid: a randomized placebo-controlled study. J Intern Med 2003; 253(2):146–152.

153. Nilsson K, Gustafson L, Hultberg B. Optimal use of markers for cobalamin and folate status in a psychogeriatric population. Int J Geriatr Psychiatry 2002; 17(10):919–925.

154. Kuzminski AM, Del Giacco EJ, Allen RH, Stabler SP, Lindenbaum J. Effective treatment of cobalamin deficiency with oral cobalamin. Blood 1998; 92(4): 1191–1198.

155. McCaddon A, Regland B, Hudson P, Davies G. Functional vitamin B12 deficiency and Alzheimer disease. Neurology 2002; 58:1395–1399.

156. Graham SM, Arvela OM, Wise GA. Long-term neurologic consequences of nutritional vitamin B12 deficiency in infants. J Pediatr 1992; 121(5 Pt 1):710–714.

157. von Schenck U, Bender-Gotze C, Koletzko B. Persistence of neurological damage induced by dietary vitamin B-12 deficiency in infancy. Arch Dis Child 1997; 77(2):137–139.

158. Renault F, Verstichel P, Ploussard JP, Costil J. Neuropathy in two cobalamin-deficient breast-fed infants of vegetarian mothers. Muscle Nerve 1999; 22(2): 252–254.

159. Emery ES, Homans AC, Colletti RB. Vitamin B12 deficiency: a cause of abnormal movements in infants. Pediatrics 1997; 99(2):255–256.

160. Cooper BA, Rosenblatt DS. Inherited defects of vitamin B12 metabolism. Annu Rev Nutr 1987; 7:291–320.

161. Carmel R, Watkins D, Goodman SI, Rosenblatt DS. Hereditary defect of cobalamin metabolism (cblG mutation) presenting as a neurologic disorder in adulthood. N Engl J Med 1988; 318(26):1738–1741.

162. Allen RH, Stabler SP, Savage DG, Lindenbaum J. Metabolic abnormalities in cobalamin (vitamin B12) and folate deficiency. Faseb J 1993; 7(14):1344–1353.

163. Bjorke Monsen AL, Ueland PM. Homocysteine and methylmalonic acid in diagnosis and risk assessment from infancy to adolescence. Am J Clin Nutr 2003; 78(1):7–21.

164. Louwman MW, van Dusseldorp M, van de Vijver FJ, Thomas CM, Schneede J, Ueland PM, et al. Signs of impaired cognitive function in adolescents with marginal cobalamin status. Am J Clin Nutr 2000; 72(3):762–769.

165. Goebels N, Soyka M. Dementia associated with vitamin B(12) deficiency: presentation of two cases and review of the literature. J Neuropsychiatry Clin Neurosci 2000; 12(3):389–394.

166. Frenkel EP, Yardley DA. Clinical and laboratory features and sequelae of deficiency of folic acid (folate) and vitamin B12 (cobalamin) in pregnancy and gynecology. Hematol Oncol Clin North Am 2000; 14(5):1079–100, viii.

167. Selhub J. Folate, vitamin B12 and vitamin B6 and one carbon metabolism. J Nutr Health Aging 2002; 6(1):39–42.

168. Wang HX, Wahlin A, Basun H, Fastbom J, Winblad B, Fratiglioni L. Vitamin B12 and folate in relation to the development of Alzheimer's disease. Neurology 2001; 56:1188–1194.
169. MRC Vitamin Study Group. Prevention of neural tube defects: results of the medical research council vitamin study. Lancet 1991; 338:131–137.
170. Czeizel AE, Dudas I. Prevention of first occurrence of neural tube defects by periconceptual vitamin supplementation. N Engl J Med 1992; 327:131–137.
171. van der Put NMJ, Steegers-Theunissen RPM, Frosst P, Trijbels FJM, Eskes TKAB, van den Heuvel LP, et al. Mutated methylene-tetrahydrofolate reductase as a risk factor for spina bifida. Lancet 1995; 346:1070–1071.
172. Kang SS, Wong PW, Bock HG, Horwitz A, Grix A. Intermediate hyperhomocysteinemia resulting from compound heterozygosity of methylenetetrahydrofolate reductase mutations. Am J Hum Genet 1991; 48(3):546–551.
173. Graf WD, Oleinik OE. The study of neural tube defects after the Human Genome Project and folic acid fortification of foods. Eur J Pediatr Surg 2000; 10(suppl I):9–12.
174. Benton D, Roberts G. Effect of vitamin and mineral supplementation on intelligence of a sample of school children. Lancet 1988; 2:140–143.
175. Malouf M, Grimley EJ, Areosa SA. Folic acid with or without vitamin B12 for cognition and dementia. Cochrane Database Syst Rev 2003; 4:CD004514.
176. Johnson KA, Bernard MA, Funderburg K. Vitamin nutrition in older adults. Clin Geriatr Med 2002; 18:773–799.
177. Rodriguez-Martin JL, Qizilbash N, Lopez-Arrieta JM. Thiamine for Alzheimer's disease. Cochrane Database Syst Rev 2001(2):CD001498.
178. Bates CJ, Pentieva KD, Prentice A, Mansoor MA, Finch S. Plasma pyridoxal phosphate and pyridoxic acid and their relationship to plasma homocysteine in a representative sample of British men and women aged 65 yearsand over. Br J Nutr 1999; 81:191–201.
179. Malouf R, Grimley EJ. The effect of vitamin B6 on cognition. Cochrane Database Syst Rev 2003; 4:CD004393.
180. Hegyi J, Schwartz RA, Hegyi V. Pellagra: dermatitis, dementia, and diarrhea. Int J Dermatol 2004; 43:1–5.
181. Simons K, Ikonen E. Functional rafts in cell membranes. Nature 1997; 387:569–572.
182. Raber J, Huang Y, Ashford JW. ApoE genotype accounts for the vast majority of AD risk and AD pathology. Neurobiol Aging 2004; 25:641–650.
183. Slooter AJ, Tang MX, van Duijn CM, Stern Y, Ott A, Bell K, et al. Apolipoprotein E cpsilon4 and the risk of dementia with stroke. A population-based investigation. JAMA 1997; 277:818–821.
184. Nicoll JA, Roberts GW, Graham DI. Amyloid beta-protein, APOE genotype and head injury. Ann NY Acad Sci 1996; 777:271–275.
185. Alberts MJ, Graffagnino C, McClenny C, DeLong D, Strittmatter W, Saunders AM, et al. ApoE genotype and survival from intracerebral haemorrhage. Lancet 1995; 346:575.
186. Cutler RG, Haughey NJ, Tammara A, McArthur JC, Nath A, Reid R, et al. Dysregulation of sphingolipid and sterol metabolism by ApoE4 in HIV dementia. Neurology 2004; 63:626–630.
187. Kitagawa K, Matsumoto M, Kuwabara K, Takasawa K, Tanaka S, Sasaki T, et al. Protective effect of apolipoprotein E against ischemic neuronal injury is mediated through antioxidant action. J Neurosci Res 2002; 68:226–232.

188. Dietschy JM, Turley SD. Thematic review series: Brain Lipids. Cholesterol metabolism in the central nervous system during early development and in the mature animal. J Lipid Res 2004; 45:1375–1397.

189. Wong WW, Hachey DL, Insull W, Opekun AR, Klein PD. Effect of dietary cholesterol on cholesterol synthesis in breast fed and formula-fed infants. J Lipid Res 1993; 34:1403–1411.

190. Cruz MLA, Wong WW, Mimouni F, Hachey DL, Setchell KDR, Klein PD, et al. Effects of infant nutrition on cholesterol synthesis rates. Pediatr Res 1994; 35:135–140.

191. Desnick RJ. Enzyme replacement and enhancement therapies for lysosomal diseases. J Inherit Metab Dis 2004; 27:385–410.

192. Peters C, Charnas LR, Tan Y, Ziegler RS, Shapiro EG, DeFor T, et al. Cerebral X-linked adrenoleukodystrophy: the international hematopoietic cell transplantation experience from 1982 to 1999. Blood 2004; 104:881–888.

193. Pentchev PG. Niemann-Pick C research from mouse to gene. Biochim Biophys Acta 2004; 1685(1–3):3–7.

194. Vanier MT, Millat G. Structure and function of the NPC2 protein. Biochim Biophys Acta 2004; 1685(1–3):14–21.

195. Loftus SK, Morris JA, Carstea ED, Gu JZ, Cummings C, Brown A, et al. Murine model of Niemann-Pick C disease: mutation in a cholesterol homeostasis gene. Science 1997; 277:232–235.

196. Park WD, O'Brien JF, Lundquist PA, Kraft DL, Vockley CW, Karnes PS, et al. Identification of 58 novel mutations in Niemann-Pick disease type C: correlation with biochemical phenotype and importance of PTC1-like domains in NPC1. Hum Mutat 2003; 22:313–325.

197. Haughey NJ, Cutler RG, Tamara A, McArthur JC, Vargas DL, Pardo CA, et al. Perturbation of sphingolipid metabolism and ceramide production in HIV-dementia. Ann Neurol 2004; 55:257–267.

198. Wolozin B, Kellman W, Ruosseau P, Celesia GG, Siegel G. Decreased prevalence of Alzheimer disease associated with 3-hydroxy-3-methyglutaryl coenzyme A reductase inhibitors. Arch Neurol 2000; 57(10):1439–1443.

199. Jick H, Zornberg GL, Jick SS, Seshadri S, Drachman DA. Statins and the risk of dementia. Lancet 2000; 356(9242):1627–1631.

200. Simons M, Keller P, Dichgans J, Schulz JB. Cholesterol and Alzheimer's disease: is there a link? Neurology 2001; 57:1089–1093.

201. von Bahr S, Movin T, Papadogiannakis N, Pikuleva I, Ronnow P, Diczfalusy U, et al. Mechanism of accumulation of cholesterol and cholestanol in tendons and the role of sterol 27-hydroxylase (CYP27A1). Arterioscler Thromb Vasc Biol 2002; 22:1129–1135.

202. Berginer VM, Berginer J, Korczyn AD, Tadmor R. Magnetic resonance imaging in cerebrotendinous xanthomatosis: a prospective clinical and neuroradiological study. J Neurol Sci 1994; 122:102–108.

203. Moghadasian MH, Salen G, Frohlich JJ, Scudamore CH. Cerebrotendinous xanthomatosis: a rare disease with diverse manifestations. Arch Neurol 2002; 59:527–529.

204. Beard J. Iron deficiency alters brain development and functioning. J Nutr 2003; 133(5 suppl 1):1468S–1472S.

205. Ortiz E, Pasquini JM, Thompson K, Felt B, Butkus G, Beard J, et al. Effect of manipulation of iron storage, transport, or availability on myelin composition and brain iron content in three different animal models. J Neurosci Res 2004; 77(5): 681–689.

206. Aoki S, Okada Y, Nishimura K, Barkovich AJ, Kjos BO, Brasch RC, et al. Normal deposition of brain iron in childhood and adolescence: MR imaging at 1.5 T. Radiology 1989; 172:381–385.

207. Scrimshaw NS. Iron deficiency. Sci Am 1991; 265(4):46–52.

208. Walter T. Effect of iron-deficiency anaemia on cognitive skills in infancy and childhood. Baillieres Clin Haematol 1994; 7(4):815–827.

209. Pollitt E, Hathirat P, Kotchabhakdi NJ, Missell L, Valyasevi A. Iron deficiency and educational achievement in Thailand. Am J Clin Nutr 1989; 50(3 suppl):687–696; discussion 696–697.

210. Sandstead HH. Causes of iron and zinc deficiencies and their effects on brain. J Nutr 2000; 130(2S suppl):347S–349S.

211. Lozoff B, Wolfe AW, Urrutia JJ, Viteri FE. Abnormal behavior and low developmental test scores in iron-deficient anemic infants. J Dev Behav Pediatr 1985; 6:69–75.

212. Lozoff B, Jimenez E, Hagen J, Mollen E, Wolf AW. Poorer behavioral and developmental outcome more than 10 years after treatment for iron deficiency in infancy. Pediatrics 2000; 105:E51.

213. Lozoff B, De Andraca I, Castillo M, Smith JB, Walter T, Pino P. Behavioral and developmental effects of preventing iron-deficiency anemia in healthy full-term infants. Pediatrics 2003; 112(4):846–854.

214. Bruner AB, Joffe A, Duggan AK, Casella JF, Brandt J. Randomised study of cognitive effects of iron supplementation in nonanaemic iron-deficient adolescent girls. Lancet 1996; 348:992–996.

215. Ahluwalia N, Sun J, Krause D, Mastro A, Handte G. Immune function is impaired in iron-deficient, homebound, older women. Am J Clin Nutr 2004; 79(3):516–521.

216. Miyajima H. Aceruloplasminemia, an iron metabolic disorder. Neuropathology 2003; 23:345–350.

217. Miyajima H, Fujimoto M, Kohno S, Kaneko E, Gitlin JD. CSF abnormalities in patients with aceruloplasminemia. Neurology 1998; 51:1188–1190.

218. Graf WD, Noetzel MJ. Radical reactions from missing ceruloplasmin. The importance of a ferroxidase as an endogenous antioxidant. Neurology 1999; 53: 446–447.

219. Kaplan RJ, Greenwood CE, Winocur G, Wolever TM. Cognitive performance is associated with glucose regulation in healthy elderly persons and can be enhanced with glucose and dietary carbohydrates. Am J Clin Nutr 2000; 72(3):825–836.

220. Greenwood CE, Winocur G. Glucose treatment reduces memory deficits in young adult rats fed high-fat diets. Neurobiol Learn Mem 2001; 75(2):179–189.

221. Sheu KF, Cooper AJ, Koike K, Koike M, Lindsay JG, Blass JP. Abnormality of the alpha-ketoglutarate dehydrogenase complex in fibroblasts from familial Alzheimer's disease. Ann Neurol 1994; 35:312–318.

222. Small GW. Neuroimaging and genetic assessment for early diagnosis of Alzheimer's disease. J Clin Psychiatry 1996; 57(suppl 14):9–13.

223. Silverman DH, Truong CT, Kim SK, Chang CY, Chen W, Kowell AP, et al. Prognostic value of regional cerebral metabolism in patients undergoing dementia

evaluation: comparison to a quantifying parameter of subsequent cognitive performance and to prognostic assessment without PET. Mol Genet Metab 2003; 80: 350–355.

224. Kalaria RN, Gravina SA, Schmidley J, Perry G, Harik SI. The glucose transporter of the human brain and bloodbrain barrier. Ann Neurol 1988; 24:757–764.

225. Martins R. Amyloid Aß precursor protein metabolism as a modulator of islet ß-cell function. J Alzheimer's Dis 2001; 3:397–399.

226. Mark RJ, Pang Z, Geddes JW, Uchida K, Mattson MP. Amyloid beta-peptide impairs glucose transport in hippocampal and cortical neurons: involvement of membrane lipid peroxidation. J Neurosci 1997; 17:1046–1054.

227. Uemura E, Greenlee HW. Amyloid beta-peptide inhibits neuronal glucose uptake by preventing exocytosis. Exp Neurol 2001; 170:270–276.

228. Jope RS, Johnson GV. The glamour and gloom of glycogen synthase kinase-3. Trends Biochem Sci 2004; 29:95–102.

229. Bhat RV, Budd Haeberlein SL, Avila J. Glycogen synthase kinase 3: a drug target for CNS therapies. J Neurochem 2004; 89:1313–1317.

230. American Diabetes Association. Standards of medical care for patients with diabetes mellitus. Diabetes Care 2002; 25:213–229.

231. Report of the Expert Committee on the Diagnosis and Classification of Diabetes Mellitus. Diabetes Care 1997; 20:1183.

232. Miles WR, Root HF. Psychologic tests applied in diabetic patients. Arch Intern Med 1922; 30:767–777.

233. Brands AMA, Kessels RPC, de Haan EHF, Kappelle LJ, Biessels GJ. Cerebral dysfunction in type 1 diabetes: effects of insulin, vascular risk factors and blood-glucose levels. Eur J Pharm 2004; 490:159–168.

234. Dejgaard A, Gade A, Larsson H, Balle V, Parving A, Parving HH. Evidence for diabetic encephalopathy. Diabet Med 1991; 8:162–167.

235. Harati Y. Diabetes and the nervous system. Endocrinol Metab Clin North Am 1996; 25:325–359.

236. Biessels GJ, van der Heide LP, Kamal A, Bleys RL, Gispen WH. Ageing and diabetes: implications for brain function. Eur J Pharmacol 2002; 441:1–14.

237. Ott A, Stolk RP, van Harskamp F, Pols HA, Hofman A, Breteler MM. Diabetes mellitus and the risk of dementia: The Rotterdam Study. Neurology 1999; 53:1937–1942.

238. Schnaider Beeri M, Goldbourt U, Silverman JM, Noy S, Schmeidler J, Ravona-Springer R, et al. Diabetes mellitus in midlife and the risk of dementia three decades later. Neurology 2004; 63:1902–1907.

239. Yaffe K, Blackwell T, Kanaya AM, Davidowitz N, Barrett-Connor E, Krueger K. Diabetes, impaired fasting glucose, and development of cognitive impairment in older women. Neurology 2004; 63:658–663.

240. Hassing LB, Grant MD, Hofer SM, Pedersen NL, Nilsson SE, Berg S, et al. Type 2 diabetes mellitus contributes to cognitive decline in old age: a longitudinal population-based study. J Int Neuropsychol Soc 2004; 10:599–607.

241. Perez A, Morelli L, Cresto JC, Castano EM. Degradation of soluble amyloid beta-peptides 1–40, 1–42, and the Dutch variant 1–40Q by insulin degrading enzyme from Alzheimer disease and control brains. Neurochem Res 2000; 25: 247–255.

242. Yan SD, Chen X, Fu J, Chen MHZ, Roher A, et al. RAGE and amyloid-beta peptide neurotoxicity in Alzheimer's disease. Nature 1996; 382:685–691.

243. Deane R, Du Yan S, Submamaryan RK, LaRue B, Jovanovic S, Hogg E, et al. RAGE mediates amyloid-beta peptide transport across the blood-brain barrier and accumulation in brain. Nat Med 2003; 9:907–913.

244. Honein MA, Moore CA, Erickson JD. Can We Ensure the Safe Use of Known Human Teratogens?: Introduction of Generic Isotretinoin in the US as an Example. Drug Saf 2004; 27:1069–1080.

245. Koren G, Pastuszak A, Ito S. Drugs in pregnancy. N Engl J Med 1998; 338: 1128–1137.

246. Kann LWC, Harris WA, et al. Youth risk behavior surveillance-United States. MMWR CDC Surveillance Summaries 1996; 45(1).

247. Isbell H, Gorodetzky C, Jasinski Dea. Effects of (-)delta 9-trans-tetrahydrocannabinol in man. Psychopharmacologia 1967; 11:184.

248. Bromberg W. Marijuana intoxication. Am J Psychiatry 1934; 91:303.

249. Borg J, Gershon S. Dose effects of smoked marihuana on human cognitive and motor functions. Psychopharmacologia 1975; 42:211.

250. Belmore S, Miller L. Levels of processing acute effects of marijuana on memory. Pharmacol Biochem Behav 1980; 13:199.

251. Roth W, Rosenbloom M, Darley Cea. Marijuana effects on TAT form and content. Psychopharmacologia 195; 43:261.

252. Sharma S, Moskowitz H. Effects of two levels of attention demand on vigilance performance under marijuana. Percept Mot Skills 1974; 38:967.

253. Heishman S, Huestis M, Henningfield J, Cone E. Acute and residual effects of marijuana: profiles of plasma THC levels, physiological, subjective and performance measures. Pharmacol Biochem Behav 1990; 37:561.

254. Clark L, Hughes R, Nakashima E. Behavioral effects of marihuana: experimental studies. Arch Gen Psychiatry 1970; 23:193.

255. Klonhoff H, Low M, Marcus A. Neuropsychological effects of marijuana. Can Med Assoc J 1973; 108:150.

256. Manno J, Kiplinger G, Haine Sea. Comparative effects of smoking marijuana or placebo on human motor and mental performance. Clin Pharmacol Ther 1970; 11:808.

257. Melges F, Tinklenberg J, Hollister Lea. Marijuana and the temporal span of awareness. Arch Gen Psychiatry 1971; 24:564.

258. Zeidenberg P, Clark W, Jaffe Jea. Effect of oral administration of delta-9-tetrahydrocannabinol on memory, speech, and perception of thermal stimulation: results with four normal human volunteer subjects: preliminary report. Compr Psychiatry 1973; 14:549.

259. Janowsky D, Meacham M, Blaine Jea. Marijuana effects on simulated flying ability. Am J Psychiatry 1976; 133:384.

260. Kiplinger G, Manno J, Rodda Bea. Dose-response analysis of the effects of tetrahydrocannabinol in man. Clin Pharmacol Ther 1971; 12:650.

261. Moskowitz H, Ziedman K, Sharma S. Visual search behavior while viewing driving scenes under the influence of alcohol and marihuana. Hum Factors 1976; 18:417.

262. Smiley A, Ziedman K, Moskowitz H. Pharmacokinetics of drug effects on driving performance: driving simulator tests of marihuana alone and in combination with

alcohol. Report to the National Institute on Drug Abuse. Los Angeles: Southern California Research Institute, 1981.

263. Brown A, Stickgold A. Self-diagnosed marijuana flashbacks. Clin Res 1974; 22:316A.
264. Keeler M, Reifler C, Lipzin M. Spontaneous recurrence of marijuana effect. Am J Psychiatry 1968; 125:384.
265. Stanton M, Mintz J, Franklin R. Drug flashbacks II. Some additional findings. Int J Addict 1976; 11:53.
266. Mendelson J, Mello N, Lex Bea. Marijuana withdrawal syndrome in a woman. Am J Psychiatry 1984; 141:1289.
267. Hollister L. Health aspects of cannabis. Pharmacol Rev 1986; 38:1.
268. Cohen S. Adverse effects of marijuana: selected issues. Ann NY Acad Sci 1981; 362:119.
269. Kolansky H, Moore W. Toxic effects of chronic marijuana use. JAMA 1972; 222:35.
270. Kolansky H, Moore W. Marijuana: can it hurt you? JAMA 1975; 232:923.
271. Smith D. The acute and chronic toxicity of marijuana. Psychoactive Drugs 1968; 2:27.
272. Soueif M. Differential association between chronic cannabis use and brain function deficits. In: Fink Me, ed. Chronic Cannabis Use. New York: Ann NY Acad Sci, 1976:282: 323.
273. Block RI, O'Leary DS, Hichwa RD, Augustinack JC, Ponto LL, Ghoneim MM, et al. Cerebellar hypoactivity in frequent marijuana users. Neuroreport 2000; 11:749–753.
274. O'Leary DS, Block RI, Koeppel JA, Flaum M, Schultz SK, Andreasen NC, et al. Effects of smoking marijuana on brain perfusion and cognition. Neuropsychopharmacology 2002; 26:802–816.
275. Soueif M. Chronic cannabis users: further analysis of objective test results. Bull Narc 1975; 27:1.
276. Mendelson J, Koehnle J, Greenberg Iea. The effects of marijuana use on human operant behavior; individual data. In: Pharmacology of Marijuana. New York: Raven Press, 1976:643–653.
277. Miles C, Congreve G, Gibbins Rea. An experimental study of the effects of daily cannabis smoking on behavior patterns. Acta Pharmacol Toxicol 1974; 34(suppl 1):1.
278. Pope H, Yurgelun-Todd D. The residual cognitive effects of heavy marijuana use in college students. JAMA 1996; 275:521.
279. Aiello LC, Wheeler P. The expensive-tissue hypothesis. The brain and the digestive system in human and primate evolution. Curr Anthropol 1995; 36:199–221.
280. Mann NJ. Paleolithic nutrition: what can we learn from the past? Asia Pac J Clin Nutr 2004; 13(suppl):S17,
281. Pascual JM, Wang D, Lecumberri B, Yang H, Mao X, Yang R, et al. GLUT1 deficiency and other glucose transporter diseases. Eur J Endocrinol 2004; 150: 627–633.
282. Gordon N, Newton RW. Glucose transporter type1 (GLUT-1) deficiency. Brain Dev 2003; 25:477–480.
283. Wolf NI, Smeitink JA. Mitochondrial disorders: a proposal for consensus diagnostic criteria in infants and children. Neurology 2002; 59:1402–1405.
284. Kish SJ. Brain energy metabolizing enzymes in Alzheimer's disease: alpha-ketoglutarate dehydrogenase complex and cytochrome oxidase. Ann NY Acad Sci 1997; 26:218–228.
285. Ames BN. Micronutrients prevent cancer and delay aging. Toxicol Lett 1998; 102–103:5–18.

286. Galli RL, Shukitt-Hale B, Youdim KA, Joseph JA. Fruit polyphenolics and brain aging: nutritional interventions targeting age-related neuronal and behavioral deficits. Ann NY Acad Sci 2002; 959:128–132.

287. Pettegrew JW, Klunk WE, Panchalingam K, Kanfer JN, McClure RJ. Clinical and neurochemical effects of acetyl-L-carnitine in Alzheimer's disease. Neurobiol Aging 1995; 16:1–4.

288. Sano M, Bell K, Cote L, Dooneief G, Lawton A, Legler L, et al. Double-blind parallel design pilot study of acetyl levocarnitine in patients with Alzheimer's disease. Arch Neurol 1992; 49:1137–1141.

289. Spagnoli A, Lucca U, Menasce G, Bandera L, Cizza G, Foiloni G, et al. Long-term acetyl-L-carnitine treatment in Alzheimer's disease. Neurology 1991; 41:1726–1732.

290. Brooks JO, Yesavage JA, Carta A, Bravi D. Acetyl L-carnitine slows decline in younger patients with Alzheimer's disease: a reanalysis of a double-blind, placebo-controlled study using the trilinear approach. Int Psychogeriatr 1998; 10: 193–203.

291. Thal L, Carta A, Clarke W, Ferris S, Friedland R, Petersen R, et al. A 1-year multicenter placebo-controlled study of acetyl-L-carnitine in patients with Alzheimer's disease. Neurology 1996; 47:705–711.

292. Thal LJ, Calvani M, Amato A, Carta A. A 1-year controlled trial of acetyl-l-carnitine in early-onset AD. Neurology 2000; 55:805–810.

293. Institute of Medicine. Dietary Reference Intakes for Vitamin A, Vitamin K, Arsenic, Boron, Chromium, Copper, Iodine, Manganese, Molybdenum, Nickel, Silicon, Vanadium, and Zinc. Washington, DC: National Academy Press, 2001.

294. Grantham-McGregor SM, Ani CC. The role of micronutrients in psychomotor and cognitive development. Br Med Bull 1999; 55(3):511–527.

295. Roy S, Arant BS. Hypokalemic metabolic alkalosis in normotensive infants with elevated plasma renin activity and hyperaldosteronism: role of dietary chloride deficiency. Pediatrics 1981; 67:423–429.

296. Chutorian AM, LaScala CP, Ores CN, Nass R. Cerebral dysfunction following infantile dietary chloride deficiency. Pediatr Neurol 1985; 1(6):335–341.

297. Kaleita T, Kinsbourne M, Menkes JH. Neurobehavioral syndrome and growth recovery following failure to thrive on chloride deficient Neo-Mull-Soy formula. Dev Med Child Neurol 1991; 33:626–635.

298. Frederickson CJ. Neurobiology of zinc and zinc-containing neurons. Int Rev Neurobiol 1989; 31:145–238.

299. Weiss JH, Sensi SL, Koh JY. Zn(2+): a novel ionic mediator of neural injury in brain disease. Trends Pharmacol Sci 2000; 21:395–401.

300. Black MM, Sazawal S, Black RE, Khosla S, Kumar J, Menon V. Cognitive and motor development among small-for-gestational-age infants: impact of zinc supplementation, birth weight, and caregiving practices. Pediatrics 2004; 113:1297–1305.

301. Brown KH, Peerson JM, Rivera JA, Allen LH. Effect of supplemental zinc on the growth and serum zinc concentrations of prepubertal children: a meta-analysis of randomized controlled trials. Am J Clin Nutr 2002; 75:1062–1071.

302. Pfeiffer CC, Braverman ER. Zinc, the brain and behavior. Biol Psychiatry 1982; 17:513–532.

303. Halas ES, Eberhardt MJ, Diers MA, Sandstead SS. Learning and memory impairment in adult rats due to severe zinc deficiency during lactation. Physiol Behav 1983; 30:371–381.

304. Sazawal S, Bentley M, Black R, Dhingra P, George S, Bhan M. Effect of zinc supplementation on observed activity in low socioeconomic Indian preschool children. Pediatrics 1996; 98:1132–1137.

305. Bentley ME, Caulfield LE, Ram M, Santizo MC, Hurtado E, Rivera JA, et al. Zinc supplementation affects the activity patterns of rural Guatemalan infants. J Nutr 1997; 127:1333–1338.

306. Friel JK, Andrews WL, Matthew JD, Long DR, Cornel AM, Cox M, et al. Zinc supplementation in very-low-birth-weight infants. J Pediatr Gastroenterol Nutr 1993; 17:97–104.

307. Castillo-Duran C, Perales CG, Hertrampf ED, Marin VB, Rivera FA, Icaza G. Effect of zinc supplementation on development and growth of Chilean infants. J Pediatr 2001; 138:229–235.

308. Ashworth A, Morris SS, Lira PI, Grantham-McGregor SM. Zinc supplementation, mental development, and behaviour in low birth weight infants in northeast Brazil. Eur J Clin Nutr 1998; 52:223–227.

309. Morley JE, Mooradian AD, Silver AJ, Heber D, Alfin-Slater RB. Nutrition in the elderly. Ann Intern Med 1988; 109:890–904.

310. Black RE, Morris SS, Bryce J. Where and why are 10 million children dying every year? Lancet 2003; 361:2226–2234.

311. Singh M. Role of micronutrients for physical growth and mental development. Indian J Pediatr 2004; 71:59–62.

312. Rayman MP. The importance of selenium to human health. Lancet 2000; 356: 233–241.

313. Schweizer U, Schomburg L, Savaskan NE. The neurobiology of selenium: lessons from transgenic mice. J Nutr 2004; 134:707–710.

314. Whanger PD. Selenium and the brain: a review. Nutr Neurosci 2001; 4:81–97.

315. Contempre B, de Escobar GM, Denef JF, Dumont JE, Many MC. Thiocyanate induces cell necrosis and fibrosis in selenium- and iodine-deficient rat thyroids: a potential experimental model for myxedematous endemic cretinism in central Africa. Endocrinology 2004; 145:994–1002.

316. Van Paesschen W, Bodian C, Maker H. Metabolic abnormalities and new-onset seizures in human immunodeficiency virus-seropositive patients. Epilepsia 1995; 36:146–150.

317. Sibai BM. Magnesium sulfate prophylaxis in preeclampsia: lessons learned from recent trials. Am J Obstet Gynecol 2004; 190:1520–1526.

318. al Zahrani A, Levine MA. Primary hyperparathyroidism. Lancet 1997; 349:1233–1238.

319. Armanini D, Vecchio F, Basso A, Milone FF, Simoncini M, Fiore C, et al. Alzheimer's disease: pathophysiological implications of measurement of plasma cortisol, plasma dehydroepiandrosterone sulfate, and lymphocytic corticosteroid receptors. Endocrine 2003; 22:113–118.

320. Baulieu EE. Neurosteroids: of the nervous system, by the nervous system, for the nervous system. Recent Prog Horm Res 1997; 52:1–32.

321. Huopio H, Shyng SL, Otonkoski T, Nichols CG. K(ATP) channels and insulin secretion disorders. Am J Physiol Endocrinol Metab 2002; 283:E207–E216.

322. Mattson MP. Pathways towards and away from Alzheimer's disease. Nature 2004; 430:631–639.

323. Stuerenburg HJ, Hansen HC, Thie A, Kunze K. Reversible dementia in idiopathic hypoparathyroidism associated with normocalcemia. Neurology 1996; 47:474–476.

324. Rosario ER, Chang L, Stanczyk FZ, Pike CJ. Age-related testosterone depletion and the development of Alzheimer disease. JAMA 2004; 292:1431–1432.

325. Pennanen C, Laakso MP, Kivipelto M, Ramberg J, Soininen H. Serum testosterone levels in males with Alzheimer's disease. J Neuroendocrinol 2004; 16:95–98.

326. Tang MX, Jacobs D, Stern Y, Marder K, Schofield P, Gurland B, et al. Effect of oestrogen during menopause on risk and age at onset of Alzheimer's disease. Lancet 1996; 348:429–432.

327. Kawas C, Resnick S, Morrison A, Brookmeyer R, Corrada M, Zonderman A, et al. A prospective study of estrogen replacement therapy and the risk of developing Alzheimer's disease: the Baltimore Longitudinal Study of Aging. Neurology 1997; 48:1517–1521.

328. Shumaker SA, Legault C, Kuller LH, Rapp SR, Thal L, Lane DS, et al. Conjugated equine estrogens and incidence of probable dementia and mild cognitive impairment in postmenopausal women: Women's Health Initiative Memory Study. JAMA 2004; 291:2947–2958.

329. Espeland MA, Rapp SR, Shumaker SA, Brunner R, Manson JE, Sherwin BB, et al. Conjugated equine estrogens and global cognitive function in postmenopausal women: Women's Health Initiative Memory Study. JAMA 2004; 291:2959–2968.

330. Gibbs RB, Gabor R. Estrogen and cognition: applying preclinical findings to clinical perspectives. J Neurosci Res 2003; 74:637–643.

331. Stromberger C, Bodamer OA, Stockler-Ipsiroglu S. Clinical characteristics and diagnostic clues in inborn errors of creatine metabolism. J Inherit Metab Dis 2003; 26:299–308.

332. Assal F, Alarcon M, Solomon EC, Masterman D, Geschwind DH, Cummings JL. Association of the serotonin transporter and receptor gene polymorphisms in neuropsychiatric symptoms in Alzheimer disease. Arch Neurol 2004; 61:1249–1253.

333. Kay AD, Milstien S, Kaufman S, Creasey H, Haxby JV, Cutler NR, et al. Cerebrospinal fluid biopterin is decreased in Alzheimer's disease. Arch Neurol 1986; 43:996–999.

334. Barford PA, Blair JA, Eggar C, Hamon C, Morar C, Whitburn SB. Tetrahydrobiopterin metabolism in the temporal lobe of patients dying with senile dementia of Alzheimer type. J Neurol Neurosurg Psychiatry 1984; 47:736–738.

335. Hevel JM, Marletta MA. Macrophage nitric oxide synthase: relationship between enzyme-bound tetrahydrobiopterin and synthase activity. Biochemistry 1992; 31:7160–7165.

336. Heales SJ, Lam AA, Duncan AJ, Land JM. Neurodegeneration or neuroprotection: the pivotal role of astrocytes. Neurochem Res 2004; 29:513–519.

337. Luth HJ, Munch G, Arendt T. Aberrant expression of NOS isoforms in Alzheimer's disease is structurally related to nitrotyrosine formation. Brain Res 2002; 953:135–143.

338. Shimohama S, Taniguchi T, Fujiwara M, Kameyama M. Changes in nicotinic and muscarinic cholinergic receptors in Alzheimer-type dementia. J Neurochem 1986; 46:288–293.

339. Hillier V, Salib E. A case-control study of smoking and Alzheimer's disease. Int J Geriatr Psychiatry 1997; 12:295–300.

340. Courtney C, Farrell D, Gray R, Hills R, Lynch L, Sellwood E, et al. Long-term donepezil treatment in 565 patients with Alzheimer's disease (AD2000): randomised double-blind trial. Lancet 2004; 363:2105–2115.

341. Reiss J. Genetics of molybdenum cofactor deficiency. Hum Genet 2000; 106:157–163.
342. Graf WD, Oleinik OE, Jack RM, Weiss AH, Johnson JL. Ahomocysteinemia in molybdenum cofactor deficiency. Neurology 1998; 51:860–862.
343. Kaye EM, Hyland K. Amino acids and the brain: too much, too little, or just inappropriate use of a good thing? Neurology 1998; 51:668–670.
344. Akil M, Brewer GJ. Psychiatric and behavioral abnormalities in Wilson's disease. Adv Neurol 1995; 65:171–178.
345. Subramanian I, Vanek ZF, Bronstein JM. Diagnosis and treatment of Wilson's disease. Curr Neurol Neurosci Rep 2002; 2:317–323.
346. Menkes JH. Disorders of copper metabolism. In: Rosenberg R, Prusiner S, DiMauro S, Barchi R, eds. The Molecular and Henetic Basis of Neurologic Disease. Boston: Butterworth-Heinemann, 1997:1273–1290.
347. Bull PC, Thomas G, Rommens JM, Forbes JR, Cox DW. The Wilson disease gene is a putative copper transporting P-type ATPase similar to the Menkes gene. Nat Genet 1993; 5:327–337.
348. Shah AB, Chernov I, Zhang HT, Ross BM, Das K, Lutsenko S, et al. Identification and analysis of mutations in the Wilson disease gene (ATP7B): population frequencies, genotype-phenotype correlation, and functional analyses. Am J Hum Genet 1997; 61:317–328.
349. Molina JA, Jimenez-Jimenez FJ, Aguilar MV, Mesegucr I, Mateos-Vega CJ, Gonzalez-Munoz MJ, et al. Cerebrospinal fluid levels of transition metals in patients with Alzheimer's disease. J Neural Transm 1998; 105:479–488.
350. McGeer EG, McGccr PL. The importance of inflammatory mechanisms in Alzheimer disease. Exp Gerontol 1998; 33:371–378.
351. Weninger SC, Yankner BA. Inflammation and Alzheimer disease: the good, the bad, and the ugly. Nat Med 2001; 7:527–528.
352. Ridker PM, Cannon CP, Morrow D, Rifai N, Rose LM, McCabe CH, et al. C-reactive protein levels and outcomes after statin therapy. N Engl J Med 2005; 352:20–28.
353. Singh VK, Guthikonda P. Circulating cytokines in Alzheimer's disease. J Psychiatr Res 1997; 31:657–660.
354. Duong T, Nikolaeva M, Acton PJ. C-reactive protein-like immunoreactivity in the neurofibrillary tangles of Alzhcimer's disease. Brain Res 1997; 749:152–156.
355. Schmidt R, Schmidt H, Curb JD, Masaki K, White LR, Launer LJ. Early inflammation and dementia: a 25-year follow-up of the Honolulu-Asia aging study. Ann Neurol 2002; 52.168–174.
356. Mintz M, Epstein LG. Neurologic manifestations of pediatric acquired immunodeficiency syndrome: clinical features and therapeutic approaches. Semin Neurol 1992; 12:51–56.
357. Schambelan M, Benson CA, Carr A, Currier JS, Dube MP, Gerber JG, et al. Management of metabolic complications associated with antiretroviral therapy for HIV-1 infection: recommendations of an International AIDS Society-USA panel. J Acquir Immune Defic Syndr 2002; 31:257–275.
358. Frisoni GB, Carabellese N, Longhi M, Geroldi C, Bianchetti A, Govoni S, et al. Is celiac disease associated with Alzheimer's disease? Acta Neurol Scand 1997; 95:147–151.
359. Collin P, Pirttila T, Nurmikko T, Somer H, Erila T, Keyrilainen O. Celiac disease, brain atrophy, and dementia. Neurology 1991; 41:372–375.

360. Zelnik N, Pacht A, Obeid R, Lerner A. Range of neurologic disorders in patients with celiac disease. Pediatrics 2004; 113:1672–1676.
361. Bruzelius M, Liedholm LJ, Hellblom M. Celiac disease can be associated with severe neurological symptoms. Analysis of gliadin antibodies should be considered in suspected cases. Lakartidningen 2001; 98:3538–3542.
362. Wills AJ. The neurology and neuropathology of coeliac disease. Neuropathol Appl Neurobiol 2000; 26:493–496.
363. Dietrich W, Erbguth F. Neurological complications of inflammatory intestinal diseases. Fortschr Neurol Psychiatr 2003; 71:406–414.
364. Thieben MJ, Lennon VA, Boeve VA, Aksamit AJ, Keegan M, Vernino S. Potentially reversible autoimmune limbic encephalitis with neuronal potassium channel antibody. Neurology 2004; 62:1177–1182.
365. Schott JM, Harkness K, Barnes J, della Rocchetta AI, Vincent A, Rossor MN. Amnesia, cerebral atrophy, and autoimmunity. Lancet 2003; 361:1266.
366. Buckley C, Oger J, Clover L, Tuzun E, Carpenter K, Jackson M, et al. Potassium channel antibodies in two patients with reversible limbic encephalitis. Ann Neurol 2001; 50:73–78.
367. Oslin DW, Cary MS. Alcohol-related dementia: validation of diagnostic criteria. Am J Geriatr Psychiatry 2003; 11(4):441–447.
368. Charness ME. Brain lesions in alcoholics. Alcohol Clin Exp Res 1993; 17:2–11.
369. Burd L, Wilson H. Fetal, infant, and child mortality in a context of alcohol use. Am J Med Genet 2004; 127C(1):51–58.
370. Streissguth AP, Landesman-Dwyer S, Martin JC, Smith DW. Teratogenic effects of alcohol in humans and laboratory animals. Science 1980; 209(4454):353–361.
371. Spohr HL, Willms J, Steinhausen HC. The fetal alcohol syndrome in adolescence. Acta Paediatr Suppl 1994; 404:19–26.
372. Streissguth AP, O'Malley K. Neuropsychiatric implications and long-term consequences of fetal alcohol spectrum disorders. Semin Clin Neuropsychiatry 2000; 5(3):177–190.
373. Ryan C, Butters N. Neuropsychology of alcoholism. In: Wedding D, Horton A, Webster J, eds. The Neuropsychology Handbook. New York: Springer, 1986.
374. Victor M. Alcoholic dementia. Can J Neurol Sci 1994; 21(2):88–99.
375. Kopelman MD. The Korsakoff syndrome. Br J Psychiatry 1995; 166:154–173.
376. Victor M, Adams RD, Collins GH. The Wernicke-Korsakoff Syndrome and Related Neurologic Disorders Due to Alcoholism and Malnutrition. Philadelphia: F.A. Davis, 1989.
377. Caine D, Halliday GM, Kril JJ, Harper CG. Operational criteria for the classification of chronic alcoholics: identification of Wernicke's encephalopathy. J Neurol Neurosurg Psychiatry 1997; 62(1):51–60.
378. Baker KG, Harding AJ, Halliday GM, Kril JJ, Harper CG. Neuronal loss in functional zones of the cerebellum of chronic alcoholics with and without Wernicke's encephalopathy. Neuroscience 1999; 91:429–438.
379. Harper CG. The incidence of Wernicke's encephalopathy in Australia: a neuropathological study of 131 cases. J Neurol Neurosurg Psychiatry 1983; 46:593–598.
380. Ganry O, Joly JP, Queval MP, Dubreuil A. Prevalence of alcohol problems among elderly patients in a university hospital. Addiction 2000; 95:107–113.

381. Rains VS, Ditzler TF. Alcohol use disorders in cognitively impaired patients referred for geriatric assessment. J Addict Dis 1993; 12:55–64.
382. Fink A, Hays RD, Moore AA, Beck JC. Alcohol-related problems in older persons. Determinants, consequences, and screening. Arch Intern Med 1996; 156(11):1150–1156.
383. Carlen PL, McAndrews MP, Weiss RT, Dongier M, Hill JM, Menzano E, et al. Alcohol-related dementia in the institutionalized elderly. Alcohol Clin Exp Res 1994; 18:1330–1334.
384. Beaudet AL, Scriver CR, Sly WS, Valle D. Genetics, Biochemistry, and Molecular Bases of Variant Human Phenotypes. 8th ed. New York: McGraw-Hill, 2001.
385. Seliger SL, Siscovick DS, Stehman-Breen CO, Gillen DL, Fitzpatrick A, Bleyer A, et al. Moderate renal impairment and risk of dementia among older adults: the Cardiovascular Health Cognition Study. J Am Soc Nephrol 2004; 15:1904–1911.
386. Antonelli Incalzi R, Marra C, Giordano A, Calcagni ML, Cappa A, Basso S, et al. Cognitive impairment in chronic obstructive pulmonary disease—a neuropsychological and spect study. J Neurol Neurosurg Psychiatry 2003; 250:325–332.
387. Kozora E, Filley CM, Julian LJ, Cullum CM. Cognitive functioning in patients with chronic obstructive pulmonary disease and mild hypoxemia compared with patients with mild Alzheimer disease and normal controls. Neuropsychiatry Neuropsychol Behav Neurol 1999; 12:178–183.

11

Drug-Induced Cognitive Impairment

Larry E. Tune

Department of Psychiatry and Behavioral Sciences,
Emory University School of Medicine, Atlanta, Georgia, U.S.A.

Drug-induced dementia is the most common reversible dementia. It is difficult to determine the prevalence for a variety of reasons: (i) Drug-induced dementia and delirium are most common in patients with pre-existing, underlying dementia. In identifying this *co-morbid* state is difficult in routine clinical practice. (ii) It is difficult to assess compliance with medications, especially when patients (particularly those with pre-existing cognitive impairments) are receiving a large number of prescription and nonprescription medications, as a result, it is hard to assign causality to medications. (iii) All dementias are routinely underdetected. Most studies suggest that drug-induced cognitive impairment as a source of co-morbidity is common. In primary care medicine this may occur in as many as 10–15% of all dementias. The two commonest manifestations of drug-induced cognitive impairments are delirium and dementia.

DRUG-INDUCED DELIRIUM

Delirium accounts for 7% of the overall neurologic consultations and for 19% of the iatrogenically induced cases of delirium (1). Drug-induced delirium may have contributed to the largest group (47%) in which no single cause was identified. The elderly are at increased risk to develop cognitive impairment because of age-related changes in pharmacokinetics and target organ response, increased use of medications, and increased premorbid cognitive impairment, many of which are associated with cholinergic deficiencies (e.g., Alzheimer's disease). In hospitalized elderly patients, the prevalence of delirium ranges from 11% to

60% depending on the type of service (2). The risk of delirium increases as a function of age (>80 years old). One of the strongest risk factors for delirium is pre-existing cognitive impairment. Pre-existing dementia increases the risk of delirium by two- to threefold, and 25–50% of delirious patients have an underlying dementia (3). Drug-induced delirium is particularly important because it is a common delirium and it is reversible and potentially preventable (2).

DRUG-INDUCED DEMENTIA

Drug-induced dementia is the commonest reversible dementia. In addition to causing dementia, medications may play a secondary role, exacerbating cognitive deficits in patients with pre-existing dementia. In a primary care setting, drugs have been reported to be the primary cause of or a contribution to cognitive impairment in 10% of patients evaluated for dementia (4–7). The drugs most commonly implicated were sedative-hypnotics, antihypertensives, and psychotrophic medications. Polypharmacy increased the risk of drug-induced dementia, with the relative odds increasing from 2.7 with two or three drugs, to 9.3 with four or five drugs, and to 13.7 with more than six drugs. To get a sense of the potential impact of this finding, 40% of nursing home residents are on nine or more medications.

    This chapter will address drug-induced dementias from two perspectives: (i) a brief, selective review of individual compounds and drug classes associated with cognitive impairment, and (ii) the problem of anticholinergic burden as a way of addressing polypharmacy by focusing on the leading putative mechanisms for drug-induced cognitive impairment.

    Cognitive side effects may be produced by a variety of medications from multiple drug classes. The most commonly implicated drugs are the anticholinergics, benzodiazepines, narcotics, neuroleptics, and sedative hypnotics. Deficits range from frank delirium to subtle cognitive changes. Impaired vigilance and slowed psychomotor speed are probably the most common compromised cognitive functions produced by centrally active drugs. Polypharmacy increases the risk of cognitive impairment. Impaired drug metabolism or elimination (e.g., hepatic or renal failure) may also predispose a patient to cognitive toxicity. Elderly patients are particularly prone to develop drug-induced cognitive deficits for both pharmacodynamic and pharmacokinetic reasons. Elderly patients with dementia are even more sensitive to adverse cognitive effects. Some central nervous system effects (e.g., sedation) may be harmful or beneficial depending on the clinical situation. When therapeutic options are limited, the benefits may outweigh relatively minor side effects. Physicians should maintain a high index of suspicion to avoid iatrogenically induced adverse cognitive deficits.

    The Appendix provides a list of the myriad of medications associated with drug-induced confusion/dementia.

Psychotropic Agents

In one early psychiatric inpatient study of psychotropic medications, 10% of the medications were discontinued due to adverse drug reaction (ADR) (8,9). Adverse "psychic" reactions accounted for 45% of these ADRs. Drug-induced delirium, agitation, and sedation were the most frequent events. The commonest causative agents were antipsychotics and antidepressants. The antimuscarinic and anticholinergic effects of tricyclic antidepressants are likely the primary cause of adverse cognitive effects in these agents (9,10). In one study, age-related delirium occurred in 8% of inpatients on tricyclic antidepressants (10). Similar prevalences (5–7%) have been found in geriatric patients in other studies (11,12). Most of the tricyclic antidepressants (e.g., amitriptyline, imipramine, clomipramine), are no longer recommended for use in treating depression in geriatric patients. In normal elderly subjects, amitriptyline impairs verbal recall (13) and produces greater cognitive impairment than trazodone (14). In one placebo-controlled study, amitriptyline and trazodone impaired choice reaction time, short-term memory, car driving, and subjective sedation, while bupropion, fluoxetine, sertraline, and paroxetine did not (15).

Selective serotonin re-uptake inhibitors (SSRIs) and reversible monoamine oxidase inhibitors (MAOI) have minimal adverse cognitive effects (16,17). SSRIs have become the antidepressants of choice in the elderly, who have increased susceptibility to the effects of the older agents. SSRIs are rarely associated with encephalopathy. Serotoninergic agents (i.e., SSRIs, tricyclic antidepressants, tryptophan) used alone or in combination with monoamine oxidase inhibitors can produce a serotonin syndrome, characterized by changes in mental status (i.e., agitation, confusion, disorientation), myoclonus, rigidity, hyper-reflexia, tremor, autonomic instability (i.e., fever, nausea, diarrhea, diapheresis, tachycardia), coma, and rarely death (18,19).

Lithium

In normal volunteers, lithium can cause psychomotor slowing (17,18). The effects on measures of memory have been more variable (20–22).

Antipsychotics

In schizophrenic patients, studies examining the cognitive effects of antipsychotics have variable results, with the majority of studies reporting improvement or no impairment (23,24). This is due in part to the fact that the primary psychotic symptoms (e.g., hallucinations, delusions) are associated with cognitive impairments. So a schizophrenic patient may improve cognitively as a result of hallucinations decreasing, but still suffer cognitive impairments from antipsychotic medications. Studies of normal volunteers have shown impairments in vigilance, psychomotor function, and response readiness as a result of exposure to phenothiazines (24). Anticholinergic medications are often coadministered with "typical" antipsychotics, and anticholinergic blood levels during neuroleptic therapy are correlated with memory impairments in schizophrenics (25). Elderly patients are at the greatest risk to develop antipsychotic-induced cognitive side effects. One study of patients with probable Alzheimer's disease treated with either haloperidol (1, 2, and 5 mg/day) or thioridazine (25, 50, and 75 mg/day) reported that Mini Mental Status Exam (MMSE) scores were not significantly reduced. MMSE scores decreased four to five points. However, in two patients when thioridazine was increased to 100–125 mg/day. In patients with probable Alzheimer's disease, haloperidol (1–5 mg daily) improved the psychiatric symptoms but lowered MMSE scores (26).

The cognitive effects of the newer atypical antipsychotics are now the topic of intensive scrutiny in patients with schizophrenia. Olanzapine, quetiapine and risperidone, ziprasidone and aripiprazole appear to produce less cognitive impairment than first generation (e.g., haloperidol) antipsychotics.

Antiparkinsonian Medications

Anticholinergic drugs improve parkinsonian symptoms but can cause cognitive impairment (27). In one study, 93% of hospitalized patients with Parkinson's disease (PD) receiving anticholinergics developed confusion compared with 46% who did not receive this type of drug (28). Trihexyphenidyl and benztropine impair memory in healthy volunteers, but amantadine does not (29–32). Dopaminergic agents can improve cognitive function in patients with PD but can also produce confusion, especially at higher dosages. At low-to-moderate dosages, direct dopamine agonists are associated with confusion. Eleven percent of patients on pergolide and 24% of patients on lisuride had to be discontinued because of confusion (29–32).

Benzodiazepines

Benzodiazepines impair psychomotor speed, vigilance, and driving performance (33,34). Anterograde memory is impaired by benzodiazepines, affecting the acquisition of both verbal and visuospatial items. Benzodiazepines impair metamemory, and treated patients may have difficulty monitoring their anterograde memory deficits.

The elderly have increased sensitivity to the adverse effects of benzodiazepines for both pharmacokinetic and pharmacodynamic reasons (35–38). The elderly are sensitive to the effects of benzodiazepine withdrawal. One study found that 52 of 103 consecutive elderly hospital patient admissions had a positive urine test for benzodiazepines (39,40); seven of the eight patients who had their benzodiazepines stopped on admission developed confusion.

Anticonvulsants

Cognitive impairments from anticonvulsants are likely due to multiple factors. These include genetic factors, the seizure disorder itself, cerebral abnormalities existing prior to the onset of epilepsy, the sequelae of the seizures, psychosocial issues, and the anti-epileptic drugs (AEDs) (41). Because AEDs reduce neuronal irritability, it is not surprising that they may reduce neuronal excitability and impair cognitive function. The older established AEDs all impair cognition, but their adverse effects are usually modest (42–44). Adverse cognitive effects are usually offset in part by the beneficial effects of reducing seizures. Factors that may increase cognitive side effects include AED dosage, higher anticonvulsant blood levels, and polypharmacy (43,45–49). Reducing the number of AEDs not only frequently improves cognition, but also may lead to a decrease in seizures (50–53).

Greater cognitive toxicity has been observed with phenobarbital and benzodiazepines. There is no convincing evidence of clinically significant differences among carbamazepine, phenytoin, and valproate (42,51,52). This conclusion is supported by a series of well-controlled randomized, double-blind, cross-over studies in patients and healthy volunteers (54–57). The Veterans Administration Cooperative Studies found few differences in cognitive function for patients treated with carbamazepine, phenobarbital, phenytoin, or primidone (58) and between carbamazepine and valproate (59). In the elderly, Craig and Tallis (60) compared phenytoin to valproate and found minimal differences.

Of the new AEDs, most studies have found few adverse cognitive effects. Gabapentin had minimal differences compared to placebo (61). Lamotrigine exhibited positive effects on psychological well-being in three studies compared to placebo or carbamazepine (62,63). One study examined cognitive function and no significant differences were found for lamotrigine compared with placebo (63). Oxcarbazepine was not different from phenytoin in a small randomized, double-blind, parallel study (64). No significant cognitive or behavioral effects were seen for tiagabine in an add-on, placebo-controlled, parallel study (65). Vigabatrin has undergone the most investigations of the new AEDs involving cognitive function. Four double-blind, randomized, add-on studies have shown few adverse effects (66–69). It should be noted, however, that the newer AED, topiramate, is known to cause mental slowing and problems with language, such as word-finding difficulties, which could be mistaken for dementia.

Antihypertensives

Neuropsychologic symptoms are common with antihypertensives. Antihypertensives have modest deleterious effects on cognition, but the neuropsychologic effects are inconsistent across drug groups (70).

Angiotensin-converting enzyme (ACE) inhibitors do not influence cognitive function and produce the least subjective side effects among the antihypertensives (11). Beta-blockers produce sedation (71) but they improve performance, perhaps because they are anxiolytic and tremor-reducing (72). In one review of beta-blocker therapy, no effects were noted in 66% of the total neuropsychological variables studied, function worsened in 18% of the subjects, and 16% improved (73).

The few studies of calcium-channel blockers (e.g., verapamil), alpha-adrenergic blockers (e.g., prazosin), and diuretics show no significant alterations in performance or behavior (70,74). Case reports have reported confusion related to calcium blockers. Diuretics have been reported to produce more subjective behavioral side effects than placebo (9,10). Clonidine has effects on neuropsychological test performance. Subjective measures of behavioral side effects (e.g., sedation, mood, quality of life) have found adverse effects for methyldopa compared with antihypertensives of other classes (70).

Cardiac Medications

Digoxin can produce delirium, dementia, and a wide array of neuropsychiatric symptoms (75). Digoxin-induced cognitive impairment is correlated with plasma levels and these may even be in therapeutic ranges (75). Quinidine and disopyramide also produce cognitive impairment probably as a result of their antimuscarinic properties (9,10). Lidocaine, lecainide, and tocainide have been associated with delirium and other neuropsychiatric symptoms (9,10).

Antihistamines

Cimetidine can cause delirium and less frequently other neuropsychiatric disorders. Reversible confusional states occurs in 0.3–4% of cases (9,10). Cognitive toxicity appears to increase as a function of age, higher dosages, intravenous administration, and hepatic or renal failure. Symptoms typically begin within a few days after initiation of therapy. Although perhaps less common, cases of cognitive toxicity have also been reported with the newer H2 antagonists (9,10).

Analgesics and Anti-Inflammatory Agents

Narcotics analgesics can impair memory and precipitate delirium (76–78). Non-steroidal anti-inflammatory drugs are rarely associated with delirium and cognitive dysfunction (79). Steroids can induce psychosis, delirium, and mood disturbance in approximately 5% of the patients; affective disorders are most common followed in frequency by psychosis or delirium (29,30). A reversible dementia has been noted to occur in 0.4% of steroid-treated patients (80).

Cyclosporine

Reports of central nervous system toxicity from cyclosporine have ranged from 0 to 27% (81–83).

Antibiotics

Neurotoxicity has been seen with antibiotics. The beta-lactams (e.g., penicillin, cephalosporins) and quinolones (e.g., ciprofloxacin) are those most commonly associated with encephalopathy (84). The risk is increased with high-dose intravenous use, reduced renal function, abnormal blood–brain barrier, and increased age. Antituberculous drugs can precipitate a niacin-deficiency encephalopathy.

Clioquinol has been associated with a transient or permanent amnesia and delayed-onset temporal lobe epilepsy (85).

Cancer Chemotherapeutic Agents

Many cancer chemotherapy drugs are associated with central nervous system toxicity (86). The effects may be irreversible as in the case of cytosine arabinoside (87). High dosages, concomitant use of head irradiation, and treatment at the age extremes increase the risk of adverse effects. Treatment with interferon for cancer or other diseases can produce a toxic encephalopathy (9,10). Many of the impairments associated with interferon are subtle and may go undetected clinically (88,89).

ANTICHOLINERGIC BURDEN IN THE ELDERLY: ONE MEANS OF ADDRESSING POLYPHARMACY

The Scope of the Clinical Syndrome

In the elderly, anticholinergic-induced cognitive impairment is important for several reasons. First, cholinergic functioning declines with age. This loss of cholinergic "reserve" may well be part of the reason that age is a major risk factor for the development of delirium. Second, cholinergic dysfunction has been implicated in a wide variety of delirium states. Third, in demented elderly patients, there is the dual loss of cholinergic function: age-associated cholinergic loss and dementia-related loss of cholinergic cell bodies.

Anticholinergics impair memory acquisition and secondarily impair memory retrieval, especially free recall. Cholinomimetics (i.e., muscarinic agonists, cholinesterase inhibitors, and nicotine) can enhance memory. Anticholinergics affect attentional mechanisms, and the cholinergic systems may control information processing. Anticholinergic effects appear to be neurotransmitter-specific. For example, amphetamine reduces the sedation of scopolamine but makes the memory deficit worse. Scopolamine-induced memory deficits are improved by the anticholinesterase physostigmine but not by a benzodiazepine antagonist (90).

That anticholinergic medications induce cognitive deficits and delirium in the elderly is supported by pharmacologic challenge studies. When scopolamine is administered to normal elderly volunteers, consistent deficits in information processing, recent memory and attention are the result. Sunderland et al. (91) administered scopolamine to Alzheimer disease patients and age-matched controls. The Alzheimer's patients were much more sensitive to scopolamine than the controls, and both groups developed significant cognitive (new learning, semantic memory), behavioral, and physiologic responses to escalating doses of scopolamine. Miller et al. (92) administered a single low dose of scopolamine to 18 cognitively intact elderly patients undergoing elective outpatient surgery. Significant impairments on the Rey auditory verbal learning test as well as the Saskatoon delirium checklist (SDC) were the result. These impairments correlated significantly with serum anticholinergic levels.

Exposure to anticholinergic medications is a risk factor for delirium in the elderly (93–95). While "anticholinergic delirium" is only one of the several types of delirium, the reason for focusing on this cause of delirium is clear. Anticholinergic delirium is a common and reversible clinical syndrome in the elderly. If one includes subsyndromal delirium and confusional states, the problem is widespread. Mulsant et al. (96) recently conducted a community-based study in which 219 elderly patients were screened for cognitive impairment with Mini Mental Stated Examination (MMSE) (97) scales and these were correlated with serum anticholinergic levels. They found that even modest anticholinergic levels were associated with cognitive impairment as determined by the score on the MMSE. Lerner et al. (98) found that 22% of 199 outpatients with Alzheimer's disease suffered from delirium during a 3-year study period, and that medication-induced delirium was one of the commonest causes. Lu and Tune (99) found that anticholinergic exposure adversely affects the course of Alzheimer's disease. All patients received the cholinesterase inhibitor donepezil at a dose of 10 mg/day. Patients ($n = 79$) were divided into two groups: those receiving one or more concomitant medications with significant anticholinergic effects ($n = 16$) and those receiving no concomitant medications with anticholinergic effects ($n = 63$). Figure 1 shows that change in MMSE scores at two years were significantly worse for patients on anticholinergic medications compared with those not on anticholinergics (t-test for equality of means, $t = 2.52$; $P = 0.017$). There were no significant differences between the two groups based on age, gender, educational level, duration of illness, or number of medical illnesses. They also found differences in the clinical progression of dementia: patients receiving anticholinergics for two years had a steeper rate of cognitive decline as evidenced by the decline in the MMSE scores.

Most recently, Perry et al. (100) examined 54 postmortem samples of patients with PD. Exposure to anticholinergic medications was assessed and the presence and number of Alzheimer disease-related amyloid plaques and neurofibrillary tangles were quantified. PD patients who were treated with anticholinergic medications longer than two years had a 2.5-fold increase in amyloid plaques and a significant increase in number of neurofibrillary tangles compared to patients with no anticholinergic exposure. While these findings need to be replicated, they may have tremendous implications for the way in which patients with Alzheimer's disease are managed and with the understanding of the possible adverse consequences of prolonged anticholinergic exposure.

ANTICHOLINERGIC BURDEN AND ITS RELATIONSHIP TO DELIRIUM/DEMENTIA

A few investigations have used scales to estimate the extent of anticholinergic exposure. The results of these attempts have been mixed. Some have found no

Change in MMSE

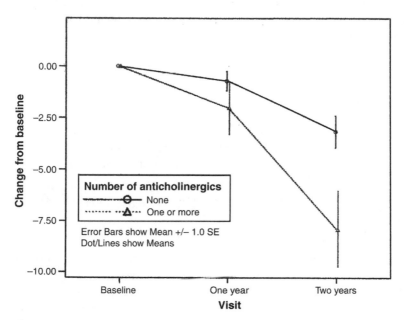

Figure 1 Comparison of MMSE scores between patients on anticholinergic medications and those not on anticholinergics.

clear association between anticholinergic exposure and cognitive impairment/delirium. These negative results might be partly explained by an under-appreciation of the extent of anticholinergicity of commonly prescribed, older medications that are not typically viewed as anticholinergic. The cumulative effects of multiple medications with subtle anticholinergic effects might go unappreciated (100,101). Other factors may contribute to these discrepant findings. First, the methods used to generate lists of which medications have anticholinergic effects have varied widely. Second, the effect of anticholinergic medications in delirium/confusional states is often confounded by and attributed to other medical factors; pre-existing dementia and medical co-morbidity are two notable confounds. Last is the sampling method itself. Many studies were cross-sectional assessments. The stronger correlations were found in studies where a patient used his or her own control method.

Two recent investigations used predictive scales (not serum anticholinergic levels) and found significant relationships between assessments of anticholinergic exposure and delirium. Egeli and Tune (102) reviewed records from 91 inpatients admitted for delirium with agitation ($n = 47$) or dementia with agitation ($n = 44$). All patients had a pre-existing diagnosis of dementia. Anticholinergic exposure was determined based on anticholinergic levels of the parent compound in an antimuscarinic radioreceptor assay, as opposed to serum anticholinergic levels. On admission, the delirious, demented patients had been prescribed significantly more anticholinergics than the nondelirious, demented patients [2.34 $\pm$ 0.20(SEM) vs. 1.81 $\pm$ 0.17; $P = 0.007$]. Total number of medications was similar for both groups.

Han et al. (103) developed a clinician-rated anticholinergic exposure score based on a list of 340 medications with known anticholinergic effects. Then, three geriatric psychiatrists employed a consensus approach to rate the relative anticholinergic effects of all of the drugs (on a 1–3 scale). Using this expanded list of anticholinergics and a "consensus" method to assess relative anticholinergic exposure, a significant correlation was found between the "anticholinergic exposure scale" and the clinical syndrome of delirium in medical inpatients.

VALIDATION OF ANTICHOLINERGIC BURDEN-INDUCED COGNITIVE IMPAIRMENT USING SERUM ANTICHOLINERGIC LEVELS

Perhaps the most difficult task in attributing a mechanism to a delirium syndrome is the fact that the exact cause of most delirium cases in geriatrics is either multifactorial or unknown. There are no formal tests to confirm either the presence or cause of delirium. One rudimentary attempt to approach anticholinergic exposure as a mechanism has been the series of studies over the last 20 years correlating the presence and severity of delirium with serum anticholinergic levels. Serum anticholinergic activity levels (SAA) are determined using a radioreceptor assay method. This test is based on competition at the muscarinic receptors between compounds present in a patient's serum and a tritiated muscarinic antagonist, 3H-quinuclidinyl benzilate (3H-QNB). The advantage of this assay is its simplicity and its ability to detect the cumulative antimuscarinic effects of multiple compounds as well as their pharmacologically active metabolites. Disadvantages of this assay are: (i) by focusing just on antimuscarinic effects, it may overlook other etiologies, especially when the true cause of the delirium involves more than one mechanism, and (ii) the assay lacks the specificity to identify specific muscarinic receptor subtypes and their individual roles in the pathogenesis of delirium. This is an important issue because some muscarinic receptor subtypes appear more closely related to cognition than others. By measuring total serum anticholinergic activity (104), the relationship between central anticholinergic activity and delirium is compelling. This could be for a number of reasons, including (i) the measurement of anticholinergic burden not only of parent compounds but also pharmacologically active metabolites, (ii) identification of drugs not commonly thought of as anticholinergic, and (iii) more remotely, the possibility that certain delirium states are associated with endogenous anticholinergic activity.

Table 1 focuses on the major studies conducted over the last 20 years using the SAA to identify an anticholinergic "signal" in patients' serum. In general, while a variety of methods were used to determine the presence and severity

Table 1 Clinical Studies Using SAA Levels

Patient group (N)	Outcome measures	Results	References
Postcardiotomy delirium	MMSE	Post-versus preoperative decline in MMSE correlated with SAA level ($r = 0.81, P < 0.001$)	(105)
Post-ECT confusional states/ delirium	MMSE, tachistoscope	Decline in MMSE significantly correlated with SAA level	(106)
Intensive Care Unit delirium	DSM-III diagnosis of delirium	Delirious patients had significantly higher SAA levels	(107)
Demented, delirious nursing home residents	Psychogeriatric dependency rating scale	Self-care impairments significantly correlated with SAA level	(108)
Delirium caused by topical homatropine ophthalmologic solution	DSM-III-R diagnosis of delirium	Delirious patients had elevated SAA levels	(109)
Normal elderly males	Ray auditory verbal learning test, SDC	Significant impairment in cognition occurred even at low SAA levels	(92)
Elderly, hospitalized medical patients	DSM-III criteria for delirium, MMSE	Delirium associated with elevated SAA levels, and delirium resolution associated with lower SAA levels	(110)
Elderly nursing home residents on anticholinergic medications	WDF, MMSE, SDC	25% reduction in anticholinergic meds significantly associated with (i) Improved performance on WDF (ii) Improved SDC score	(111)
Delirious, elderly medically ill inpatients	CPS, CAM, DSI	Delirium independently associated with elevated SAA levels	(112,113)
Elderly medically ill inpatients	CAM	Delirium patients had significantly elevated SAA versus nondelirium patients	(114)

Abbreviations: SAA, serum anticholinergic activity level; MMSE, Mini Mental Stated Examination; ECT, electroconvulsive therapy; SDC, Saskatoon delirium checklist; WDF, Wechsler digit span forward; CPS, cognitive performance scale; DSI, delirium symptom interview; CAM, confusion assessment method.

of delirium states, SAA levels have correlated with the presence and severity of delirium in various postoperative patient groups, hospitalized elderly medical inpatients, demented nursing home residents, and delirium following electroconvulsive therapy.

CONCLUSIONS

The problem of "anticholinergic burden" and its consequences simply cannot be overestimated in geriatrics. It is a well-documented, widespread cause of delirium and cognitive morbidity in elderly patients. What is needed are more studies correlating either drug exposure with delirium (12) or serum anticholinergic levels and confusional states. Especially anticholinergic reduction intervention studies like that of Tollefson et al. (111) are needed. By simply reducing anticholinergic burden by 25% in a small sample of nursing home residents, significant improvements in measures of cognition, attention, and delirium were found a few weeks later. More speculatively, prolonged anticholinergic exposure may play a negative role in the course of Alzheimer's disease (9,10) and perhaps PD (100). This latter issue needs to be addressed as soon as possible.

REFERENCES

1. Moses H, Kaden I. Neurologic consultations in a general hospital. Am J Med 1986; 81:955–958.
2. Tune L. Delirium. In: Coffey CE, Cummings JL, eds. Textbook of Geriatric Neuropsychiatry. 2nd ed. Washington, DC, 2000:441–452.
3. Erkinjuntti T, Wikstrom J, Palo J, et al. Dementia among medical inpatients: evaluation of 2000 consecutive admissions. Arch Intern Med 1986; 146:1923–1926.
4. Larson EB, Kukull WA, Buckner D, et al. Adverse drug reactions associated with global cognitive impairment in elderly persons. Ann Intern Med 1987; 107:169–173.
5. Larson EB, Reifler BV, Featherstone HJ, et al. Dementia in elderly outpatients: a prospective study. Ann Intern Med 1984; 100:417–423.
6. Larson EB, Reifler BV, Sumi SM, et al. Diagnostic tests in the evaluation of dementia: a prospective study of 200 elderly outpatients. Arch Intern Med 1986; 146: 1917–1922.
7. Larson EB, Reifler BV, Sumi SM, et al. Diagnostic evaluation of 200 elderly outpatients with suspected dementia. J Gerontol 1985; 40:526–534.
8. Grohmann R, Strobel C, Rother E, et al. Adverse psychic reactions to psychotropic drugs—a report from the AMUP study. Pharmacopsychiatry 1993; 26:84–93.
9. Schor JD, Levkoff SE, Kipsitz LA, et al. Risk factors for delirium in hospitalized elderly. JAMA 1992; 267:827–831.
10. Momson RL, Katz IR. Drug-related cognitive impairment: current progress and recurrent problems. Ann Rev Gerontol Geriatr 1989; 9:232–279.
11. Bulpitt CJ, Fletcher AE. Cognitive function and angiotensin-coverting enzyme inhibitors in comparison with other antihypertensive drugs. J Cardiovasc Pharmacol 1992; 19(suppl 6):S100–S104.

12. Meyers BS, Bei-Tal V. Psychiatric reactions during tricyclic treatment of the elderly reconsidered. J Clin Psychophamacol 1983; 3:2–6.

13. Branconnier RJ, Cole JO, Ghazvinian S. Treating the depressed elderly patient: The comparative behavioral pharmacology of mianserin and amitriptyline. Adv Biochem Psychopharm 1982; 32:195–212.

14. Cadieux RJ. Azapirones: An alternative to benzodiazepines for anxiety. Am Fam Physician 1996; 53:2349–2353.

15. Bums M, Moskowitz H, Jaffe J. A comparison of the effects of trazodone and arnitripty line on skills performance by geriatric subjects. J Clin Psych 1986; 47:252–254.

16. Knegtering H, Eijick M, Huijsman A. Effects of antidepressants on cognitive functioning of elderly patients: A review. Drugs Aging 1994; 5:192–199.

17. Arnado-Boccara I, Gougoulis N, Poirier Littre MF, et al. Effects of antidepressants on cognitive function: A review. Neurosci Biobehav Rev 1995; 19:479–493.

18. Oxman IE. Antidepressants and cognitive impairment in the elderly. J Clin Psych 1996; 57(suppl 5):38–44.

19. Sternberg H. The serotonin syndrome. Am J Psych 1991; 148:F705–F713.

20. Judd LL, Hubbard B, Janowsk' DS, et al. The effect of lithium carbonate on the cognitive functions of normal subjects. Arch Gen Psych 1977; 34:355–357.

21. Reus VI, T argum SD, Weingartner H, et al. Effects of lithium carbonate on memory processes of bipolar affectively ill patients. Psychopharmacology 1979; 63:39–42.

22. Squire LR, Judd LL, Janowsky DS, et al. Effects of lithium carbonate on memory and other cognitive functions. Am J Psych 1980; 137:1042–1046.

23. Weingartner H, RudOlfer MV, Linnoila M. Cognitive effects of lithium treatment in normal volunteers. Psychopharmacology 1985; 86:472–474.

24. Goldberg TE, Weinberger DR. Effects of neuroleptic medications on the cognition of patients with schizophrenia: a review of recent studies. J Clin Psych 1996; 57:62–65.

25. King DJ. The effect of neuroleptics on cognitive and psychomotor function. Br J Psych 1990; 157:799–811.

26. Tune LE, Strauss ME, Lew MF, et al. Serum levels of anticholinergic drugs and impaired recent memory in chronic schizophrenic patients. Am J Psych 1982; 139:1460–1462.

27. Steele C, Lucas MJ, Tune L. Halopelidol versus thioridazine in the treatment of behavioral symptoms in senile dementia of the Alzheimer's type: Preliminary findings. J Clin Psych 1986; 47:310–312.

28. Meco G, Casacchia M, Lazszari R, et al. Mental impairment in Parkinson's disease: the role of anticholinergic drugs. Acta Psychiatr Belg 1984; 84:325–355.

29. Perlick D, Stastny P, Katz I, et al. Memory deficits and anticholinergic levels in chronic schizophrenia. Am J Psych 1986; 143:230–232.

30. Lewis DA, Smith RE. Steroid-induced psychiatric syndromes. J Affect Disord 1983; 5:319–332.

31. McEvoy JP. A double-blind crossover comparison of antiparkinson drug therapy: Amantadine versus anticholinergics in 90 normal volunteers, with an emphasis on differential effects of memory function. J Clin Psych 1987; 48:20–23.

32. Lieberman AN, Goldstein M, Gopinathan G, et al. Further studies with pergolide in Parkinson disease. Neurology 1985; 32:1181–1184.

33. McEvoy JP, McCue M, Spring B, et al. Effects of amantadine and trihexyphenidyl on memory in elderly normal volunteers. Am J Psych 1987; 144:573–577.
34. Taylor JL, Tinklenberg JR. Cognitive impairment and benzodiazepines. In: Meltzer HY, ed. Psychopharmacology: The Third Generation of Progress. New York: Raven Press, 1987:1449–1454.
35. Barbee JG. Memory, benzodiazepines, and anxiety: Integration of theoretical and clinical perspectives. J Clin Psych 1993; 54(suppl 10):86–97.
36. Meyers BR. Benzodiazepines in the elderly. Med Clin North Am 1982; 66: 1017–1035.
37. Pomara N, Deptula D, Singh R, et al. Cognitive toxicity of benzodiazepines in the elderly. In: Salzman C, Lebowitz B, eds. Anxiety in the Elderly: Treatment and Research. New York: Springer-Verlag, 1991:175–196.
38. Francis J. Delirium in older patients. J Am Geriatr Soc 1992; 40:829–838.
39. Pomara N, Stanley B, Block R, et al. Increased sensitivity of the elderly to the central depressant effects of diazepam. J Clin Psych 1985; 46:183–187.
40. Foy A, Drinkwater V, March S, et al. Confusion after admission to hospital in elderly patients using benzodiazepines. BMJ 1986; 293:1072.
41. Francis J, Martin D, Kapoor WN. A prospective study of delirium in hospitalized elderly. JAMA 1990; 263:1097–1101.
42. Lennox WG. Brain injury, drugs and environment as causes of mental decay in epilepsy. Am J Psych 1992; 99:174–180.
43. Meador KJ. Cognitive side effects of antiepileptic drugs. Can J Neurol Sci 1994; 21(suppl 3):S12–S16.
44. Meador KJ. Cognitive effects of epilepsy and of antiepileptic medications. In: Wyllie E, ed. The Treatment of Epilepsy: Principles and Practice, 2nd ed. Baltimore: Williams & Wilkins, 1991:1121–1130.
45. Meador KJ, Loring DW. Cognitive effects of antiepileptic drugs. In: Devinsky O, Theodore W, eds. Epilepsy and Behavior. New York: John Wiley & Sons, 1991:151–170.
46. Arnan MG, Welty JS, Paxton JW, et al. Effect of sodium valproate on psychomotor performance in children as a function of dose, fluctuations in concentration, and diagnosis. Epilepsia 1987; 28:115–124.
47. Dekaban AS, Lehman EJB. Effects of different dosages of anticonvulsant drugs on mental performances in patients with chronic epilepsy. Acta Neurol Scand 1975; 52:319–330.
48. Golinger RC, Peet T, Tune L. Association of elevated plasma anticholinergic activity with delirium in surgical patients. Am J Psych 1987; 144:1218–1220.
49. Reynolds EH, Travers RD. Serum anticonvulsant concentrations in epileptic patients with mental symptoms. Br J Psych 1974; 124:440–445.
50. Thompson PI, Trimble MR. The effect of anticonvulsant drugs on cognitive function: Relation to serum levels. J Neurol Neurosurg Psych 1983; 46:227–233.
51. Ludgate J, Keating J, O'Dwyer R, et al. An improvement in cognitive function following polypharmacy reduction in a group of epileptic patients. Acta Neurol Scand 1985; 71:448–452.
52. Grubb BP. Digitalis delirium in an elderly woman. Digitalis Toxicity 1987; 18: 329–330.
53. Prevey ML, Mattson RH, Cramer JA. Improvement in cognitive functioning and mood state after conversion to valproate monotherapy. Neurology 1989; 39: 1640–1641.

54. Shorvon SD, Reynolds EH. Reduction in polypharmacy for epilepsy. BMJ 1979; 2:1023–1025.
55. Meador KJ, Loring DW, Abney OL, et al. Effects of carbamazepine and phenytoin on EEG and memory in healthy adults. Epilepsia 1991; 34:153–157.
56. Meador KJ, Loring DW, Allen ME, et al. Comparative cognitive effects of carbamazepine and phenytoin in healthy adults. Neurology 1991; 41:1537–1540.
57. Meador KJ, Loring DW, Huh K, et al. Comparative cognitive effects of anticonvulsants. Neurology 1990; 40:391–394.
58. Meador KJ, Loring DW, Moore EE, et al. Comparative cognitive effects of phenobarbital, phenytoin and valproate in healthy adults. Neurology 1989; 45:1494–1499.
59. Smith DB, Mattson RH, Cramer JA, et al. Results of a nationwide Veterans Administration cooperative study comparing the efficacy and toxicity of carbamazepine, phenobarbital, phenytoin, and primidone. Epilepsia 1987; 28(suppl 3): S50–S58.
60. Prevey ML, Delaney RC, Cramer JA, et al. Valproate versus carbamazepine: Comparison of effects on cognitive functioning. Epilepsia 1992; 33:110.
61. Craig I, Tallis R. The impact of sodium valproate and phenytoin on cognitive function in elderly patients: Results of a singleblind randomized comparative study. Epilepsia 1994; 35:381–390.
62. Leach JP, Girvan J, Paul A, et al. Gabapentin and cognition: A double-blind, dose-ranging, placebo-controlled study in refractory epilepsy. J Neurol Neurosurg Psych 1997; 62:372–376.
63. Brodie M, Richens A, Yuen A WC, UK Lamotrigine/Carbamazepine Monotherapy Trial Group. Double-blind comparison of lamotrigine and carbamazepine in newly diagnosed epilepsy. Lancet 1995; 345:476–479.
64. Smith D, Baker G, Davies G, et al. Outcomes of add-on treatment with lamotrigine in partial epilepsy. Epilepsia 1993; 34:312–322.
65. Aikia M, Kalviainen R, Sivenius J, et al. Cognitive effects of oxcarbazepine and phenytoin monotherapy in newly diagnosed epilepsy: one year follow-up. Epilepsy Res 1992; 11(3):199–203.
66. Dodrill CB, Arnett JL, SommelVille K, et al. Cognitive and quality of life effects of differing dosages of tiagabine in epilepsy. Neurology 1997; 48:1025–1031.
67. Dodrill CB, Arnett JL, SommelVille KW, et al. Evaluation of the effects of vigabatrin on cognitive abilities and quality of life in epilepsy. Neurology 1993; 43:2501–2507.
68. Dodrill CB, Arnett JL, SommelVille KW, et al. Effects of differing dosages of vigabatrin (Sabril) on cognitive abilities and quality of life in epilepsy. Epilepsy 1995; 36:164–173.
69. Gillham RA, Blacklaw J, McKee PJW, et al. Effect of vigabatrin on sedation and cognitive function in patients with refractory epilepsy. J Neurol Neurosurg Psych 1993; 56:1271–1275.
70. Grunewald RA, Thompson PI, Corcoran R, et al. Effects of vigabatrin on partial seizures and cognitive function. J Neurol Neurosurg Psych 1994; 57:1057–1063.
71. Muldoon MF, Manuck SB, Shapiro AP, et al. Neurobehavioral effects of antihypertensive medications. J Hypertens 1991; 9:549–559.

72. Frcka G, Lader M. Psychotropic effects of repeated doses of enalapril, propranolol and atenolol in normal subjects. Br J Clin Pharm 1988; 25:67–73.
73. Gengo FM, Kalonaros GC, McHugh WB. Attenuation of response to mental stress in patients with essential tremor treated with metroprolol Arch Neurol 1986; 43: 687–689.
74. Dimsdale J, Newton R, Joist T. Neuropsychological side effects of beta blockers. Arch Intern Med 1989; 149:514–525.
75. Omvik P, Thaulow E, Herland OB, et al. Double-blind, parallel, comparative study on quality of life during treatment with amlodipine or enalapril in mild or moderate hypertensive patients: a multicenter study. J Hypertension 1993; 11:103–113.
76. Tucker AR, Ng KT. Digoxin-related impairment of learning and memoir in cardiac patients. Psychopharmacology 1983; 81:86–88.
77. Eisendrath SJ, Goldman B, Douglas J, et al. Meperidine-induced delirium. Am J Psych 1987; 13:1062–1065.
78. Kaiko RF, Foley KM, Grabinski PY, et al. Central nervous system excitatory effects of meperidine in cancer patients. Ann Neurol 1983; 21:180–185.
79. Marcantonio ER, Juarez G, Goldman L, et al. The relationship of postoperative delirium with psychoactive medications. JAMA 1994; 272:1518–1522.
80. Hoppmann RA, Peden JG, Ober SK. Central nervous system side effects of non-steroidal anti-inflammatory drugs. Arch Intern Med 1991; 151:1309–1313.
81. Weingartner H, Eckardt M, Molchan S, et al. Neuropsychological factors in mental disorders and their treatments. Psychopharm Bull 1992; 28:331–340.
82. Atkinson K, Biggs J, Darveniza P, et al. Cyclosporine-associated central nervous system toxicity after allogeneic bone marrow transplantation. Transplantation 1987; 38:34–37.
83. De Groen PC, Aksamit AJ, Rakela J, et al. Central nervous system toxicity after liver transplantation. N Eng J Med 1987; 317:861–866.
84. Wilczek H, Ringden O, Tyden G. Cyclosporine-associated central nervous system toxicity after renal transplantation. Transplantation 1985; 39:110.
85. Thomas RJ. Neurotoxicity of antibacterial therapy. South Med J 1994; 87:869–874.
86. Farwell JR, Lee YJ, Hirtz DG, et al. Phenobarbital for febrile seizures—effects on intelligence and on seizure recurrence. N Engl J Med 1990; 322:364–369.
87. Silberfarb PM. Chemotherapy and cognitive defects in cancer patients. Ann Rev Med 1983; 34:35–46.
88. Gottlieb D, Bradstock K, Koutts J, et al. The neurotoxicity of high-dose cytosine arabinoside is age-related. Cancer 1987; 60:1439–1441.
89. Adams F, Quesda J, Guttennan J. Neuropsychiatric manifestations of human leukocyte interferon therapy in patients with cancer. JAMA 1984; 252:938–941.
90. The Medical Letter, Vol. 44 (Issue 1134), July 2, 2002.
91. Meadar KJ. Iatrogenic disorders: cognitive side effects of medications. Neurology Clinics 1988; 6(1):141–158.
92. Sunderland T, Tariot P, Cohen RM, et al. Anticholinergic sensitivity in patients with dementia of the Alzheimer type and age-matched controls: a dose response study. Arch Gen Psych 1987; 44:418–426.
93. Miller PS, Richardson JS, Jyu CA, et al. Association of low serum anticholinergic levels and cognitive impairment in elderly presurgical patients. Am J Psych 1988; 145:342–345.
94. Tune LE. Serum anticholinergic activity levels and delirium in the elderly. Seminars Clin Neuropsych 2000; 5(2):149–153.

95. Mewaldt SP, Ghoneim MM. The effects and interactions of scopolamine, physostigmine and methamphetamine on human memory. Pharm Biochem Behav 1983; 10:205–210.
96. Mulsant BH, Pollack BG, Kirschner M, et al. Serum anticholinergic activity in a community based sample of older adults: relationship with cognitive performance. Arch Gen Psych 2003; 60:198–203.
97. Folstein ME, Folstein SE, McHugh PR. "Mini-mental state." A practical method for grading the cognitive state of patients for the clinician. Psych Res 1975; 12(3):189–198.
98. Lerner AJ, Hedera P, Koss E, et al. Delirium in Alzheimer's Disease. Alzheimer Disease & Associated Disorders 1997; 11:16–20.
99. Lu CJ, Tune L. Chronic exposure to anticholinergic medications adversely affects the course of Alzheimer Disease. Am J Geriatric Psych 2003; 11:458–461.
100. Perry EK, Kilford L, Lees A, et al. Increased Alzheimer pathology in Parkinson's disease related to antimuscarinic drugs. Ann Neurol 2003; 54:235–238.
101. Tune L, Carr S, Cooper TC, et al. Anticholinergic effects of drugs commonly prescribed in the elderly:potential means for assessing risk of delirium. Am J Psych 1993; 149:139–143.
102. Tune L, Egeli S. Acetylcholine and delirium. Dementia & Geriatric Cognitive Disorder. 1999; 10(5):32–34.
103. Han L, McCusker J, Cole M, Abrahamowicz M, Primeau F, Elie M. Use of medications with anticholinergic effects predicts clinical severity of delirium in older medical inpatients. Arch Int Med 2001; 161(8):1099–1105.
104. Tune L, Coyle JT. Serum levels of anticholinergic drugs in the treatment of acute extrapyramidal side effects. Arch Gen Psych 1980; 37:293–297.
105. Tune L, Holland A, Folstein M, et al. Association of postoperative delirium with raised serum anticholinergic levels Lancet; 1981; ii:651–653.
106. Mondimore F, Damlouji N, Folstein, et al. Post-ECT confusional states associated with elevated serum anticholinergic levels. Am J Psych 1983; 140:930–931.
107. Gollinger RC, Peet T, Tune L. Association of elevated plasma anticholinergic activity with delirium in surgical patients. Am J Psych 1987; 144:1218–1220.
108. Rovner B, David A, Lucas-Blaustein MJ, et al. Self care capacity and anticholinergic drug levels in nursing home patients. Am J Psych 1988; 145:107–109.
109. Tune LE, Bylsma FW, Hilt DC. Anticholinergic delirium caused by topical homatropine ophthalmologic solution: confirmation by anticholinergic radioreceptor assay in two cases. J Neuropsych 1992; 4(2):195–197.
110. Mach JF, Dysken M, Kuskowski M, et al. Serum anticholinergic activity in hospitalized older persons with delirium: a preliminary study. J Am Geriatric Soc 1995; 43:491–495.
111. Tollefson G, Montague-Close J, Lancaster SP. The relationship of serum anticholinergic to mental status performance in an elderly nursing home population. J Neuropsych Clin Neurosci 1991; 3:314–319.
112. Flacker J, Lipsitz LA. Serum anticholinergic activity changes with acute illness in elderly medical patients. Am J Geriatric Psych 1988; 6:47–54.
113. Livingston RL, Zucker DK, Isenberg K, et al. Tricyclic antidepressants and delirium. J Clin Psych 1983; 44:173–176.
114. Mussi C, Ferrari R, Ascari S, et al. Importance of serum anticholinergic activity in the assessment of elderly patients with delirium. J Geriatric Psych Neurol 1999; 12:82–86.

Appendix

DRUGS THAT MAY CAUSE PSYCHIATRIC SYMPTOMS

Some Drug Classes

Drug	Reactions	Comments
Amphetamine-like drugs	Bizarre behavior, hallucinations, paranoia, agitation, anxiety, mania, nightmares	Usually with overdose or abuse; can occur with inhaler abuse; depression on withdrawal
Anabolic steroids	Psychosis, mania, depression, anxiety, aggressiveness, paranoia	Most reports based on abuse
Angiotensin-converting enzyme (ACE) inhibitors	Mania, anxiety, hallucinations, depression, psychosis	Many reports
Antichollinergics and atropine	Confusion, memory loss, disorientation, depersonalization, delirium, auditory and visual hallucinations, fear, paranoia, agitation, bizarre behavior	More frequent in elderly and children with high doses; can occur with transdermal scopolamine
	Sudden incoherent speech, delirium, with high fever, flushed dry skin, hallucinations, retrograde amnesia	From eye drops, particularly when mistaken for nose drops
Antidepressants, tricyclic	Mania or hypomania, delirium, hallucinations, paranoia, irritability, dysphoria	Patients with bipolar disorder at highest risk for mania; antichollinergic effects may cause delirium in elderly
Antiepileptics	Agitation, confusion, delirium, depression, psychosis, aggression, mania, toxic encephalopathy, nightmares	Usually with high doses or high plasma concentrations

(Continued)

Some Drug Classes (*Continued*)

Drug	Reactions	Comments
Barbiturates	Excitement, hyperactivity, visual hallucinations, depression, delirium-tremens-like syndrome	Especially in children and elderly, or on withdrawal
Benzodiazepines	Rage, hostility, paranoia, hallucinations, delirium, depression, nightmares, anterograde amnesia, mania, disinhibition	During treatment or on withdrawal; may be more common in elderly
Beta-adrenergic blockers	Depression, psychosis, delirium, anxiety, nightmares, hallucinations	With oral or ophthalmic preparations; incidence of depression may be overestimated
Calcium-channel blockers	Depression, delirium, confusion, psychosis, mania	Several reports
Cephalosporins	Euphoria, delusions, depersonalization, illusions	Renal disease is a risk factor
Corticosteroids (prednisone, cortisone, ACTH, others)	Psychosis, delirium, mania, depression	1–3% incidence; may be dose-related; can occur on withdrawal
Corticosteroids, inhaled	Hyperactivity, aggression, disinhibition	Several reports
Dopamine receptor agonists	Hallucinations, paranoia, delusions, confusion, mania, hypersexuality, anxiety, depression, nightmares	During treatment or on withdrawal
Estrogens	Panic attacks, depression	Several reports
Fluoroquinolone antibiotics	Psychosis, confusion, agitation, depression, hallucinations, paranoia, Tourette-like syndrome, mania	Many reports
Histamine H_1-receptor blockers	Hallucinations	Especially with overdose of first generation drugs
Histamine H_2-receptor blockers	Delium, confusion, psychosis, mania, aggression, depression, nightmares	Especially elderly and seriously ill

(*Continued*)

Some Drug Classes *(Continued)*

Drug	Reactions	Comments
HMG-CoA reductase inhibitors ("statins")	Anxiety, depression, obsessions, delusions	Several reports
Monoamine oxidase (MAO) inhibitors	Mania or hypomania	
Nonsteroidal anti-inflammatory drugs (NSAIDs)	Depression, paranoia, psychosis, confusion, anxiety	Probably more common with indomethacin; one case of auditory hallucinations with celecoxib *(Celebrex)*
Opioids	Nightmares, anxiety, agitation, euphoria, dysphoria, depression, paranoia, psychosis, hallucinations, dementia	Usually with high doses; also occurs with intrathecal morphine; especially in elderly
Procaine derivatives (procainamide, procaine penicillin G)	Fear of imminent death, hallucinations, illusions, delusions, agitation, mania, depersonalization, psychosis	Probably due to procaine
Salicylates	Agitation, confusion, hallucinations, paranoia	Chronic intoxication
Sulfonamides	Confusion, disorientation, depression, euphoria, hallucinations	Several reports
Thiazide diuretics	Depression, suicidal ideation	After weeks to months of use

Note: Also available with other brand names or generically.

Some Individual Drugs

Drug	Reactions	Comments
Acetazolamide (*Diamox**)	Depression, delirium, confusion, stupor	Especially elderly, or with renal disease, hypoalbuminernia or concurrent salicylates[17]
Acyclovir (*Zovirax**)	Hallucinations, fearfulness, confusion, insomnia, hyperacusia, paranoia, depression	At high doses, particularly in patients with chronic renal failure

(Continued)

Some Individual Drugs (*Continued*)

Drug	Reactions	Comments
Amantadine (*Symmetrel**)	Illusions, visual hallucinations, delusions, depression	Risk increases with duration of therapy; more common in elderly
Asparaginase (*Elspar*)	Confusion, depression, paranoia	May occur frequently
Baclofen (*Lioresal**)	Hallucinations, paranoia, nightmares, mania, depression, anxiety, confusion	Sometimes with high doses, but usually after sudden withdrawal
Bupropion (*Wellbutrin**)	Psychosis, agitation, anxiety, nightmares, mania	Agitation, anxiety most common
Buspirone (*BuSpar**)	Vivid dreams, delirium, mania, panic attack	In a few patients
Caffeine	Anxiety, confusion, psychotic symptoms	With excessive doses; anxiety on withdrawal
Chlorambucil (*Leukeran*)	Hallucinations, lethargy, seizures, stupor, coma	With high doses
Chloroquine (*Aralen**)	Confusion, delusions, hallucinations, mania	Several reports
Clarithromycin (*Blaxin*)	Mania	Many reports
Clonidine (*Catapres⁺*)	Depression, delirium, psychosis, hallucinations	May resolve with continued use
Clozapine (*Clozaril**)	Delirium	Less with slow dose titration; psychosis following abrupt withdrawal
Cyclobenzaprine (*Flexeril**)	Hallucinations	Especially in elderly
Cycloserine (*Seromycin**)	Agitation, depression, psychosis, anxiety	Many reports
Cytarabine (*Cytosar-U*)	Confusion	Especially with high doses
Dapsone	Insomnia, agitation, hallucinations, mania, depression	Several reports; may occur even with low doses
DEET (*Oil**)	Mania, hallucinations	With excessive or prolonged use
Dextromethorphan (*Robitussin**)	Psychosis	Several reports with high doses

(*Continued*)

Some Individual Drugs (*Continued*)

Drug	Reactions	Comments
Digoxin (*Lanoxin**)	Delirium, depression, psychosis, mania, visual hallucinations	Dose-dependent; elderly at higher risk
Disopyramide (*Norpace**)	Hallucinations, psychosis, paranoia, panic, depression	Within 24–48 hr after starting
Disulfiram (*Antabuse*)	Catatonia, delirium, depression, psychosis	Not related to alchohol reactions
Dronabinol (*Marinol*)	Anxiety, psychosis, confusion	Most disturbing in the elderly
Efavirenz (*Sustiva*)	Vivid dreams or nightmares, hallucinations, anxiety depression, psychosis, confusion	Several reports
Erythropoietin (*Epogen**)	Visual hallucinations	Reported in dialysis and bone marrow transplant patients
Ganciclovir (*Cytovene*)	Psychosis, delirium, confusion	Several reports
Ilostamide (*Ilex*)	Encephalopathy, hallucinations, emotional liability, confusion, psychosis	Several reports, especially in elderly
Interleukin-2 (*Proleukin*)	Hallucinations, confusion	Especially with high doses
Interferon alpha (*Roferon-A**)	Irritability, emotional liability, depression, agitation, paranoia	Depression also on withdrawal
Isoniazid (*INH**)	Psychosis, hallucinations, mania	Several reports
Isotretinoin (*Accutane*)	Depression, suicidality	Several reports
Ketamine (*Ketalar**)	Nightmares, hallucinations, delirium, emotional liability	Acute; frequent with usual doses
Levodopa (*Sinemet**)	Hallucinations, delusions, mania, depression, anxiety, panic attacks, confusion, nightmares	Dose-dependent; anxiety may occur in off phase
Lidocaine (*Xylocaine**)	Hallucinations, psychosis, paranoia, delusions, agitation, anxiety	Several reports

(Continued)

Some Individual Drugs (*Continued*)

Drug	Reactions	Comments
Mefloquine (*Lariam*)	Vivid dreams or nightmares, hallucinations, encephalopathy, depression, confusion, psychosis, aggression, agitation, anxiety	Vivid dreams and nightmares are frequent
Methyldopa (*Aldomet**)	Depression, amnesia, nightmares, psychosis	Incidence of depression may be overestimated
Methylphenidate (*Ritalin**)	Hallucinations, anxiety, ancephalopathy	In children and adults
Methysergide (*Sansert*)	Depersonalization, hallucinations, agitation, depression	Several reports
Metoclopramide (*Reglan**)	Depression, anxiety, mania	Several reports; confusion in elderly
Metronidazole (*Flagyl**)	Depression, agitation, emotional liability, confusion, hallucinations	Many reports
Nevirapine (*Viramune*)	Hallucinations, delirium, psychosis	Several reports
Ondansetron (*Zofran*)	Panic attack, dysphoria	Occurs rarely
Pilocarpine (*Pilocar**)	Confusion, agitation, memory loss	Topical ocular use especially in elderly and demented patients
Propafenone (*Rythmol**)	Agitation, delusions, disorientation, mania, paranoia	Several reports
Pseudoephedrine (*Sudafed**)	Hallucinations, paranoia, psychosis	Reported in children with usual doses
Quinidine	Confusion, agitation, psychosis	Usually dose-related
Selegiline (*Eldepryl**)	Hallucinations, mania, nightmares, behavioral disturbance, confusion, hypersexuality, delusions	Several reports
Sildenafil (*Viagra*)	Aggression, confusion, delusions, hallucinations, mania, paranoia	Several reports

(*Continued*)

Some Individual Drugs (*Continued*)

Drug	Reactions	Comments
Sumatriptan (*Imitrex*)	Panic-like somatic symptoms	Especially with history of anxiety
Theophylline	Mutism, hyperactivity, anxiety, mania	With high serum concentrations
Tizanidine (*Zanaflex*)	Hallucinations	Reported in 3% of patients in cilinical trials
Trazodone (*Desyrel**)	Delirium, hallucinations, paranoia, mania	Several reports
Trimethoprim-sulfamethoxazole (*Bactrim**)	Delirium, psychosis, depression, hallucinations	Several reports
Venlafaxine (*Effexor*)	Visual hallucinations, mania	Few reports
Vinblastine (*Velban**)	Depression, anxiety	May occur commonly and is dose-related
Vincristine (*Oncovin**)	Hallucinations, depression	May be dose-related
Zaleplon (*Sonata*)	Visual illusions, anxiety, depression, hallucinations	
Zolpidem (*Ambien*)	Psychosis, hallucinations, sensory distortions	Women may be at greater risk; higher doses may increase risk

Note: Brand names are in italics.
*Also available with other brand names or generically.

12

Cognitive Impairment in Depression

Irene Hegeman Richard

Department of Neurology, University of Rochester Medical Center, Rochester, New York, U.S.A.

INTRODUCTION

Major depressive disorder may be associated with complaints of memory impairment, difficulty thinking and concentrating, and an overall reduction in cognitive abilities. Subjective complaints of altered cognition may be accompanied by impaired performance on objective measures (mental status exam and neuropsychological testing). Tests on which performance is frequently impaired involve attention, mental processing speed, spontaneous elaboration, and analysis of detail (1). Particularly in elderly persons, it is often difficult to determine whether cognitive deficits are better accounted for by a dementia or by a major depressive episode (2). However, it is important to remember that depression is quite common in dementia, particularly early in the disease process (3).

In this chapter, the cognitive deficits associated with depression will be reviewed and compared with those caused by dementia. The complex relationship between depression and dementia will be explored and the issue of whether or not cognitive abilities are differentially affected in young versus old depressed patients will be examined. Finally, there will be a brief discussion of issues related to the treatment of depression in patients with cognitive impairment.

The term most often used when referring to reversible cognitive deficits caused by psychiatric conditions has been "pseudodementia." This term was originally used to describe any patient who had cognitive disturbance caused by any psychiatric impairment (including depression, psychosis, conversion, and personality disorders) (4). The term pseudodementia is sometimes made more specific by using the adjective "depressive" pseudodementia. Folstein et al. (5) used the phrase "dementia syndrome of depression" when describing a group of depressed patients with decreased Mini Mental Status Examination (MMSE) scores that improved with resolution of depression. The phrase "cognitive impairment of depression" is probably better to use than terms containing the word "dementia" (since the relationship between dementia and depression is already complex and confusing enough).

DEPRESSIVE SUBTYPES AND COGNITIVE IMPAIRMENT

Not all depressed patients have cognitive deficits and the degree of cognitive impairment does not necessarily correlate with the severity of the depression. Most evidence suggests that a subgroup (or certain subgroups) of depressed patients are more likely to develop cognitive impairment.

Austin et al. (6) demonstrated that patients with melancholic depression had more cognitive impairments than non-melancholic patients. Melancholic patients were impaired in their tasks of memory, selective attention and set-shifting, while non-melancholic subjects were largely unimpaired in their cognitive performance.

Melancholic depression is a subtype of depression characterized by a unique profile of features. According to DSM-IV (2), in order to use the "melancholic features specifier" a patient must experience either (i) anhedonia (a loss of pleasure in all, or almost all, activities) and/or (ii) a lack of reactivity to usually pleasurable stimuli (does not feel better, even temporarily, when something good happens). In addition, the patient must experience three or more of the following: (i) a distinct quality of the depressed mood (different than sadness or the feeling experienced after the death of a loved one), (ii) depression regularly worse in the morning, (iii) early morning awakening, (iv) marked psychomotor retardation or agitation, (v) significant anorexia or weight loss, and (vi) excessive or inappropriate guilt.

Massman et al. (7) compared memory test profiles of unipolar depressives ($n = 40$) and bipolar depressives ($n = 9$) with those of patients with a prototypical subcortical dementia (Huntington's disease, HD), patients with a prototypical cortical dementia (Alzheimer's disease, AD), and normal controls. In a discriminant function analysis that well differentiated the HD, AD, and normal subjects, it was found that 28.6% of the depressed patients were classified as performing like HD patients (DEP-HD subjects), 49.0% were classified as normals (DEP-N subjects), none were classified as performing like AD patients, and 22.4% were not well classified. The authors concluded that their findings provide support for the hypothesis that subcortical dysfunction occurs in patients with depression, but only for a subgroup of depressed patients.

THE CLINICAL EVALUATION: PROFILE OF COGNITIVE DEFICITS IN DEPRESSION AND DISTINCTIONS FROM DEMENTIA

History

The history can be of great help in distinguishing between depression- and dementia-related cognitive impairment. Rabins et al. (8) validated criteria for diagnosing reversible dementia caused by depression. Eighteen patients fulfilling DSM-III criteria for both major depression and dementia were matched by age and sex to patients with a diagnosis of irreversible dementia and patients with a diagnosis of major depression alone. A past history of depression, self-reports of depressed mood, self-blaming, hopeless and somatic delusions, appetite disturbance, and subacute onset identified the patients suffering from cognitive impairment caused by depression. Two-year follow-up confirmed the initial diagnosis and demonstrated that co-existing cognitive impairment and major depression are not usually precursory to a progressive dementing illness.

The following components of the history may be helpful in distinguishing cognitive impairment of depression from dementia:

1. *Rate of Onset*: In general, the onset of depressive cognitive impairment is relatively abrupt (or subacute), whereas that associated with dementia is more gradual and insidious (2,9,10). The symptoms of depression usually precede those of cognitive loss (11).

2. *Somatic Complaints and Vegetative Symptoms*: Elderly depressed patients tend to have many physical complaints, and, if psychotic, are more likely to experience somatic delusions. Depressed patients are more likely to experience disturbances of "vegetative" functions (e.g., appetite disturbance) (12).

3. *Subjective Complaints of and Distress Related to Cognitive Impairment*: It has long been noted that depressed patients are more likely to complain about their cognitive deficits and experience distress related to perceived impairments. The complaints may be out of proportion to the objective findings. Some investigators have specifically examined this issue.

Wang et al. (13) examined the associations of subjective memory complaint in old age with objective test performance, past and subsequent cognitive decline, and depression. A total of 543 Chinese men and women aged 65 years and older were examined twice during a 3-year period. Examinations consisted of neurological histories and examinations as well as administration of the cognitive abilities screening instrument (CASI) and the geriatric depression scale-short version (GDS-S). Subjective memory complaints were associated with poorer objective memory performance even after controlling the effect of depression and demographic data, but did not predict faster cognitive decline or dementia over three years.

Riedel-Heller et al. (14) examined the prevalence of memory complaints and assessed the validity of memory complaints for detecting cognitive impairment in 349 randomly selected non-institutionalized individuals, aged 75 and over. Twenty individuals who suffered from moderate or severe dementia according to DSM-III-R were excluded. Memory complaints were measured by means of a single item question. The MMSE and the short neuropsychological battery of the SIDAM (structured interview for the diagnosis of dementia of Alzheimer type, Multi-infarct dementia, and dementias of other etiology according to ICD-10 and DSM-III-R) were used to test cognitive performance. One in three individuals aged 75 and over complained about memory deficits. The MMSE was not significantly related to memory complaints, whereas poorer performance on two of eight tests regarding specific areas of cognitive function (immediate recall, short-term memory) were found to be significantly associated with memory complaints. Despite these statistically significant associations, it was noted that memory complaints do not have diagnostic validity in detecting cognitive impairment on the individual level. These authors concluded that memory self-assessment should not be used as a substitute measure of cognitive performance. They noted that relying solely on memory complaints would miss individuals in need and allocate resources to worried but cognitively healthy persons.

Neuropsychological Testing

Neuropsychological testing cannot always distinguish cognitive impairments related to depression from those secondary to dementia. However, there tend to be qualitative and quantitative differences in performance which, when combined with other clinical information, can help with the diagnosis. Overall, the pattern of cognitive impairment in depression has been described as "subcortical," characterized most frequently by problems with attention, rapid mental processing, spontaneous verbal elaboration, and memory retrieval (1). On the other hand, cortical functions, including language, tend to be spared.

There are some aspects of the neuropsychological performance that help to distinguish the cognitive impairment seen in depression from that seen in dementia (cortical or subcortical). Inconsistent cognitive performance is frequently seen in depression (4). Depressed patients often do poorly on some tests of memory and intelligence but unexpectedly well on others. There may also be inconsistency between the degree of cognitive deficits on objective evaluations (e.g., memory testing) and the cognitive capacities demonstrated during "informal" encounters (e.g., conversations in which the patient provides very detailed accounts of recent events). Depressed patients often do not put forth full effort and tend to give "don't know" answers, rather than guessing or confabulating (11,15,16).

Another distinguishing feature of depression-related cognitive impairment is that depressed patients rarely experience the nocturnal worsening of cognitive functions ("sundowning") so often observed in demented patients. In fact, patients who have major depression with melancholia frequently exhibit improvement as the day goes on. Moffoot et al. (17) assessed 20 depressed patients and 20 controls with a battery of neuropsychological tests. A morning pattern of neuropscyhological impairment in the depressed patients affected attention and concentration/working memory, episodic memory, reaction time, and the speed of simultaneous match to sample. The depressed patients had significantly improved neuropsychological function in the evening, along with diurnal improvement in mood.

Specific Cognitive Functions Affected in Depression: Attention, Memory, and Speed

Attentional difficulties are seen in depression (7,18–20) and may result in problems with other aspects of testing since attention is a prerequisite to many other cognitive tasks.

In the literature, memory disturbances are the most frequently discussed cognitive impairment associated with depression. Most studies suggest that depressed patients can learn new information but that they may have problems with registration (due to poor attention) and spontaneous recall (but do well with recognition or cued recall) (7,16). Unlike many patients with dementia, they do not have problems with retention (once information is learned, they do not forget rapidly) (12). It has been hypothesized that memory dysfunction in depression results from "weak or incomplete encoding strategies" (21) reflecting insufficient or poorly sustained effort, although automatic memory processes remain intact (22,23). Thus, the new information is learned but not in such a way as to facilitate retrieval, so much of what was learned must wait for the stimulus of cueing or a recognition format to help it become manifest (19).

Research by Murray et al. (24) suggests that, although positive and negative trait words were adequately encoded in memory, depressed patients were better able to retrieve "negative" words (i.e., words with a sad or bad affective content). Research by one group suggests that, with increasing age, depression may affect learning and recognition (25) (see discussion that follows later).

Depression is frequently associated with "psychomotor" slowing. This implies that patients have slowing of their mental processing speed, as well as slowing of their motor function. According to DSM-IV (2), depressed patients who meet criteria for psychomotor retardation must exhibit motor slowing of sufficient severity to be observed by others.

Some have suggested that psychomotor retardation is a secondary result of changes in attention, arousal or motivation (26,27), while others view the motor change as a "core" behavioral pattern (28). There appears to be a correlation between psychomotor retardation and cognitive deficits in depression (29). The finding of psychomotor retardation in depression emphasizes the importance of viewing major depressive disorder (particularly depression with melancholic features) as a syndrome, including impairments in not only mood, but cognitive, motor, and vegetative functions (2,6).

Cognitive Functions Preserved in Depression: Orientation, Language, and Construction

Unlike many demented patients, depressed patients usually remain oriented since incidental learning (establishing memories through daily experiences) generally remains intact.

While Alzheimer's disease (AD) is characterized by cortical deficits including aphasia, apraxia and agnosias, the presence of language disturbances is extremely rare in depression (12,16,29,30). An age-related effect was found on learning and recognition in depression, and also an age-related impairment in naming (see discussion below).

Constructional ability is frequently impaired in dementia. Even early in their illness, dementia patients may show severe impairment on both copy and recall trials of drawing tests and on constructional tasks, despite appropriate effort. The performance of depressed patients may be careless or incomplete due to apathy, low energy level, and poor motivation but, if given enough time and encouragement, they may make a recognizable and often fully adequate response (12,31).

Cognitive Functions Sometimes Affected in Depression: Executive Function

Executive functions include planning, sequencing, organizing, and abstracting. The frontal lobes are thought to be responsible for these processes. Impairment in frontal or "executive" functions has been reported even in dysphoric college students (32), but is most frequently reported in severely depressed patients (33–35) or in older patients, particularly those with a poorer prognosis (36,37).

Alexopolus et al. (36) investigated the relationship of executive function and memory impairment to relapse, recurrence, and course of residual symptoms in elderly subjects with major depression. Executive dysfunction (abnormal initiation and perseverations) was associated with relapse and recurrence of depression. Neither memory impairment nor other factors, including disability, medical burden, social support and history of previous episodes, influenced the outcome of depression. It has been noted that patients who experience executive dysfunction may represent a subtype of cognitively impaired depressives (38). It has also been noted that executive dysfunction is correlated with white matter lesions (39).

Rating Scales

In general, there is no universally accepted rating scale that can distinguish between dementia- and depression-related cognitive impairment. However, one group of researchers (40) proposed the use of a new scale to diagnose "pseudo-dementia." They administered the checklist to 128 patients who were referred to their clinic for the differential diagnosis of dementia versus pseudodementia.

The "gold standard" diagnosis was that performed by a psychiatrist 18 months later. The checklist contains 44 questions with "yes" or "no" answers that were noted in the literature to differentiate between organic dementia and depressive pseudodementia. The checklist contains 44 questions and covers the areas of history, clinical data, insight, and performance. An 18-item shortened questionnaire was able to classify 98% (43/44 cases) of dementia cases and 95% (60/63) of depression patients correctly. The authors suggested that depressive pseudodementia may be classified into two subtypes: Type I is a group of patients who have depressive symptoms with subjective memory complaints without measurable intellectual deficits. Type II is a group of patients who have depressive symptoms and show poor cognitive performance based on poor concentration not due to organic disorder.

Biomarkers and Laboratory Tests

There are no routinely used laboratory tests that can distinguish between depression and dementia in the cognitively impaired patient.

Rosen (41) suggests that, at an early stage of clinical evaluation, EEG may be useful in the discrimination of organic dementia from pseudodementia, because EEG is usually normal in depression but abnormal in AD.

One polysomnographic study (42) examined parameters of sleep continuity, architecture, and REM sleep to differentiate dementia from depression. The authors investigated 35 dementia of the Alzheimer-type (DAT) patients, 39 old-age depressed (OAD) patients, and 42 healthy controls for two consecutive nights in the sleep laboratory. The DAT patients were in relatively early/mild stages of the disease, the severity of depression in the OAD group was moderate to severe. Depressed patients showed characteristic "depression-like" EEG sleep alterations, that is, a lower sleep efficiency, a higher amount of nocturnal awakenings and decreased sleep stage 2. Sleep continuity and architecture in DAT was less disturbed. Nearly all REM sleep measures significantly differentiated the diagnostic groups. OAD patients showed a shortened REM latency, increased REM density and a high rate of sleep onset REM periods (SOREM), whereas in DAT, REM density was decreased in comparison with control subjects. To assess the discriminative power of REM sleep variables, a series of discriminant analyses were conducted. Overall, 86% of the patients were correctly classified, using REM density and REM latency measures. The authors suggest that REM density as an indicator of phasic activity appears to be more sensitive as a biological marker for the differentiation of OAD and DAT than REM latency.

LOCALIZATION

Many authors have suggested that the cognitive impairments in depression resemble those seen in "subcortical" dementias and reflect a functional disconnection between subcortical structures and the frontal lobes. Particular emphasis has been placed on prefrontal and cingulate cortical regions.

Prefrontal cortical deficits include difficulty initiating voluntary responses, shifting attention, and cognitive set, inhibiting context-inappropriate responses, and maintaining information in working memory. Merriam et al. (43) provided evidence for prefrontal cortical dysfunction in depression using the Wisconsin card sorting test (WCST). This widely used neuropsychological index of prefrontal cortical function was administered to 79 patients with major depression who had been unmedicated for at least 28 days, 47 patients with schizophrenia who had never received antipsychotic medication, and 61 healthy comparison subjects. Depressed patients demonstrated significant deficits on multiple WCST measures compared with healthy individuals. Deficits were correlated with the severity of depression and were less severe than those demonstrated by patients with schizophrenia.

As noted earlier, the study by Austin et al. (6) suggests that depressed patients with melancholia are particularly vulnerable to cognitive impairment. Their study involved 77 depressed subjects and 28 controls. Unlike the cognitively intact non-melancholic patients, the melancholic patients were impaired on tasks of memory, selective attention, and set-shifting. This profile of cognitive impairment reflects dysfunction of the frontal lobes. In their discussion, the authors cite a framework suggested by Alexander et al. (44) who proposed the existence of a number of fronto-subcortical neural networks impacting upon motor function, cognition, and mood. The authors comment that the results of their studies support the dysfunction of the anterior cingulate in patients with melancholic depression, citing Mayberg et al. (45), who postulated that the dorsal anterior cingulate (AC) (in conjunction with the dorsolateral prefrontal cortex) modulates the cognitive and psychomotor aspects of depression while the ventral AC is thought to modulate vegetative, autonomic and affective aspects of depression, via the modulation of the subgenual prefrontal cortex.

Using functional imaging, Mayberg et al. (46) have provided compelling evidence implicating the dorsolateral prefrontal cortex, particularly in the right hemisphere, as a key brain structure in emotion/cognition interactions in negative mood states. In one study, they found that reciprocal changes involving subgenual cingulate and right prefrontal cortex occur with both transient and chronic changes in depressed mood. The authors note that the presence and maintenance of functional reciprocity between these regions with shifts in mood in either direction suggest that these regional interactions are obligatory and probably mediate the well-recognized relationships between mood and attention seen in both normal and pathological conditions.

ETIOLOGY

Although there is clear evidence that depressed patients may experience cognitive impairment, the precise etiology of cognitive dysfunction is not known. This is not surprising since the etiology of depression itself remains elusive.

A study by O'Brien et al. (47) suggests that the vulnerability of some depressed patients to developing cognitive impairment during a depressive episode is *not* related to AD-type neuropathological changes. Neuropathological assessments were performed on 11 subjects (five with cognitive impairment) who died during episodes of major depression. No Lewy bodies were found and plaque and tangle counts were within normal limits for age. There were no significant differences in plaque and tangle counts between the cognitively impaired and intact groups.

Although the study by O'Brien et al. (47) also demonstrated no difference between their two small groups on the basis of vascular pathology, other studies support the notion that white matter ischemic disease predisposes some patients to the development of depression-related cognitive impairment. Kramer-Ginsberg et al. (48) conducted a study in which 41 elderly subjects with major depression and 38 healthy elderly controls underwent MRI scans and neuropsychological testing. Depressed patients with moderate to severe white matter hyperintensities demonstrated worse performance on tests of executive function, memory, and language than did depressed patients without such lesions and normal elderly subjects with or without deep white matter changes. The authors suggest that the presence of deep white matter changes may predispose individuals to cognitive impairment but that the cognitive impairment may only become manifest during depression, perhaps due to state-related changes in cerebral metabolism.

There is substantial evidence linking dysfunction of the hypothalamic–pituitary axis (HPA) to depression. Van Londen et al. (49) studied medication-free patients with major depression and found that global intellectual functioning (on neuropsychological testing) was negatively correlated with mean baseline plasma concentrations of cortisol and that certain aspects of cognitive function were positively correlated with high mean plasma vasopressin concentrations. No association was found between neuropsychological performance and plasma concentrations of oxytocin. The authors suggest that vasopressin independently enhances memory, directly or indirectly through increasing arousal and attention.

THE RELATIONSHIP BETWEEN DEPRESSION AND DEMENTIA

There appears to be a definite but ill-defined relationship between dementia and depression. Jorm (50) explored this relationship and, based on this meta-analysis, concluded that depression was associated with an increased risk of subsequent dementia in both case control and prospective studies. This author noted that further work is needed to examine depression as a prodrome of vascular dementia, depression as an early reaction to perceived cognitive decline, the effects of depression on the threshold for manifesting dementia, and depression as a source of hippocampal damage through a glucocorticoid cascade. In this section, the possibilities that (i) depression may be a cause of dementia, and (ii) depression may be an early sign of preclinical AD will be explored.

In support of the theory that depression may cause dementia (or contribute to it) are the results of a controlled cohort study by Kessing (51), which revealed a possible association between the number of depressive episodes and the cognitive outcome. Patients who were hospitalized with an affective diagnosis, and who fulfilled criteria for a primary affective unipolar or bipolar disorder according the ICD-10, were compared with age- and gender-matched controls. Interviews and assessments of cognitive function were made in the euthymic phase. About 118 unipolar patients, 28 bipolar patients, and 58 controls were included. Patients with recurrent episodes were significantly more impaired than patients with a single episode and more impaired than controls. It was the number of depressive episodes that correlated with cognitive decline rather than the number of manic or mixed episodes. They noted that the mean age of the unipolar patients was greater than 65 years and included the caveat that the association between the number of episodes and cognitive outcome may not be valid for younger patients.

Another line of evidence supporting the notion that depression might actually cause dementia relates the known effects of glucocorticoids on the hippocampus. McEwen (52) notes that the hippocampus displays structural plasticity, involving ongoing neurogenesis of the dentate gyrus, synaptogenesis under control of estrogens in the CA1 region, and dendritic remodeling caused by repeated stress or elevated levels of exogenous glucocorticoids in the CA3 region. In all three forms of structural plasticity, excitatory amino acids participate along with circulating steroid hormones. This author hypothesizes that structural plasticity of the hippocampus in response to repeated stress starts out as an adaptive and protective response, but ends up as being damaging if the imbalance in the regulation of the key mediators is not resolved.

Maurice et al. (53) report that steroids, synthesized in peripheral glands or centrally in the brain, exert an important role as modulators of neuronal activity by interacting with different receptors or ion channels. In addition to the modulation of GABA(A), NMDA or cholinergic receptors, neuroactive steroids interact with an atypical intracellular receptor, the sigma 1 protein. At the cellular level, sigma 1 agonists modulate intracellular calcium mobilization and extra-cellular calcium influx, NMDA-mediated responses, acetylcholine release, and alter monoaminergic systems. At the behavioral level, the sigma 1 receptor is involved in learning and memory processes, the response to stress, depression, neuroprotection, and pharmacodependence. In their review, they detail the consequences of these interactions, focusing on recent results on memory and depression.

Arguing against the idea that depression causes dementia are results from a study by Bassuk et al. (54) in which the relationship between depressive symptoms and subsequent cognitive decline in a community-dwelling elderly population was examined. About 2812 elderly subjects underwent four in-home visits over a 12-year period. Cognitive function was assessed with the short portable mental status questionnaire (SPMSQ). Response was scored as high, medium, and low and cognitive decline was defined as a transition to a lower category. Depressive symptoms were measured with the center for epidemiological studies depression scale. They found that an elevated level of depressive symptoms was associated with an increased risk of cognitive decline only among *medium* SPMSQ performers. The researchers concluded that while depressive symptoms (particularly dysphoric mood) presage future cognitive losses among elderly persons with moderate cognitive impairments, the depressive symptoms did not clearly precede (and may in fact have been due to) cognitive decline. They conclude that the data do not provide support for the hypothesis that depressive symptoms are associated with the onset or rate of cognitive decline among cognitively intact elderly persons.

Along these lines, several studies reporting that depressive symptoms are common in "preclinical AD" suggest that depressive symptoms are a manifestation of early AD, rather than a cause of it. Visser et al. (55) conducted a prospective, observational cohort study to assess the prevalence of depression in subjects with preclinical AD and to investigate the possibility of differentiating subjects with preclinical AD and depression from subjects with depression-related cognitive impairment. The subjects consisted of non-demented subjects with cognitive impairment older than 55 years ($n = 111$). Data were collected at baseline, two years, and five years. Twenty-five subjects had preclinical dementia with Alzheimer's-type dementia at follow-up. Sixty percent of these subjects ($n = 15$) were depressed at baseline. Subjects with depression and preclinical AD had at baseline a poorer performance on the cognitive tasks and were older than the subjects with depression-related cognitive impairment. Age and memory performance were the best predictors for AD in the depressed subjects. The specificity of these predictors for the diagnosis of future AD in depressed subjects was 94%, sensitivity was 90%, positive predictive value was 90%, and negative predictive value was 94%. The authors concluded that depression is common in preclinical AD and that depressed subjects with preclinical AD can be accurately differentiated from subjects with depression-related cognitive impairment by age and the severity of the memory impairment.

A prospective study by Yaffe et al. (56) included 5781 elderly community-dwelling women. The geriatric depression scale (short form) was used to assess depressive symptoms and the cognitive evaluations included trails B, digit symbol, and a modified MMSE. These authors concluded that depressive symptoms in older women are associated with poor cognitive function and subsequent cognitive decline. They noted that the number of depressive symptoms is associated with the extent of cognitive impairment and subsequent decline. Other researchers have found no correlation between the degree of depression and the severity of cognitive impairments (57).

A study by Berger et al. (58) also supports the idea that depressive symptoms are a manifestation of preclinical AD. The authors examined preclinical depressive symptoms three years before the diagnosis of AD. They found that depressive symptoms are elevated preclinically in AD and that this elevation is not simply due to self-perceived cognitive difficulties. They compared incident AD patients and non-demented individuals in terms of baseline mood- and motivation-related symptoms of depression, and assessed whether depressive symptoms in preclinical AD are related to self-perceived memory problems. Participants came from a population-based longitudinal study on aging and dementia. The sample consisted of 222 people older than 74 years who were followed for a 3-year interval. Thirty-four individuals had developed AD at follow-up, whereas 188 remained non-demented. Dementia diagnosis was made according to DSM-IIIR criteria. Depressive symptoms were assessed by the comprehensive psychopathological rating scale. The incident AD patients had more depressive symptoms than the non-demented persons at baseline.

It should be noted that in this study, there was a dominance of motivation-related symptoms of depression (e.g., lack of interest, loss of energy, concentration difficulties) in preclinical AD. Perhaps the profile of depressive symptoms (e.g., apathy and decreased energy versus depressed mood and hopelessness) may help to distinguish those depressed patients manifesting early AD from those who will not develop progressive cognitive decline.

Evidence to date suggests that older age, greater degree of cognitive and functional impairment, and residual cognitive deficits after effective treatment of the mood disorder are predictors of subsequent dementia. Butters et al. (59) examined changes in cognitive function following treatment of late-life depression. Their sample included 45 non-demented, elderly depressed patients who achieved remission after 12 weeks of antidepressant therapy and 20 elderly comparison subjects. They found that elderly depressed patients with cognitive impairment may experience improvement in specific domains following antidepressant therapy, but may not necessarily reach normal levels of performance, particularly in memory and executive functions. This subgroup of late-life depression patients is likely at high risk of developing progressive dementia.

THE IMPACT OF AGE ON COGNITIVE IMPAIRMENT IN DEPRESSION

Some studies, but not others, have suggested that cognitive impairment may preferentially occur in elderly as compared to younger depressed patients.

King et al. (25) compared neuropsychological test performance among elderly depressed patients ($n = 23$), AD patients ($n = 20$), and healthy controls ($n = 23$). Depressed subjects were deficient relative to controls on most tasks, including naming and cued memory. There was a greater negative influence of age on the performance of depressed subjects (relative to controls) on some tasks. The naming and verbal recognition deficits in the elderly depressed group were significant and distinct from what was expected on the basis of some studies of younger depressives. These were not viewed as early manifestations of AD because all patients were followed clinically for at least 18 months and none evidenced progressive functional decline. Despite their significant deficits, depressed patients were clearly distinguishable from AD patients. The authors suggest that the combined effects of age and depression produce a pattern of deficits that is distinct from that of younger depressives, but less severe than that of AD patients, and note that their results confirm results of Speedie et al. (60) of a confrontation naming deficit in elderly depressives (a deficit previously thought to be an indicator of progressive neuropathology). The naming impairment was seen with increasing age, apparent only when using regression techniques to study the effects of age as a continuous variable.

A second important finding in the study by King et al. (25) was the deficient performance of subjects on delayed word list recognition. This is a cued memory task designed to minimize retrieval demands and to maximize the subject's ability to demonstrate learning. These results suggest a true deficiency in learning (acquisition or encoding), rather than a deficit in the retrieval of information. Although the depressed subjects did have impaired verbal recognition memory, observation of their performance revealed that they were able to benefit from cues, whereas AD subjects appeared to be guessing. The authors suggest that the presence of significant naming and verbal recognition memory deficits calls for a broader view than only a subcortical dementia picture.

Tarbuck and Paykel (61) investigated the effects of age and depression on cognitive function and concluded that older subjects were not more severely affected by depression than the younger subjects. The researchers examined two groups of inpatients with major depression (aged under and over 60 years), when depressed and after recovery from depression. The pattern of impairment associated with depression was different from that associated with older age: depression affected performance on more complex tasks, whereas age was associated particularly with slowing on timed tests. This study did not suggest that the impairment from baseline due to the depression is greater in older than younger subjects. The changes associated with depression affected particularly complex tasks that require a greater degree of internal processing and conscious effort.

TREATMENT OF DEPRESSED PATIENTS WITH COGNITIVE IMPAIRMENT

Although the older generation of tricyclic antidepressants (e.g., amitriptyline) may negatively impact cognition due to anticholinergic side effects, the later generation of tricyclics (e.g., nortriptyline) are much less apt to do this. The newer antidepressants, including the commonly prescribed selective serotonin re-uptake inhibitors (SSRIs) are very well tolerated in this regard. In fact, Nebes et al. (62) found that paroxetine (an SSRI with anticholinergic properties) does not worsen cognitive function, even in elderly subjects with pre-existing cognitive deficits.

In patients for whom antidepressant medications have proven ineffective or are contraindicated, electroconvulsive therapy (ECT) may be beneficial. Given the fact that side effects of ECT include delirium and memory disturbances, it is logical to question whether or not this form of treatment should be used for depressed patients who have cognitive impairment. Studies of elderly, cognitively impaired depressed patients (including those with concomitant depression and dementia) suggest that although ECT can be associated with transient cognitive worsening during the course of the treatment, this therapy is associated with significantly improved cognition by discharge (63,64).

Wilkinson (63) studied the relationship between age and the outcome of ECT in 78 patients (aged 18–88 years) who had major depression with melancholia or psychosis. Sixty-eight subjects were evaluated for change in cognitive performance before and after treatment. Strongly positive correlations between increasing age, response to ECT, and improved cognitive function were demonstrated. The author noted that ECT remains an important treatment for depression in old age, where the greatest benefits may be seen.

Based on their prospective follow-up study of 81 inpatients with major depression, Brodaty et al. (65) concluded that depressive outcome and adverse effects of ECT are largely independent of age. They did note, however, that older patients receiving ECT appear to have a higher risk of developing dementia, possibly related to cerebrovascular disease. The authors compared ECT outcome among three age groups (under 65, 65–74, and 75 years and over) on the Hamilton rating scale for depression (HRSD), global assessment of functioning scale (GAF), and clinical outcome rating scale. Assessments were performed before ECT, immediately after ECT, one to three years later and, for patients suspected of having dementia, five years later. At post-ECT and follow-up, improvement on HRSD and clinical outcome ratings were comparable for patients in the three age groups. At follow-up, 35.7% of the oldest group had dementia. Patients who did and did not develop dementia were clinically indistinguishable prior to ECT. The number and severity of common adverse events were similar pre- and post-ECT and were not associated with age.

Rao and Lyketsos (64) performed a chart review of 31 patients with a discharge diagnosis of "dementia with depression" treated with ECT over a 5-year period. Admission and discharge ratings were made on the MMSE and the Montgomery-Asberg depression rating scale (MADRS) as part of the clinical routine. All patients suffered from dementia: 55% had vascular dementia, 13% AD, and 32% degenerative dementia of uncertain etiology. The patients received between 1 and 23 ECT treatments (mean 9, SD 5.7). At discharge, there was a statistically significant mean decline on the MADRS of 12.28 points ($p < 0.01$). Forty percent had scores less than 10 (normal). While 49% of patients developed delirium, by discharge there was also a significant mean increase (improvement) in MMSE of 1.62 points ($p < 0.02$). The authors suggest that ECT is an effective treatment for depression in patients with dementia, leading to improvements in both mood and cognition. They note that multiple ECT treatments may be necessary before a significant improvement in mood is achieved.

In their prospective, multicenter study involving 268 patients, Tew et al. (66) compared characteristics and treatment outcomes of adult (59 and younger), young-old (60–74 years), and old-old (75 years and older) patients treated with ECT for major depression. Patients were treated with suprathreshold right unilateral or bilateral ECT in a standardized manner. Despite a higher level of physical illness and cognitive impairment, even the oldest patients with severe major depression tolerated ECT in a manner similar to that of the younger patients and demonstrated similar or better acute response.

SUMMARY

Depression is a syndrome that can affect cognition in addition to mood, motor, and vegetative functions. Frequently affected cognitive functions include attention, memory (recall), and psychomotor speed. Not all depressed patients develop cognitive deficits and some evidence suggests that cognitive impairment is more frequent in melancholic depression.

In elderly patients, it may be difficult to distinguish the cognitive impairment from depression from that due to dementia. A thorough history and neuropsychological evaluation is important in this regard. Aspects of the history that point toward depression rather than dementia include the following: personal history of affective illness, abrupt or subacute onset, depressive symptoms preceding cognitive decline, significant distress related to cognitive impairment, and/or complaints of cognitive impairment out of proportion to actual deficits, somatic complaints and diminished appetite.

Both qualitative and quantitative differences between depressed and demented patients in neuropsychological testing have been observed. Depressed patients tend to have inconsistent performance, may give poor effort, and frequently answer "I don't know" rather than guessing. They tend to have problems with attention, psychomotor speed, and certain aspects of memory. Depression may affect spontaneous recall but should not impair learning or recognition. Orientation, language, and constructional abilities should be normal. There is some suggestion that naming and recognition may be affected with increasing age, but not to the degree that they are in dementia.

Executive functions may be affected in depression. This has been reported mostly in severe depression and in the elderly. Elderly patients with executive dysfunction are more apt to have white matter hyperintensities on MRI imaging and they tend to have a worse prognosis with regard to their depression.

The cognitive impairment of depression has been described as having a "subcortical" pattern. Evidence that suggests that frontal-subcortical circuitry is disturbed include neuropsychological testing and functional imaging studies. It appears as though the prefrontal and cingulate cortical regions play a key role.

The etiology of depression-related cognitive impairment is not known but it does not appear to be due to AD-type neuropathology. There is some evidence to suggest that white matter lesions may play a role in the vulnerability of some elderly patients to develop cognitive impairment during depressive episodes.

There appears to be a relationship between depression and dementia, but the precise nature of this relationship remains to be determined. While there is some evidence to suggest that depression may cause or contribute to dementia, there is substantial evidence to support the notion that depression may be a manifestation of early AD.

The role that increasing age may play in the prevalence, severity, and profile of cognitive impairment in depression continues to be explored. Some researchers suggest that depression in the elderly has unique features (e.g., problems with naming and recognition), whereas others suggest that age does not affect the way in which depression impacts cognition.

The cognitive impairment of depression is generally reversible with appropriate treatment of the depression, including antidepressant medications, or, in certain cases, ECT. Patients who have residual cognitive impairments, despite effective treatment mood, may be at an increased risk of dementia.

REFERENCES

1. Caine ED. Pseudodementia: current concepts and future directions. Arch Gen Psych 1981; 38:1359–1364.
2. American Psychiatric Association. Diagnostic and Statistical Manual of Mental Disorders. 4th ed. Washington, DC: American Psychiatric Publishing, 1994.
3. Reifler BV, Larson EB, Hanley R. Coexistence of cognitive impairment and depression in geriatric outpatients. Am J Psychiatr 1982; 139:623–626.
4. Wells CE. Pseudodementia. Am J Psychiatr 1979; 136:895–900.
5. Folstein MF, Folstein SE, McHugh PR. "Mini-mental state": a practical method for grading the cognitive state of patients for the clinician. J Psychiatr Res 1975; 12:189–198.
6. Austin MP, Mitchell P, Wilhelm K, et al. Cognitive function in depression: a distinct pattern of frontal impairment in melancholia? Psychol Med 1999; 29:73–85.
7. Massman PJ, Delis DC, Butters N, Dupont RM, Gillin JC. The subcortical dysfunction hypothesis of memory deficits in depression: neuropsychological validation in a subgroup of patients. J Clin Exp Neuropsychol 1992; 14:687–706.
8. Rabins PV, Merchant A, Nestadt G. Criteria for diagnosing reversible dementia caused by depression: validation by 2-year follow-up. Br J Psychiatr 1984; 144:488–492.
9. Kiloh LG. Pseudo-dementia. Acta Psychiatr Scand 1969; 37:336–351.
10. Roth M, Myers DH. The diagnosis of dementia. Br J Psychiatr 1975(special publication); 9:87–99.
11. Post F. Dementia, depression, and pseudodementia. In: Benson DR, Blumer D, eds. Psychiatric Aspects of Neurologic Disease. New York: Grune & Stratton, 1975.

12. Lezak MD. Neuropsychological Assessment. 3rd ed. New York: Oxford University Press, 1995.
13. Wang SJ, Fuh JL, Teng EL, et al. Subjective memory complaint in relation to cognitive performance and depression: a longitudinal study of a rural Chinese population. J Am Geriatr Soc 2000; 48:295–299.
14. Riedel-Heller SG, Matschinger H, Schork A, Angermeyer MC. Do memory complaints indicate the presence of cognitive impairment? Results of a field study. Eur Arch Psychiatr Clin Neurosci 1999; 249:197–204.
15. Kaszniak AW, Sadeh M, Stern LZ. Differentiating depression from organic brain syndromes in older age. In: Chaisson-Stewart GM, ed. Depression in the Elderly: An Interdisciplinary Approach. New York: Wiley, 1985.
16. McPherson SE. Neuropsychological Evaluation, Section 49.5b, Chapter 49 (Geriatric Psychiatry) In: Kaplan HK, Sadock BJ, eds. Comprehensive Textbook of Psychiatry VI. Vol. 2. Baltimore: Williams & Wilkins, 1995:2556.
17. Moffoot APR, O'Carroll JB, Carroll S, Dick H, Ebmeier KP, Goodwin GM. Diurnal variation of mood and neuropsychological function in major depression with melancholia. J Affective Disord 1994; 32:257–269.
18. Brand N, Jolles J. Information processing in depression and anxiety. Psychological Med 1987; 17:145–153.
19. Caine ED. The neuropsychology of depression: the pseudodementia syndrome. In: Grant I, Adams KM, eds. Neuropsychological Assessment of Neuropsychiatric Disorders. New York: Oxford University Press, 1986.
20. Niederehe G. Depression and memory impairment in the aged. In: Poon LW, ed. Handbook for Clinical Memory Assessment of Older Adults. Washington DC: American Psychological Association, 1986.
21. Weingartner H, Cohen RM, Murphy DL, et al. Cognitive processes in depression. Arch Gen Psychiatr 1981; 38:42–47.
22. Weingartner H. Psychobiological determinants of memory failures. In: Squire L, Butter N, eds. Neuropsychology of Memory. New York: Guilford Press, 1984.
23. Weingartner H. Automatic and effort-demanding cognitive processes in depression. In: Poon LW, ed. Handbook for Clinical Memory Assessment of Older Adults. Washington, DC: American Psychological Association, 1986.
24. Murray LA, Whitehouse WG, Alloy LB. Mood congruence and depressive deficits in memory: a forced-recall analysis. Memory 1999; 7:175–196.
25. King DA, Caine ED, Conwell Y, Cox C. The neuropsychology of depression in the elderly: a comparative study of normal aging and Alzheimer's disease. J Neuropsychiatry Clin Neurosci 1991; 3:163–168.
26. Swann AC, Katz MM, Bowden CL, Berman NG, Stokes PE: Psychomotor performance and monoamine function in bipolar and unipolar affective disorders. Biol Psychiatr 1999; 45:979–988.
27. Lemke MR, Puhl P, Koethe N, Winkler T: Psychomotor retardation and anhedonia in depression. Acta Psychiatr Scand 1999; 99:252–256.
28. Sachdev P, Aniss AM. Slowness of movement in melancholic depression. Biol Psychiatr 1994; 35:253–262.
29. Lemelin S, Baruch P. Clinical psychomotor retardation and attention in depression. J Psychiatr Res 1998; 32:81–88.

30. Mesulam M-M. Principles of Behavioral Neurology, Philadelphia: FA Davis Company, 1985.

31. Jones RD, Tranel D, Benton A, Paulsen J. Differentiating dementia from "pseudodementia" early in the clinical course: Utility of neuropsychological tests. Neuropsychology 1992; 6:13–21.

32. Channon S. Executive dysfunction in depression: the Wisconsin Card Sorting Test. J Affective Disord 1996; 39:107–114.

33. Jones B, Henderson M, Welch CA. Executive functions in unipolar depression before and after electroconvulsive therapy. Int J Neurosci 1988; 38:287–297.

34. Raskin A, Friedman AS, DeMascio A. Cognitive and performance deficits in depression. Psychopharmacol Bull 1982; 18:196–202.

35. Silberman EK, Weingartner H, Post RM. Thinking disorder in depression. Arch Gen Psychiatr 1983; 40:775–780.

36. Alexopolus GS, Meyers BS, Young RC, et al. Executive dysfunction and long-term outcomes of geriatric depression. Arch Gen Psychiatr 2000; 57:285–290.

37. Kalayam B, Alexopoulos Gs. Prefrontal dysfunction and treatment response in geriatric depression. Arch Gen Psychiatr 1999; 56:713–718.

38. Lockwood KA, Alexopoulos GS, Kakuma T, Van Gorp WG. Subtypes of cognitive impairment in depressed older adults. Am J Geriatr Psychiatr 2000; 8:201–208.

39. Boone KB, Miller Bl, Lesser IM, Merhinger CM, Hill-Gutierrez E, Goldberg M, Berman NG. Neuropsychological correlates of white matter lesions in healthy elderly subjects. Arch Neurol 1992; 49:549–554.

40. Yousef G, Ryan WJ, Lambert T, Pitt B, Kellett J. A preliminary report: a new scale to identify the pseudodementia syndrome. Int J Geriatr Psychiatr 1998; 13:389–399.

41. Rosen I. Electroencephalography as a diagnostic tool in dementia. Dementia & Geriatric Cognitive Disorders 1997; 8:110–116.

42. Dykierek P, Stadtmuller G, Schramm P, Bahro M, van Calker D, Braus DF, Steigleider P, Low H, Hohagen F, Gattaz WF, Berger M, Riemann D. The value of REM sleep parameters in differentiating Alzheimer's disease from old-age depression and normal aging. J Psychiatric Res 1998; 32:1–9.

43. Merriam EP, Thase ME, Haas GL, Keshavan MS, Sweeney JA. Prefrontal cortical dysfunction in depression determined by Wisconsin Card Sorting Test performance. Am J Psychiatr 1999; 156:780–782.

44. Alexander GE, DeLong MR, Strick PL. Parallel organisation of functionally segregated circuits linking basal ganglia and cortex. Ann Rev Neurosci 1986; 9:357–381.

45. Mayberg HS, Brannan SK, Mahurin RK, et al. Cingulate function in depression: a potential predictor of treatment response. NeuroReport 1997; 8:1057–1061.

46. Mayberg HS, Liotti M, Brannon SK, et al. Reciprocal limbic-cortical function and negative mood: converging PET findings in depression and normal sadness. Am J Psychiatr 1999; 156:675–682.

47. O'Brien J, Thomas A, Ballard C, Brown A, Ferrier N, Jaros E, Perry R. Cognitive impairment in depression is not associated with neuropathologic evidence of increased vascular or Alzheimer-type pathology. Biol Psychiatr 2001; 49:130–136.

48. Kramer-Ginsberg E, Greenwald BS, Krishnan KRR, et al. Neuropsychological functioning and MRI signal hyperintensities in geriatric depression. Am J Psych 1999; 156:438–444.

49. Van Londen L, Goekoop JG, Zwinderman AH, Lanser JB, Wiegant VM, De Wied D. Neuropsychological performance and plasma cortisol, arginine vasopressin and oxytocin in patients with major depression. Psychol Med 1998; 28:275–284.
50. Jorm AF. Is depression a risk factor for dementia or cognitive decline? A review. Gerontology 2000; 46:219–227.
51. Kessing LV. Cognitive impairment in the euthymic phase of affective disorder. Psychological Med 1998; 28:1027–1038.
52. McEwen BS. Plasticity of the hippocampus: adaptation to chronic stress and allostatic load. Ann NYAcad Sci 2001; 933:265–277.
53. Maurice T, Urani A, Phan VL, Romieu P. The interaction between neuroactive steroids and the sigma1 receptor function: behavioral consequences and therapeutic opportunities. Brain Res—Brain Res Rev 2001; 37:116–132.
54. Bassuk SS, Berkman LF, Wypij D. Depressive symptomatology and incident cognitive decline in an elderly community sample. Arch Gen Psych 1998; 55:1073–1081.
55. Visser PJ, Verhey FR, Ponds RW, Cruts M, Van Broeckhoven CL, Jolles J. Course of objective memory impairment in non-demented subjects attending a memory clinic and predictors of outcome. Int J Geriatr Psych 2000; 15:363–372.
56. Yaffe K, Blackwell T, Gore R, Sands L, Reus V, Browner WS. Depressive symptoms and cognitive decline in nondemented elderly women: a prospective study. Arch Gen Psych 1999; 56:425–430.
57. Li Y, Meyer JS, Thornby J. Depressive symptoms among cognitively normal versus cognitively impaired elderly subjects. Int J Geriatr Psych 2001; 16:455–461.
58. Berger AK, Fratiglioni L, Forsell Y, Winblad B, Backman L. The occurrence of depressive symptoms in the preclinical phase of AD: a population based study. Neurology 1999; 53:1998–2002.
59. Butters MA, Becker JT, Nebes RD, Zmuda MD, Mulsant BH, Pollock BG, Reynolds CF 3rd. Changes in cognitive functioning following treatment of late-life depression. Am J Psych 2000; 157:1949–1954.
60. Speedie L, Rabins P, Pearlson G, et al. Confrontation naming deficit in dementia of depression. J Neurpsych Clin Neurosci 1990; 2:59–63.
61. Tarbuck AF, Paykel ES. Effects of major depression on the cognitive function of younger and older subjects. Psychol Med 1995; 25:285–296.
62. Nebes RD, Pollock BG, Mulsant BH, Butters MA, Zmuda MD, Reynolds CF 3rd. Cognitive effects of paroxetine in older depressed patients. J Clin Psych 1999; 60(suppl 20):26–29
63. Wilkinson AM, Anderson DN, Peters S. Age and the effects of ECT. Int J Geriatr Psych 1993; 8:401–406.
64. Rao V, Lyketsos CG. The benefits and risks of ECT for patients with primary dementia who also suffer from depression. Int J Geriatr Psych 2000; 15:729–735.
65. Brodaty H, Hickie I, Mason C, Prenter L. A prospective follow-up study of ECT outcome in older depressed patients. J Affect Disord 2000; 60:101–111.
66. Tew JD Jr, Mulsant BH, Haskett RF, Prudic J, Thase ME, Crowe RR, Dolata D, Begley AE, Reynolds CF 3rd, Sackeim HA. Acute efficacy of ECT in the treatment of major depression in the old-old. Am J Psych 1999; 156:1865–1870.

Index

About the Editor

Roger Kurlan is Professor of Neurology and Chief of the Cognitive and Behavioral Neurology Unit, University of Rochester Medical Center, Rochester, New York. He is the author or coauthor of numerous articles published in highly regarded journals of neurology and psychiatry, as well as editor of the *Handbook of Tourette's Syndrome and Related Tic and Behavioral Disorders, Second Edition* (Taylor & Francis Group). Dr. Kurlan is also a frequent presenter at national conferences on movement disorders and cognitive and behavioral disorders. He received the M.D. degree from Washington University School of Medicine, St. Louis, Missouri.